MATERNAL AND CHILD NUTRITION

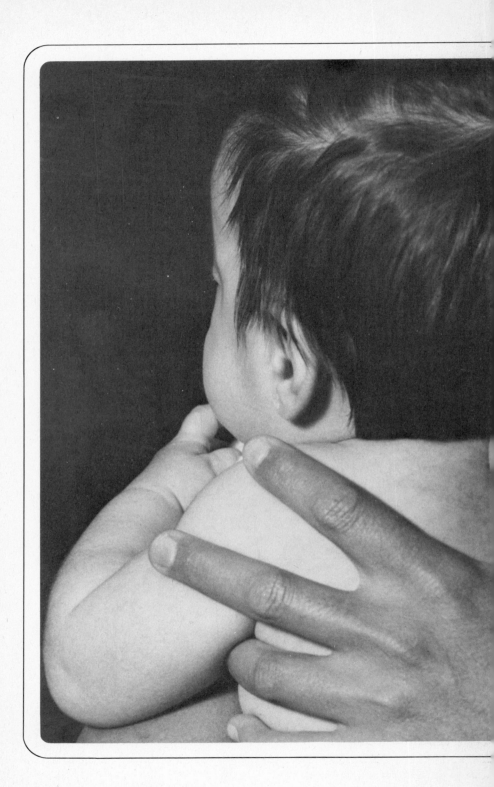

MATERNAL AND CHILD NUTRITION

S. J. RITCHEY
Professor, Human Nutrition and Foods
Virginia Polytechnic Institute and State University
Blacksburg, Virginia

L. JANETTE TAPER
Associate Professor, Human Nutrition and Foods
Virginia Polytechnic Institute and State University
Blacksburg, Virginia

1817

HARPER & ROW, PUBLISHERS, New York
Cambridge, Philadelphia, San Francisco
London, Mexico City, São Paulo, Sydney

Cover photo: John Scheiber

RG
559
.R57

Photo Credits: Facing title page, John Scheiber. *Chapter 1:* page xvi, © Arms, Jeroboam: page 3, from *Food to Grow On: The Teenager vs. Nutrition.* Courtesy of Tupperware® Home Parties, a division of Dart Industries, Inc. *Chapter 2:* page 44, Simon, Stock, Boston; page 58, provided by the authors; page 65, Virginia Extension Service. *Chapter 3:* page 76, © Bodin, Stock, Boston. *Chapter 4:* page 102, © Joel Gordon, 1975. *Chapter 5:* page 138, © Joel Gordon, 1980; page 140, Michigan Extension Service. *Chapter 6:* page 176, Leo de Wys, Inc.; page 178, from *Food to Grow On: From Toddler to Twelve.* Courtesy of Tupperware® Home Parties, a division of Dart Industries, Inc.; page 181, provided by the authors; page 190, from *Food to Grow On: From Toddler to Twelve.* Courtesy of Tupperware® Home Parties, a division of Dart Industries, Inc.; page 193, from *Food to Grow On: From Toddler to Twelve.* Courtesy of Tupperware® Home Parties, a division of Dart Industries, Inc. *Chapter 7:* page 212, © Joel Gordon, 1980; page 237, from *Food to Grow On: Nutrition Begins When You Do.* Courtesy of Tupperware® Home Parties, a division of Dart Industries, Inc. *Chapter 8:* page 252, Leo de Wys, Inc.; page 254, Beech-Nut Foods Corp.; page 255, Beech-Nut Foods Corp.; page 257, Wisconsin Extension Service. *Chapter 9:* page 292, Wolinsky, Stock, Boston. *Chapter 10:* page 324, © Joel Gordon, 1979; page 353, from *Food to Grow On: The Teenager vs. Nutrition.* Courtesy of Tupperware® Home Parties, a division of Dart Industries, Inc. *Chapter 11:* page 364, Skytta, Jeroboam. *Chapter 12:* page 388, © Wu 1979, Jeroboam.

Sponsoring Editor: Fred Henry
Project Editor: Beena Kamlani
Designer: Michel Craig
Production Manager: Jeanie Berke
Photo Researcher: Mira Schachne
Compositor: Lexigraphics, Inc.
Printer and Binder: R.R. Donnelley & Sons Company
Art Studio: Vantage Art, Inc.

MATERNAL AND CHILD NUTRITION

Library of Congress Cataloging in Publication Data
Ritchey, S. J.
  Maternal and child nutrition.

  Includes bibliographical references.
    1. Pregnancy—Nutritional aspects.   2. Infants—
Nutrition.   3. Children—Nutrition.   I. Taper,
L. Janette.   II. Title. [DNLM: 1. Child nutrition.
2. Infant nutrition.   3. Nutrition—In pregnancy.
4. Fetus—Physiology. WS 115 R598m]
RG559.R57 1982   618.2'4   82—6275
ISBN 0—06—453519—3   AACR2

CONTENTS

Photo Credits   iv

Preface   xiii

CHAPTER 1 NUTRITIONAL HEALTH OF THE ADULT FEMALE   1
- **Nutritional Status of the Preconceptional Woman**   2
- **Nutrient Requirements of the Preconceptional Woman**   5
  - *Recommended Dietary Allowances for the Adult Female*   5
  - *Energy Requirements*   6
  - *Energy-Supplying Nutrients*   9
  - *Vitamins*   16
  - *Minerals*   22
  - *Water*   28
- **Planning Food Intake for the Preconceptional Female**   30
- **Dietary Counseling for the Young Woman**   36
- **Summary**   38
- **Study Questions and Topics for Individual Investigation**   39
- **References**   40

CHAPTER 2 PREGNANCY AND LACTATION   45
- **The Female Reproductive System**   46
- **Physiological Development and Changes During Pregnancy**   47
- **The Placenta**   48
  - *Amniotic Sac*   48

Period of Intrauterine Growth   49
Hormonal Aspects of Pregnancy   51
Immunological Functions of the Placenta   51
Transport of Materials Across the Placenta   51
  Transport of Gases   52
  Water   52
  Electrolytes   53
  Minerals   54
  Glucose   54
  Amino Acids   54
  Proteins   54
  Lipids   54
  Fat-Soluble Vitamins   54
  Water-Soluble Vitamins   54
  Fetal Metabolic End Products   55
Changes in the Maternal System During Pregnancy   55
  Blood Volume and Composition   55
  Changes in the Cardiovascular System   56
  Changes in the Respiratory System   56
  Changes in the Kidney Function   56
  Changes in the Alimentary Function   56
  Changes in Weight and Water Retention   57
Increased Nutritional Needs During Pregnancy   58
  Energy   59
  Protein   59
  Vitamins A, D, and E   60
  Thiamin, Riboflavin, and Niacin   60
  Folacin   60
  Vitamin B_6   60
  Vitamin B_{12}   60
  Calcium, Phosphorus, and Magnesium   60
  Sodium and Potassium   60
  Iron   60
  Iodine   61
  Zinc   61
Sources of Nutrients During Pregnancy   61
The Lactating Mother   64
Mammary System   64
Early Stages of Breast-Feeding   65
Increased Nutrient Needs During Lactation   66
  Energy   66
  Protein   67
  Calcium   67
  Trace Minerals   67
  Fat-Soluble Vitamins   67

Water-Soluble Vitamins 67
Sources of Nutrients During Lactation 68
Fluid 69
Foods to Avoid 69
Nutrient Supplements 69
Drugs 70
Summary 70
Study Questions and Topics for Individual Investigation 72
References 73

**CHAPTER 3 PHYSIOLOGICAL DEVELOPMENT
OF THE FETUS AND INFANT** 77
Cellular Growth of the Fetus 78
**Structural and Functional Differentiation During the
Fetal Period** 80
Body Growth 80
Development of the Fetal Respiratory System 83
Development of the Fetal Kidney 84
Development of the Fetal Liver 84
Development of the Fetal Heart 85
Development of the Fetal Brain 86
Development of the Fetal Gastrointestinal Tract 87
Accumulation of Nutrients by the Fetus 89
Metabolism and the Use of Nutrients 90
Carbohydrate 90
Lipid 91
Types of Adipose Tissue 94
Protein and Amino Acids 94
Vitamin Absorption 95
Mineral Absorption 95
Nutrient Transport 96
Hormonal Development and Control 96
Summary 98
Study Questions and Topics for Individual Investigation 99
References 99

**CHAPTER 4 NUTRITIONAL COMPLICATIONS
OF PREGNANCY** 103
Malnutrition and Physical Growth 104
Malnutrition and Brain Development 108
The Anemias of Pregnancy 110
Iron 110
Folic Acid 111
Vitamin B_{12} 112

The Toxemias of Pregnancy 112
Maternal Weight Gain 114
Teenage Pregnancy 118
The Use of Drugs in Pregnancy 120
  Antibiotics 121
  Hormones 122
  Anticoagulants 123
  Tranquilizers 123
  Narcotics 123
  Hallucinogens 123
  Alcohol 124
  Cigarettes 124
  Vitamins 124
  Need for Education and Research 125
The Use of Oral Contraceptives—Nutritional
  Complications 125
Summary 127
Study Questions and Topics for Individual Investigation 129
References 130

CHAPTER 5 PATTERNS OF POSTNATAL GROWTH
  AND DEVELOPMENT 139
Patterns of Growth 139
Development of Organs and Systems 143
  Enzyme Systems 143
  Muscle 143
  Cutaneous Structures 145
  Skeleton 145
  Central Nervous System 146
  Development of Sensory Characteristics 148
  Circulatory System 148
  Hemopoietic System 148
  Lymphatic System 152
  Respiratory System 152
  Digestive System 152
  Urinary System and Water Balance 153
Growth Standards 154
  Use of Growth Charts 155
  Interpretation of Growth Charts 156
  Useful Physical Measurements 156
  Lean Body Mass 166
  Cessation of Growth 167
  Obese Children 167
Summary 171
Study Questions and Topics for Individual Investigation 172
References 172

CHAPTER 6 DEVELOPMENT OF FOOD HABITS 177
   The Development of Food Habits in Children 178
   Factors Affecting the Development of Food Habits 183
   Recent Changes in National Food Habits 186
   Factors Facilitating Change in Food Habits 189
     Food Advertising 189
     Working Women 191
     Fast-Food Restaurants 192
     Snacking 193
     Vending Machines 194
   Food Habits Shaped by Dietary Fads 195
     Natural, Organic, and Health Foods 195
     Zen-Macrobiotic Diet 196
     Vegetarianism 196
     Dietary Supplements 197
     Weight Control 198
   Better Food Habits Through Nutrition Education 204
   Summary 205
   Study Questions and Topics for Individual Investigation 207
   References 208

CHAPTER 7 MILK IN THE INFANT DIET 213
   Nutrient Requirements 213
     Protein and Amino Acids 216
     Carbohydrate 217
     Fat 218
     Calories 219
     Vitamins 221
     Minerals 224
   Breast-Feeding 227
     Nutrient Content of Breast Milk 227
     Immunological Properties of Breast Milk 232
     Further Advantages of Breast-Feeding 233
     Possible Disadvantages of Breast-Feeding 235
   Infant Formulas 237
   Milk Feeding Following Weaning 243
   Should Milk Drinking by Children be Discouraged? 244
   Summary 245
   Study Questions and Topics for Individual Investigation 246
   References 247

CHAPTER 8 SOLID FOODS IN THE INFANT DIET 253
   Early Feedings 253
   Three Meals a Day 255
   Discovering Foods 256

Introducing Solid Foods   **257**

Commercial Baby Foods   **259**

Commercially-Prepared versus Home-Prepared Infant Foods   **268**

Health Problems Related to Food Intake During the Early Years   **272**

Undernutrition and Related Problems   *272*

Overnutrition and Related Problems   *274*

Nutritional Management of the Low Birth-Weight Infant   **278**

Summary   **284**

Study Questions and Topics for Individual Investigation   **285**

References   **286**

CHAPTER 9 NUTRITIONAL PROBLEMS IN THE INFANT AND CHILD   **293**

General Nutritional Guidelines   **294**

Energy and Protein   *294*

Fats   *294*

Carbohydrate   *295*

Vitamins and Minerals   *295*

Electrolytes   *295*

Fluids   *295*

Special Formulas and Supplements   **295**

Malabsorption Syndromes   **296**

Cystic Fibrosis   *296*

Sucrase-Isomaltase Deficiency   *296*

Glucose-Galactose Malabsorption   *296*

Celiac Sprue   *296*

Lactose Intolerance and Malabsorption   *299*

Allergies   **300**

Milk Allergy   *300*

Wheat Allergy   *300*

Desensitizing the Allergic Person   *301*

Inborn Errors of Metabolism   **301**

Diabetes Mellitus   *301*

Galactosemia   *303*

Glycogen Storage Diseases   *305*

Phenylketonuria   *305*

Tyrosinemia   *306*

Homocystinuria   *308*

Maple Syrup Urine Disease   *309*

Gout   *310*

Familial Hyperlipoproteinemia   *311*

Cardiac Disease   **314**

Handicapping Conditions   **314**

Hyperbilirubinemia   **317**

Summary 317
Study Questions and Topics for Individual Investigation 319
References 319

**CHAPTER 10 NUTRITION DURING CHILDHOOD
AND ADOLESCENCE 325**
Growth Patterns During Childhood 326
Nutritional Needs During Growth 327
  Energy 327
  Protein and Amino Acids 333
  Fat-Soluble Vitamins 336
  Water-Soluble Vitamins 337
  Minerals 337
Evaluation of Nutrient Intakes and Nutritional Status 340
  Calculation of Nutrient Intakes 340
  Assessment of Nutrient Intake Data 341
Biochemical Evaluation of Nutritional Status 343
Guides for Adequate Food Intakes 345
Specific Concerns Related to Nutrition During the
Growing Years 348
  Obesity in the Rapidly Growing Young Person 349
  Teenage Pregnancy 354
  Nutrition for the Athlete 357
Summary 359
Study Questions and Topics for Individual Investigation 360
References 360

CHAPTER 11 NUTRITION AND DENTAL HEALTH 365
Development of Teeth 365
Composition of Teeth 368
Saliva 370
Oral Diseases 371
  Host Factors 373
  Microbial Factor 373
  Diet or Food 373
Nursing Bottle Syndrome 381
Prevention of Dental Disease 382
Summary 383
Study Questions and Topics for Individual Investigation 384
References 385

**CHAPTER 12 NUTRITION PROGRAMS
FOR MOTHER AND CHILD 389**
Food Programs of the USDA 389
  School Lunch Program 390
  School Breakfast Program 395

Special Milk Program   *396*
Special Nonschool Food Service Program   *396*
Food Programs for Mothers and Children   **397**
Commodity Distribution Program   **400**
Food Stamp Program   **400**
Nutrition Education in Government Feeding Programs   **401**
Reliable Sources of Nutrition Information   **403**
Government Agencies   *404*
Professional and Other Organizations   *408*
Summary   **410**
Study Questions and Topics for Individual Investigation   **411**
References   **413**

Glossary   **417**

Index   **425**

PREFACE

The health of the mother and growing child has been a focus of interest of health professionals for many years. In recent years, nutritional scientists and others have recognized the important role of nutrition in the growth, development, and health of both mother and child. Government and private agencies have given attention to the problems and difficulties during the critical periods of pregnancy, lactation, growth, and development. Nutrition has long been recognized as essential for physical growth, but recently mental and emotional development have been associated with nutrition during the very early periods of fetal and postnatal life.

Students of nutrition need to recognize that proper growth is a manifestation of adequate nutrition of the mother both prior to and during pregnancy. Students should have a basic knowledge of the physiological and genetic events that occur during the processes of conception, pregnancy, and growth and the importance and implications of these processes for nutritional health. In this book we relate nutrition to physiological development of the entire human being. We review the numerous potential problems that may result from inappropriate nutrient intake. We demonstrate that good nutrition is affected by food intake that is a result of eating habits. Finally, we review current education and support programs available to the mother and child.

Throughout all this we make an effort to provide the most recent information without the depth of a scientific review or a journal article. We try to avoid broad-sweeping statements that cannot be documented and may, indeed, be more myth than fact. We hope that readers, both professionals and students, will find the book understandable and useful. For this book to be useful in college and university courses concerned with maternal and child nutrition, users should have a prior basic understanding of the principles of nutrition and sufficient background in biology and chemistry to handle the physiological concepts relating nutrition to development.

We owe many persons for their assistance, patience, and support. We especially thank the following: John Woods and Earl Shepherd, the editors, who kept us moving in the appropriate direction; Emily Wikstrom, our faithful typist who transcribed our scribbling into readable sentences; those who generously permitted reproduction of materials from other publications; and those who reviewed early drafts and provided guidance and direction for subsequent improvements.

S. J. Ritchey
L. J. Taper

MATERNAL
AND
CHILD NUTRITION

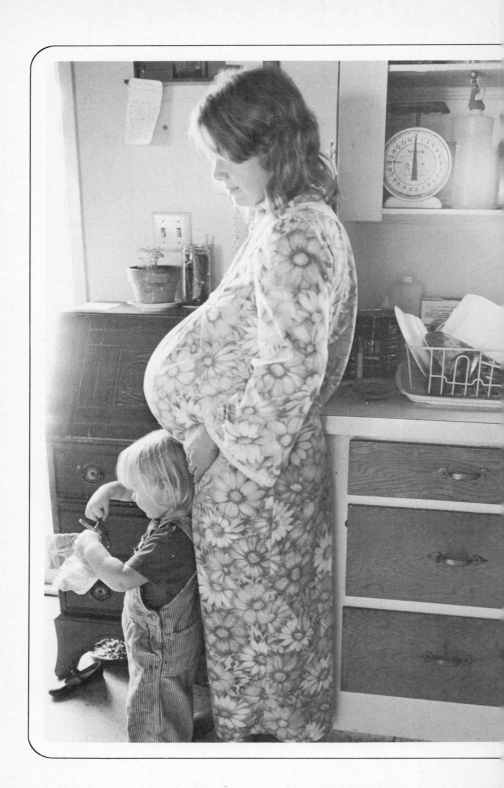

CHAPTER 1

NUTRITIONAL HEALTH OF THE ADULT FEMALE

We have little available literature to help us understand the nutritional needs of women, and especially those of women during the reproductive years (**1, 2**).* Therefore, throughout this text we are concerned with the relationship of nutrition to health in women at different stages during the life cycle. We discuss the preconceptional nutriture of the mother and the relationship of nutrition during pregnancy to the outcome of that pregnancy and the subsequent health of the infant. We also cover nutrition throughout the various physiological stages of growth and development. Traditionally, the medical concept of what constitutes good maternity care has focused on three phases: the prenatal period, actual childbirth, and the immediate postpartum period. Wishik (**3**) suggests that a fourth stage be added—that of preparing young women for a good start in their reproductive life history.

The subject of nutrition for the preconceptional woman is a vital one. The adult female often comes to the point of pregnancy with only fragmentary knowledge about the importance of nutrition to her health and the health of her future children. Parents and potential parents, however, are becoming more aware of the need for good nutrition. So as a young woman develops the desire to become pregnant and rear a healthy baby she, at the same time, becomes more concerned about her own health and the health and well-being of the child.

Good nutrition is never an easy goal to achieve. Yet good nutrition is a positive force that affects health and the quality of life throughout the life cycle. The concept of ideal nutritional health suggests that all the essential nutrients are supplied to and used efficiently by the individual on a long-term basis. So the

*Boldface numbers in parentheses refer to reference at the end of each chapter.

nutritional history of the pregnant woman is equally as important as the nature of her diet during pregnancy. It plays a significant role in determining the outcome of pregnancy and the health of the infant. Unfortunately, lifelong poor nutrition can be a major factor in causing the poor outcome of pregnancy. Therefore, more consideration should be given to the nutritional needs of women during the years before childbearing to decrease the number who enter pregnancy in poor physical health.

The most desirable nutritional condition is based on a sound knowledge of the principles of nutrition by both adult women and those health professionals who work with them prior to and during pregnancy. This chapter addresses the nutritional needs of women and emphasizes the importance of nutrition for the best reproductive conditions. The essential nutrients and their function and major sources are reviewed, since knowledge about nutrition begins with an understanding of nutrients and their roles in the body. We suggest that readers with a fundamental knowledge of nutrition merely scan this section and use it as a reference. Other sections of the chapter, focusing on nutrition counseling and practical application, should intensify interest in an area too often neglected—the preconceptional nutriture of the mother.

NUTRITIONAL STATUS OF THE PRECONCEPTIONAL WOMAN

The woman entering her childbearing years reflects a host of influences to which she has been exposed throughout her own fetal period, infancy, childhood, and adolescence. The habits, attitudes, and values she developed during her earlier years will affect her nutritional status as she comes to maturity. McGanity (**4**) states that if potential mothers and fathers are indeed made and nurtured from their own conception through childhood, then growth and development during the first 17 years of life are critical. The consequences of inadequate maternal nutrition represent a major health problem for society (**5**). Unfavorable consequences range from failure to conceive to failure of the newborn infant to achieve adequate growth and development and encompass fetal failure and problems in childbirth. The unfavorable outcome of pregnancy and its relation to maternal nutrition is discussed in greater depth in Chapter 4.

How well are young women being prepared for their first pregnancy? The University of Texas Medical branch in Galveston has gathered cross-sectional and longitudinal data on over 3000 young women from birth to 25 years of age (**4**). The study covers dietary, anthropometric, clinical, and biochemical evidence of poor nutrition and its consequences. It shows that a relatively large percentage of infants, teenagers, and pregnant and/or lactating women studied ingested less than 50 percent of the recommended dietary allowance (RDA) for several nutrients. Nutrients ingested in low amounts by teenagers and pregnant and/or lactating women included calcium, iron, vitamin A, vitamin C, and niacin. Ten to 38 percent of children from birth to 16 years of age were at risk for at least one nutrient factor as shown by clinical signs of poor nutrition. Clinical signs of nutritional deficiencies of vitamin C, riboflavin, and iron or B vitamins were observed in persons 16 years of age and over. Researchers conducting this

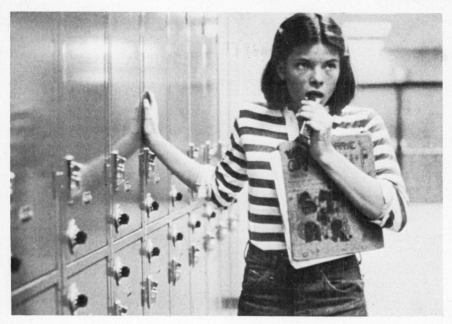

Long term nutritional health of the female is important to the health of her future children.

survey regard it as no surprise that many young women enter their first pregnancy with several nutritional handicaps which could decrease reproductive performance and affect maternal and fetal outcome. Other studies lead to similar conclusions (**6**). A significant number of young women enter their reproductive years in poor nutritional health. These young women obviously are not in a desirable condition to superimpose a pregnancy on already deficient nutrient reserves.

The nutritional vulnerability of women of childbearing age is such that they are regarded as one of the high-risk groups in the United States (**4, 7**). A recent survey of the American population, the first Health and Nutrition Examination Survey (HANES) (**8, 9**), found that the major nutrition-related health problems in women of childbearing age were largely subclinical in nature and included iron-deficiency anemia, endemic goiter, and possible calcium-phosphorus imbalance. The prevalence of iron-deficiency anemia is widespread regardless of race and income level (Table 1.1). Goiter was reported in girls aged 6–11, becoming most prevalent in young adults, and then decreasing with age (**7**). The following table summarizes the incidence of goiter in women of childbearing age (Table 1.2).

Calcium-phosphorus imbalance, as indicated by hyperirritability of the neuromuscular system, was found more often in black than in white adolescents regardless of income (**7**). The problem appeared to be related to lower intakes of calcium.

TABLE 1.1   HEMOGLOBIN AND HEMATOCRIT
IN WOMEN AGED 18−44 BY INCOME AND RACE

	INCOME		INCOME	
	Below Poverty Level		Above Poverty Level	
	White	Black	White	Black
Hemoglobin (g/100 ml)	13.6	12.7	14.0	13.2
Percentage low values	6.8	21.5	4.6	14.1
Hematocrit (percentage)	40.4	38.4	41.4	40.0
Percentage low values	16.3	26.7	10.1	19.7

Source: Reproduced with permission from F. W. Lowenstein in *Nutritional Disorders of American Women,* ed. M. Winick (**7**). Copyright © 1977 by John Wiley & Sons, Inc., New York.

TABLE 1.2   PREVALENCE OF
GOITER IN AMERICAN FAMILIES

Race	Age	Income	Percentage of prevalence
Black	Adolescents	High	15.8
Black	18−24	Marginal	13.4
White	18−24	Marginal	12.1

Source: Data from several sources.

Numerous researchers recognize that the use of hormonal agents for contraception may result in altered nutritional needs in women of childbearing age (**10−13**). The following table summarizes the nutritional changes associated with the use of oral contraceptives (Table 1.3). Possible nutritional problems related to the use of oral contraceptives are discussed in greater depth in Chapter 4.

Why do many young women suffer from a poor nutritional status? Frequently they lack adequate knowledge of good nutrition and its relationship to health. More often, young women's busy lives prevent them from paying enough attention to good nutrition. The pressures and tensions of everyday living are sufficient without worrying about what to eat. So as long as they feel all right, young people may not give enough attention to their eating habits.

Eating is not just a matter of hunger. It is closely related to social activities and feelings about appearance, independence, and acceptance. None of these has anything to do with the major function of food—that of nourishing our bodies. Each person has reasons for eating in a particular way. The high school student at 17 and the young career woman at 25 will each bring her own unique perspective to a discussion of individual eating habits. Both these women have developed food habits that could affect the health of the next generation. As a student of child development and nutrition, the reader may someday be in a position to guide young women in the selection of a diet best suited for their health and that of their

TABLE 1.3 NUTRITIONAL ABERRATIONS
ATTRIBUTED TO CONTRACEPTIVE STEROIDS

Nutrient	Effect
Folacin	Serum level decreased
	Erythrocyte level decreased
	Megaloblastic anemia (rare)
Vitamin B_{12}	Lowered serum level
Riboflavin	Lowered erythrocyte level
	Glossitis (rare)
Vitamin B_6	Altered tryptophan metabolism
	Plasma PLP[1] decreased
	Depression
Ascorbic acid	Decreased leukocyte content
	Decreased platelet level
Vitamin A	Increased plasma level
Iron	Increased serum level
	Increased TIBC[2]
Copper	Increased plasma level
	Increased ceruloplasmin
Zinc	Decreased plasma zinc

Source: Reproduced with permission from D. A. Roe in *Nutritional Disorders of American Women,* ed. M. Winick (**10**). Copyright © 1977 by John Wiley & Sons, Inc., New York
[1]Pyridoxal phosphate.
[2]Total Iron Binding Capacity.

unborn children. The following sections deal with the nutrient requirements of the preconceptional woman, dietary counseling, and practical application. They should help future health professionals visualize their roles and the important contributions they can make in the area of preconceptual nutrition.

NUTRIENT REQUIREMENTS OF THE PRECONCEPTIONAL WOMAN

The following section discusses the essential nutrients with special reference to the needs of the female of childbearing age. Nutrients are not discussed in depth. Rather, a review approach is used to provide the reader with a brief overview of the nutrients mentioned throughout this book. Again, readers with a sound background in nutrition may decide to omit this section.

Recommended Dietary Allowances for the Adult Female

Recommended dietary allowances (RDAs) are amounts of the various essential nutrients suggested for daily consumption by healthy persons. In the United States, RDAs are established by a committee of the Food and Nutrition Board (FNB) of the National Research Council. They were first published in 1943 and are revised about every five years. The latest edition was published in 1980.

RDA values are estimates of the amount of each nutrient that healthy persons should eat daily to meet physiological needs. These values are thought to be large enough to meet the physiological needs of those persons with the highest requirements. Therefore, RDA values for most nutrients (except energy) are much higher than the average requirements of the population. Energy allowances are calculated to meet the average needs of a healthy population.

Nutrient requirements and allowances change with age, sex, and physiological state. The RDA values are determined, therefore, for different age, weight, and sex groupings. After infancy, the nutrient allowances are given for age groups of three- to four-year intervals. Up to age 10 no distinction is made between the needs for boys and girls. Above age 10, however, separate nutrient allowances are given for boys and girls. Additional requirements are also listed for pregnant and nursing women.

Present information is inadequate about many of the nutrients that humans require for good health. There is little information, for instance, on the possible long term effects of excessive intakes of certain nutrients or marginal intakes of others. RDA values are not synonymous with individual nutritional requirements but should serve to insure that the daily food supply provides each of the essential nutrients in sufficient amounts to keep the probability of nutritional inadequacy low. The RDAs for the adult female are shown in Table 1.4.

Energy Requirements

Energy is required for the many metabolic processes essential for life, physical activity, growth of the fetus during pregnancy, lactation, and growth and development of the child. Energy needs of the adult vary with body size, with the amount and severity of physical activity, with physiological state, and to a lesser degree, with climate. An understanding of the effect of each of these factors on energy is necessary to make sound judgments about the energy needs of an individual. One basis for estimating the energy needs of any given person is a change in body weight in relation to the desirable weight for height and body build. A gain in weight is, for most persons, a clear indication that energy consumption is in excess of energy needs. Likewise, loss of weight is the result of energy intake below needs.

In contrast to other nutrients for which RDAs are set, the energy allowance is established at a level thought to be associated with good health of average persons in each age group and a given activity category. Therefore, the recommendations for energy represent the average needs of people in each category rather than intakes high enough to meet the upper limits of variability of almost all people of a specific age and sex. Energy allowances for adult females are shown in Table 1.5. In the United States, people are presumed to live in an environment with a mean temperature of 20° C. Energy allowances can be adjusted to account for increased physical activity, for body size, and, rarely, for climate. Adjustment must also be made for the special energy demands of pregnancy and lactation.

TABLE 1.4 RECOMMENDED DAILY DIETARY ALLOWANCES (RDAs) FOR THE ADULT FEMALE POPULATION

	Age Range		
	15–18	19–22	23–50
Energy (kcal)	2100	2100	2000
Protein (g)	46	44	44
Vitamin A (mcg R.E.)[1]	800	800	800
Vitamin D (mcg)[2]	10	7.5	5
Vitamin E (mgα T.E.)[3]	8	8	8
Ascorbic Acid (mg)	60	60	60
Folacin (mcg)	400	400	400
Niacin (mg N.E.)[4]	14	14	13
Riboflavin (mg)	1.3	1.3	1.2
Thiamin (mg)	1.1	1.1	1.0
Vitamin B_6 (mg)	2.0	2.0	2.0
Vitamin B_{12} (mcg)	3.0	3.0	3.0
Calcium (mg)	1200	800	800
Phosphorus (mg)	1200	800	800
Iodine (mcg)	150	150	150
Iron (mg)	18	18	18
Magnesium (mg)	300	300	300
Zinc (mg)	15	15	15

Source: From Food and Nutrition Board (FNB), *Recommended Dietary Allowances,* 9th edition. National Academy of Sciences, Washington, 1980 (**14**).

[1] Retinol equivalents (R.E.). 1 R.E. = 1 μg retinol or 6 μg carotene. See text for calculation of vitamin A activity of diets as retinol equivalents.

[2] As cholecalciferol. 10 μg cholecalciferol = 400 international units (IU) vitamin D.

[3] α-tocopherol equivalents. 1 mg D-α-tocopherol = 1 α-T.E. See text for variation in allowances and calculation of vitamin E activity of the diet as α-tocopherol equivalents.

[4] One Niacin equivalent (N.E.) = 1 mg niacin or 60 mg dietary tryptophan.

Each individual expends considerable energy simply maintaining life. Basal energy use is related to body size. Persons of larger (or smaller) body size require proportionately more (or less) total energy per unit of time for activities, such as walking, that involve moving mass over distance. The hourly resting metabolic rate of these persons will also be slightly higher or lower than the average. It has been customary to include basal metabolism as one of the factors affecting the overall energy requirement for an individual. *Basal metabolism,* or basal metabolic rate, refers to energy expenditure at a specific time. In practice, the major interest has been in "resting metabolism," that is, the metabolism of a person in a normal life situation while at rest and under conditions of thermal neutrality.

TABLE 1.5 RECOMMENDED ENERGY INTAKES, MEAN HEIGHTS AND WEIGHTS FOR ADULT WOMEN[1]

Age (years)	Weight (kg)	(lb)	Height (cm)	(in)	Energy Needs (with range) (kcal)[2]
19–22	55	120	163	64	2100 (1700–2500)
23–50	55	120	163	64	2000 (1600–2400)
51–75	55	120	163	64	1800 (1400–2200)
76+	55	120	163	64	1600 (1200–2000)
Pregnancy					+300
Lactation					+500

Source: From Food and Nutrition Board, Recommended Dietary Allowances, 9th edition. National Academy of Sciences, Washington, 1980 (**14**).

[1]Data in this table have been assembled from the desirable weight for the mean height of adult females (64 in.) between the ages of 18 and 34 years as surveyed in the U.S. population (Department of Health, Education and Welfare [DHEW] and National Center for Health Statistics [NCHS] data). Energy allowances for the younger age groups are for women doing light work. The allowances for the two older groups represent mean energy needs over these age spans, allowing for a 2 percent decrease in basal metabolic rate per decade and for a reduction in activity of 200 kilocalories (kcal) per day for women between 51 and 75 years and 400 kcal for women over 75 based on a variation in energy needs of ±400 kcal at any one age emphasizing the wide range of energy intakes appropriate for any group of people.

[2]The accepted international unit of energy is the joule (J). 1 kcal = 4.184 kilojoules (kJ).

Activity, a major variable affecting energy expenditure, ranges from very light or sedentary to very heavy. For most adult females in the United States, the level of activity is likely to be light or moderate, although there will be exceptions. The following guide may be useful in estimating energy expenditures for various activity levels for the adult females weighing 58 kg (**14**).

Activity	*Kcal/minute*
Very light	up to 2.0
Light	2.0–3.9
Moderate	4.0–5.9
Heavy	6.0–10.0

Total energy needs can be estimated by adding basal energy needs and energy used in activity. In general, the adult energy requirement for weight maintenance with moderate activity is about 1.6 times the basal energy expenditure for women.

Energy needs of adults generally decline with age as both metabolic resting rate and activity decline. Resting metabolism declines at a rate of about 2 percent each decade. The decline in activity is less predictable. Energy allowances can usually be reduced by approximately 10 percent for the adult between 51 and 75 years of age and for persons beyond age 75 years by approximately 20−25 percent of the amount required by the younger adult. There will be exceptions based on activity levels.

The physiological state of an individual influences energy requirements. During pregnancy, additional energy is needed to build new tissue in the placenta and fetus, to provide for the increased work load associated with movement of the mother, and to support an increase in the resting metabolic rate. Additional energy is also required during lactation and is proportional to the quantity of milk produced.

Although climate affects the human body's energy use, the influence is minimal and can generally be ignored. Energy needs for work, however, are approximately 5 percent higher in colder climates (mean temperature < 14° C) than in very warm climates. People tend to avoid activity at high temperatures (> 37° C), but wherever people are required to be physically active in extreme heat, energy allowances may need to be slightly increased.

The general goal for the healthy woman is maintenance of body weight within an acceptable range, and adjustments in energy intake and/or activity level can usually achieve that objective.

The adult female should understand the need to maintain desirable weight prior to pregnancy as excess weight can be a detrimental and complicating factor during pregnancy. The health of both the mother and the fetus can be affected adversely by the mother's excess weight. A more comprehensive discussion of the problems associated with obesity during pregnancy occurs in a later chapter; here, we touch on the general problem of obesity in the adult female.

The risks of adult obesity were summarized recently in hearings before the Senate Select Committee on Nutrition and Human Needs (**15**). These risks included increased incidence of heart disease, hypertension, complications following surgery, hypoventilation, insulin antagonism, gynecological irregularities, and toxemia of pregnancy. This information indicated that about 20 percent of American women from 35 to 44 and about 30 percent of those from 44 to 55 are obese (**16**). In some affluent populations 60 percent of the women above 50 are classified as obese (**17**). Numerous review papers and books are available on the types, causes, potential remedies, and associated problems of obesity for additional insight into this major health problem (**18−20**).

Energy-Supplying Nutrients

Carbohydrates.   Carbohydrates can be classified into three major groups on the basis of their chemical structures. These are monosaccharides, which are simple sugars; disaccharides, two simple sugars linked together; and polysaccharides, which are complex carbohydrates composed of many simple sugar units linked together.

Of the monosaccharides, the least complex carbohydrates, the most important ones from a nutritional viewpoint are the six carbons called "hexoses."

The three most common hexoses are glucose, fructose, and galactose. The structures of these hexoses are as shown here:

```
        H                       CH₂OH                      H
        |                         |                        |
      C = O                     C = O                     C = O
        |                         |                        |
     H-C-OH                    OH-C-H                    H-C-OH
        |                         |                        |
     OH-C-H                     H-C-OH                    OH-C-H
        |                         |                        |
     H-C-OH                     H-C-OH                    OH-C-H
        |                         |                        |
     H-C-OH                     CH₂OH                    H-C-OH
        |                                                   |
      CH₂OH                                               CH₂OH

     Glucose                    Fructose                  Galactose
```

Glucose is commonly found in fruits and vegetables. Fructose is found in fruits, vegetables, and cane sugar. Galactose is found in milk. These three hexoses are the end products of all digestible carbohydrates. During metabolism fructose and galactose are converted to glucose in the liver.

Disaccharides include sucrose, lactose, and maltose. Each of these yields two monosaccharides on digestion. Sucrose, formed by the linkage of glucose and fructose, is the most widely distributed in foods. In its pure form it is ordinary table sugar. Lactose, made up of glucose and galactose, is found in milk. Maltose, a polymer of two glucose molecules, results from the partial breakdown of starch.

Polysaccharides, the most complex carbohydrates, are made up of large numbers of glucose molecules linked together. The principal polysaccharides are starch, cellulose, hemicellulose, and glycogen. Starch, the most common digestible polysaccharide, is found in the cells of grains, fruits, and certain vegetables. It is the storage form of energy in plants and, on digestion, eventually yields glucose. Cellulose and hemicellulose, integral components of plant cell wall structure, are resistant to the digestive enzymes that break down other polysaccharides and, therefore, yield a minimum of carbohydrate to humans. These nondigestible carbohydrates are the major components of dietary fiber. They provide bulk in the diet and regulate the process of digestion and the elimination of waste products from the digestive tract. Although controversial, the intake of fiber is regarded as a positive factor in the maintenance of good health (**21**). Glycogen is the storage form of carbohydrate in the animal and the human. Because of the limited amount that exists in our diet, however, it is not a major source of energy, although it is readily utilized by the tissues.

Carbohydrate is synthesized in body tissues from other sources of carbon (fat and protein), so a specific dietary need has not yet been established for it. However, it is desirable to include carbohydrate in the diet. This prevents the excessive use of body protein as an energy source, the loss of cations and dehydration that accompany protein breakdown, and the development of ketosis. As little as 100 g of carbohydrate per day (400 kcal) will prevent excessive protein breakdown, and probably as little as 40 g per day will prevent ketosis. The FNB (14) suggests a carbohydrate intake of 50–100 g of digestible carbohydrate per day. This intake level will prevent undesirable metabolic reactions associated with fasting or high fat diets (22).

In the past carbohydrate was the predominant source of energy in the human diet. Now, however, carbohydrate and fat contribute almost equally to the energy content of the American diet, with carbohydrate providing 46 percent and fat 41 percent of total caloric intake. The consumption of sugars and other sweeteners increased rapidly during the early part of this century. Since 1925, though, sugar consumption has remained fairly constant at approximately 17 percent of total energy intake. The consumption of complex carbohydrates in the form of fresh fruits and vegetables and unrefined grain products has decreased from 43 percent of dietary food energy in 1909 to approximately 29 percent today (23). The following table summarizes some changes in the consumption of carbohydrate sources in recent years (Table 1.6).

The continuing change in the consumption pattern of carbohydrates is a cause for concern (21). The consumption of refined carbohydrates is implicated in the increased incidence of heart disease and the development of dental caries.

We have no specific requirement now for dietary fiber in the form of complex carbohydrates. Recent research suggests that a relationship may exist between inadequate intake of dietary fiber and the development of certain disease conditions (24). These include cancer of the colon, appendicitis, diverticular disease, and coronary heart disease.

Carbohydrate, in the form of concentrated sweets, is high in calories but provides few other nutrients. On the other hand, other carbohydrate foods, fruits

TABLE 1.6 CHANGES IN PER CAPITA CONSUMPTION OF FOODS CONTAINING COMPLEX CARBOHYDRATES AND "NATURALLY OCCURRING" SUGARS BETWEEN 1947–1949 AND 1976

	Change per Capita/Year (lb)
Vegetables	−12
Flour and cereals	−31
Fruits (noncitrus)	−30
Potatoes	−21
Citrus fruits	+10.5
Dark green and yellow vegetables	−6.3

Source: Based on Nutritional Review Consumer and Food Economics [CFE] (Adm.) 299–11, January 1977, Agricultural Research Service, U.S. Department of Agriculture.

and vegetables, cereals, and cereal products are relatively rich in other nutrients. In addition, the enrichment of flour, breads, and, to some extent, cereals and other grain products with B-vitamins (thiamin, niacin, riboflavin) and iron increases the nutrient content of these carbohydrate foods.

Lipids.   Lipids or fats consist of a molecule of glycerol and from one to three fatty acids. Each of the three hydroxyl (OH) groups of glycerol can combine with a fatty acid. Fats are classified according to the number of fatty acids esterified to the glycerol molecule and thus may be mono-, di-, or triglycerides. The majority of fats are present in food as triglyceride and are stored in the body in this form. The structure of glycerol and an example of a triglyceride, where R represents the individual fatty acids, are shown next.

$$
\begin{array}{ll}
\begin{array}{c}
\text{H} \\
| \\
\text{H} - \text{C} - \text{OH} \\
| \\
\text{H} - \text{C} - \text{OH} \\
| \\
\text{H} - \text{C} - \text{OH} \\
| \\
\text{H} \\
\text{Glycerol}
\end{array}
&
\begin{array}{c}
\qquad\qquad\quad \text{O} \\
\qquad\qquad\quad /\!/ \\
\text{CH}_2 - \text{C} - \text{R} \\
| \qquad\quad \text{O} \\
| \qquad\quad /\!/ \\
\text{CH} - \text{C} - \text{R} \\
| \qquad\quad \text{O} \\
| \qquad\quad /\!/ \\
\text{CH}_2 - \text{C} - \text{R} \\
\text{Triglyceride}
\end{array}
\end{array}
$$

Fatty acids are straight-chain carbon compounds with a methyl group (CH_3) at one end and a carboxyl group (COOH) at the other. The general formula for fatty acids is $CH_3 (CH_2)_n COOH$. They can be classified as saturated or unsaturated based on the degree of hydrogenation of the carbon atoms within the chain. Fatty acids are classified as polyunsaturated when two or more carbon atoms do not have the maximum number of hydrogen atoms attached. Linoleic acid is an example of this type:

$$CH_3(CH_2)_4CH = CHCH_2CH = CH(CH_2)_7COOH$$

Fats can also be classified as saturated or unsaturated on the basis of the relative amounts of saturated and unsaturated fatty acids they contain. Saturated fats are solid at room temperature and are present in both animal and plant tissue but chiefly in animal tissue. Unsaturated fats are present in oils found in plant seeds and fish oils. As a rule fats of plant origin are unsaturated, the only major exception being coconut oil that is highly saturated. All naturally occurring fats are mixtures of saturated, monounsaturated or polyunsaturated fats.

The primary function of fat in the diet is to provide a concentrated form of energy to the body. Fats provide an average of 9 kcal per gram, more than twice as much energy per unit of weight as either carbohydrate or protein. In addition, fats carry the fat-soluble vitamins A, D, E, and K into the body and improve their absorption from the intestinal tract. Normal deposits of fat tissue beneath the skin help to regulate and maintain body temperature by exerting an insulating effect and thus preventing excessive heat loss. Layers of fat tissue also provide protection for various internal body organs. Fats improve the palatability of food and provide flavor, as many of the flavor components of foods are associated with the fat portion. Fats provide satiety value in the diet, since they are digested more slowly than carbohydrates and protein and, therefore, delay the onset of hunger. They also improve the absorption of certain minerals from the intestinal tract.

Humans require fat in the diet as a source of the essential fatty acid, linoleic acid, and as a source of the fat soluble vitamins. This requirement for fat-soluble vitamins and essential fatty acid can be met by including 15–25 g of fats and oils in the daily diet. The requirement for essential fatty acid is in the range of 1–2 percent of total calories consumed.

The fat content of American diets varies considerably and has increased over the years (Figure 1.1), although the intake has decreased slightly in recent years. In 1910 the average American consumed 125 g of nutrient fat per day, 32 percent of the total caloric intake. Today, the average consumption of fat has increased to 147 g per person per day or approximately 41 percent of the total caloric intake. Some common sources of fat are butter, margarine, shortening, cooking and salad oils, cream, most cheeses, mayonnaise, salad dressing, nuts, bacon, and other fatty meats. Meats, whole milk, eggs, and chocolate contain some natural fat; and many popular snacks, baked goods, pastries, and other desserts are made with fat or are cooked in fat. The percentage of calories contributed by fat is high in most foods of animal origin. The predominant monounsaturated fats in the diet are olive and peanut oils, and polyunsaturated fats are represented by soybean, cottonseed, safflower, and palm oils.

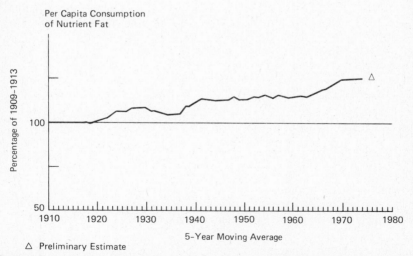

Figure 1.1 *Per capita consumption of nutrient fat.* (*Source:* From U.S.D.A., Handbook of Agricultural Charts. Agricultural Handbook No. 504, 1976 [**25**]).

The American diet is probably higher in fat content than is compatible with good health. Recently, the relationship of the amount and type of fat in the diet to the incidence of coronary heart disease has been a cause of concern (**9, 10, 14, 21, 26, 27**). Coronary heart disease is a significant cause of death in the United States, and available evidence concludes that the cause may well be in the diet. An increased intake of polyunsaturated fat and a decreased intake of saturated fat could be beneficial in preventing the development of coronary heart disease. The effect, however, of dietary changes on coronary heart disease in humans is not fully understood. Although it is difficult to define precisely a reasonable allowance for fat or a pattern of fatty acids in the diet, the American Heart Association recommends that no more than 35 percent of the total caloric intake be in the form of fat and that less than 10 percent of total caloric intake come from saturated fats (**14**).

Proteins.   Proteins, the large complex molecules made up of amino acids, differ from carbohydrates and fats in that they contain nitrogen in addition to carbon, hydrogen, and oxygen. Amino acids are the basic units of protein structure, and 22 amino acids are commonly found in foods. A wide variety of protein molecules can be made from these 22 amino acids. Protein molecules differ in the numbers, kinds, and proportions of amino acids they contain. The spatial arrangement of each amino acid chain also differs for different proteins and increases the number of possible proteins. Body proteins contain all 22 amino acids, but only 14 are synthesized by the body. The remaining eight amino acids are called "essential amino acids," because it is essential that they be supplied in the diet. The eight essential amino acids are isoleucine, leucine, tryptophan, lysine, methionine, phenylalanine, threonine, and valine. A ninth amino acid, histidine, is considered essential for infants, and recent evidence shows that histidine is also essential for the human adult (**28**).

All the essential amino acids must be present in adequate amounts in the diet if dietary protein is to be utilized fully for growth and maintenance.

A dietary protein is called a "complete protein" if it contains all the essential amino acids in the amounts required by the body. If it is low or totally lacking in one or more of the eight essential amino acids it is called an "incomplete protein." In general, the proteins of animal products tend to be complete, but those of plant products are incomplete. For example, most grains are low in the essential amino acid lysine. Most legumes are low in the essential amino acid methionine. Protein quality is an expression of how well the amino acid pattern of a dietary protein matches the pattern of amino acids required by the human body. Animal protein, therefore, tends to be higher quality protein than that of plant origin. The protein quality of incomplete proteins can be improved by combining proteins whose amino acid patterns complement one another. For example, both cereal grains and legumes provide protein of marginal quality. However, when grains and legumes are eaten together, the methionine provided by the cereal grain supplements the low methionine provided by the legume. Similarly, the lysine provided by the legume makes up for the low amount of lysine present in the cereal grain. When eaten together, the amino acid balance of both is improved and a better quality protein is provided.

The primary function of dietary protein is to supply the essential amino acids required for synthesis of body protein and for the growth, maintenance, and repair of body tissue. Dietary protein is also the source of nitrogen for the synthesis of nonprotein nitrogen-containing compounds such as nucleic acids, hormones, and certain nitrogen-containing lipids. Proteins in the blood play a role in the regulation of fluid balance in the body, and plasma proteins assist in the maintenance of body pH, which is essential for normal cellular metabolism. Protein provides energy at the average level of 4 kcal per gram. When too little carbohydrate or fat is consumed or when an excess amount of protein is ingested, the body's energy supply comes from the carbon portion of the protein.

Protein requirements by the body represent the sum of the needs for the essential amino acids and sufficient utilizable nitrogen for the synthesis of body protein and other nitrogen-containing compounds essential for health. Factors affecting the amount of protein required include protein quality, energy value of the diet, carbohydrate content of the diet, stage of growth and physiological state of the individual, and variability among individuals. The current daily allowance for the adult female, based on a reference woman weighing 55 kg, is 44 g (**14**).

The FNB further estimates the needs for the essential amino acids. Those estimated requirements are expressed on a body weight basis for a reference woman (55 kg in body weight) (Table 1.7). Approximately 20 percent of the dietary nitrogen as essential amino acids will generally meet the needs of the healthy adult.

TABLE 1.7 ESTIMATED AMINO ACID REQUIREMENTS OF THE ADULT AND PATTERN FOR HIGH QUALITY PROTEIN

	Adult need (mg/kg/day)	Need for adult woman[1] (mg)	Pattern for protein (mg/g of protein)
Histidine	—	—	17
Isoleucine	12	696	42
Leucine	16	928	70
Lysine	12	696	51
Sulfur-containing amino acids[2]	10	580	26
Aromatic amino acids[3]	16	928	73
Threonine	8	464	35
Tryptophan	3	174	11
Valine	14	812	48

Source: From Food and Nutrition Board, Recommended Dietary Allowances, 9th edition. National Academy of Sciences, Washington, 1980 (**14**).
[1] Estimated to weigh 55 kg. From FNB (**14**).
[2] Methionine and cystine.
[3] Phenylalanine and tyrosine.

Important amounts of protein are found in meat, poultry, fish, milk, cheese, eggs, dry beans, dry peas, and nuts. Breads, cereals, vegetables, and fruits contain relatively smaller amounts of protein.

Vitamins

Vitamins are chemically unrelated organic compounds required in relatively minute amounts for normal growth and maintenance of life. The absence of certain vitamins from the diet will result in characteristic deficiency symptoms. Fat-soluble vitamins are carried in fat or oil. These include vitamins A, D, E, and K. Others are soluble in water and are classified as "water soluble." Vitamin C and the B-complex vitamins are water soluble. The water-soluble vitamins are excreted and are not generally stored in the body.

Vitamin A.   Vitamin A, retinol, is found in animal tissue as the free alcohol or ester form. No free or esterified vitamin A is found in plant tissue, but certain substances known as "carotenoids" or "carotenes" are present in the tissues of green and yellow vegetables. Carotenes can be converted to vitamin A in the liver and intestinal wall. Vitamin A is calculated in terms of retinol equivalents (R.E.). The FNB (**14**) establishes the daily allowance for vitamin A for the adult female to be 800 R.E.

Vitamin A is essential for growth and the maintenance of health in the human. It is necessary for maintaining the integrity of epithelial tissue lining the respiratory, alimentary, and genitourinary tracts. Vitamin A also plays a role in the maintenance of good vision by protecting the cornea and conjunctiva of the eye from degenerative changes. It is a component of "visual purple" or "rhodopsin" that is the photosensitive pigment of the retinal rods responsible for vision in dim light. It is also shown to play a role in bone metabolism, detoxication mechanisms, and cholesterol synthesis, but these functions are not as clearly defined as the role in the visual cycle.

Vitamin A is stored in the liver and can be toxic if taken in excessive amounts. Toxic levels are 200,000–400,000 international units (IU) of vitamin A per day taken over an extended time. The Food and Drug Administration (FDA) has, therefore, placed a restriction on the amount of vitamin A that can be included in commercial vitamin preparations. Large amounts of carotene are not toxic. An excess of dietary carotene, however, may not be converted to vitamin A rapidly enough and will be deposited in the skin giving it a yellowish color.

Liver is a major source of vitamin A. Significant amounts are also found in eggs, butter, margarine, whole milk, and cheese made with whole milk. Carotene is found in largest amounts in dark green (collards, kale, leafy greens, etc.) and deep yellow vegetables (carrots, sweet potatoes, winter squash) and deep yellow fruits (apricots).

Vitamin D.   Vitamin D is responsible for the prevention of rickets and is often called the "antirachitic vitamin." Vitamin D exists in several forms. The two most important in human nutrition are ergocalciferol (vitamin D_2) and cholecalciferol (vitamin D_3). Ergosterol, a form of vitamin D found in plant tissue, is activated by sunlight to form ergocalciferol. Cholecalciferol is formed in human epidermal cells exposed to sunlight and ultraviolet radiation. The active forms of the vitamin are 25-hydroxycholecalciferol and 25-hydroxyergocalciferol. These are converted from cholecalciferol (vitamin D_3) and ergocalciferol (vitamin D_2) in the liver. The formation of an even more active form—1, 25-dihydroxycholecalciferol—occurs in the kidney. The synthesis of the active forms appear to be regulated by the availability of calcium through a feedback mechanism.

The primary function of vitamin D is the mineralization of bone. Vitamin D stimulates the intestinal absorption of calcium and phosphorus, the mobilization of calcium from bone, and the reduction of calcium excretion through the kidney. It functions in a hormonelike manner to maintain the level of calcium in the blood plasma by controlling the movement of calcium to and from bone. A deficiency of vitamin D in the diet will result in the failure of teeth and bones to calcify or harden properly. Disorders in bone development can lead to the disease osteomalacia (adult rickets) in adult females. This osteomalacia is characterized by decreased bone density.

Vitamin D is not widely distributed in nature. The chief source of vitamin D is the activation of the provitamin in the skin through ultraviolet radiation. In temperate climates, the amount synthesized in this manner may not be sufficient to meet the body's requirements, and vitamin supplements are often prescribed. Few foods contain much vitamin D naturally. Small amounts are present in egg yolk, butter, and liver, with larger amounts occurring in sardines, salmon, herring, and tuna and fish liver oils. Milk is commonly fortified with vitamin D, since it is the major source of calcium and phosphorus in the diet.

The FNB (**14**) sets an RDA of vitamin D at 5 mcg or 200 IU for the normal adult female. Intakes above 2000 IU per day may result in toxic conditions, whose symptoms include loss of appetite, nausea, diarrhea, and general apathy. These excess amounts result in hypercalcemia and tissue damage in both infants and adults, as well as calcification of soft tissues and an abnormal increase in blood calcium and phosphorus. Because of these dangers the FDA has established regulations to control the addition of vitamin D to commercial preparations.

Vitamin E.   Vitamin E is a group of chemically related compounds known as "tocopherols." It exists in three forms: alpha-, beta-, and gamma-tocopherol, with the alpha form being the most active biologically.

Vitamin E functions as an antioxidant and is essential for the prevention of degenerative changes in certain tissues. It prevents the formation of toxic peroxides of unsaturated fatty acids that may damage cells. This vitamin plays a role in certain enzyme systems, although it is not known if the vitamin is an integral part of such enzyme systems or serves as an antioxidant to protect the enzyme system itself. It acts to preserve the easily oxidized vitamins A and C and plays a role in maintaining the integrity and proper functioning of reproductive, vascular, and muscular tissues in certain species.

Miracle claims for the vitamin recently increased its popularity. Some of these claims are that vitamin E prolongs life and protects against certain diseases, including cancer, heart disease, and ulcers. Current scientific evidence, however, does not support the suggestion that excess intakes of vitamin E will contribute to better health.

The FNB (**14**) recommends a daily intake of 8 mg of D-α-tocopherol. Vitamin E is abundant in vegetable oils, whole grain cereals, and green leafy vegetables. In general the average American diet of fruits, vegetables, vegetable oil, milk, meat, and eggs regularly supplies enough vitamin E to meet recommended requirements. The requirement for vitamin E is influenced by the kind and amount of fat in the diet, with the need increasing as the amount of polyunsaturated fat increases. However, oils supplying large amounts of polyunsaturated fats also supply large amounts of vitamin E. A dietary deficiency of vitamin E, therefore, is rare. Vitamin E deficiency may occur, however, in cases of fat malabsorption, and a long-term deficiency causes an increase in the fragility of the red blood cells.

Vitamin K.   Vitamin K, the coagulation vitamin, occurs in nature in two forms, phylloquinone (vitamin K_1) and menaquinone or vitamin K_2. A third form is the synthetic compound menadione, vitamin K_3.

Vitamin K functions primarily to promote the normal clotting of blood and to prevent hemorrhage. It is essential for the formation of prothrombin, a precursor of thrombin, that is necessary for normal clot formation and may be involved in the formation of other blood clotting factors. It may also be involved in the respiratory chain of oxidative phosphorylation.

A vitamin K deficiency will cause an increase in blood clotting time. However, this deficiency is rarely seen in the human, since vitamin K is synthesized by intestinal bacteria and is also widely distributed in plants. Green leafy vegetables such as turnip greens, spinach, and broccoli are high in vitamin K. Cauliflower, peas, and cereals also contain vitamin K. The amount of vitamin K present in the average American diet, plus that available from bacterial synthesis in the body appears to be adequate to meet the needs of the majority of individuals. There is no established RDA for vitamin K, although a range of estimated safe intakes has been set at 70–140 mcg per day (**14**).

A vitamin K deficiency can occur if there is a decrease in the intestinal synthesis of the vitamin or a decrease in intestinal absorption. The use of certain antibiotic drugs may interfere with the metabolism of intestinal bacteria and availability of vitamin K.

Vitamin B-Complex.   Several vitamins, all soluble in water, including thiamin, riboflavin, niacin, vitamin B_6, folacin, vitamin B_{12}, pantothenic acid, and biotin, make up the B-complex group. The biochemical function of each of these vitamins tends to be better known than those of the fat-soluble group, and deficiency symptoms are reasonably well defined for the B-complex group. Deficiencies are no longer a major public health problem in the developed countries of the world. A few deficient individuals, however, may be reported on any large scale nutrition survey. Subclinical or borderline deficiencies may be present in a larger percentage of the population and may cause problems for individuals during stress periods. Although excessive intakes are not warranted, the importance of adequate B-complex vitamins cannot be emphasized too much for pregnant and lactating mothers and for growing children.

Thiamin. Vitamin B_1 or thiamin exists as (1) the free compound or its salts, (2) a thiamin-protein complex, or (3) thiamin pyrophosphate or cocarboxylase.

Symptoms of a mild thiamin deficiency include increased hypersensitivity, loss of appetite, fatigue, and general weakness. An extreme deficiency of thiamin leads to the disease beriberi, characterized by damage to the nervous and cardiovascular systems. A form of beriberi known as "dry beriberi" is accompanied by wasting of muscle tissue and is most common among adults.

Thiamin is found in enriched cereals, whole grain cereals, milk, legumes, and meat. Allowances for thiamin are usually related to energy intake, and an intake of 0.5 mg per 1000 kcal or 1.0 mg per day is recommended for the adult female (**14**).

Riboflavin. Riboflavin, or vitamin B_2, exists in the free form or as various chemical complexes with protein, phosphoric acid, or nucleic acid. It is a constituent of two coenzymes: flavin mononucleotide (FMN) and flavin adenine dinucleotide (FAD). These coenzymes play a role in tissue respiration and oxidation by serving as carriers of hydrogen and electrons in the electron transport system leading to the formation of high-energy adenosine triphosphate (ATP). Riboflavin also plays a role in the conversion of tryptophan to niacin.

Symptoms of a riboflavin deficiency include dermatitis, cheilosis (drying and cracking of lips), angular stomatitis (inflammation of mucous membranes of mouth), and damage to the conjunctiva of the eye. Riboflavin requirements are related to caloric intake, and the RDA (**14**) is established at 0.6 mg per 100 kcal or 1.2 mg of riboflavin per day for the adult female who consumes approximately 2000 kcal daily. Riboflavin is supplied by meats, milk, and whole grain or enriched breads and cereals.

Niacin. Niacin, the antipellagra vitamin, can exist free in nature but occurs chiefly as an integral part of several enzyme systems. It is a component of the two coenzymes: nicotinamide adenine dinucleotide (NAD) and nicotinamide adenine dinucleotide phosphate (NADP). Like the flavin coenzymes, NAD and NADP function in tissue respiration by serving as carriers of hydrogen or electrons in the electron transport system. Reduced NADP (NADPH) is required for the synthesis of fatty acids.

Pellagra, a disease characterized by rough or inflamed skin, nervousness, mental depression, and intestinal disorders, is caused by a niacin deficiency.

Niacin recommended intakes are related to caloric intake and are established as 6.6 mg per 1000 kcal or 13 mg of niacin per day for the adult woman. Niacin can be found in whole grain and enriched cereals, meat and meat products, and peas and beans. Tryptophan, one of the essential amino acids, can be converted to niacin in the body, and 60 mg of tryptophan is equivalent to 1 mg of niacin. Foods containing animal protein are, therefore, good sources of potential niacin.

Vitamin B_6.   Vitamin B_6 is a collective term referring to three pyridine compounds; pyridoxine, pyridoxal, and pyridoxamine. The phosphorylated pyridoxal form serves as a coenzyme in many of the reactions of amino acid metabolism. These include transamination, decarboxylation, desulfhydration, amine oxidation, and deamination. Vitamin B_6 also plays a role in the metabolism of unsaturated fatty acids and carbohydrates.

A deficiency of vitamin B_6 can cause skin lesions, including glossitis (inflammation of the tongue), dermatitis, stomatitis, and cheilosis. Microcytic anemias responsive to vitamin B_6 have been reported. Lack of vitamin B_6 also causes loss of appetite, convulsions, and hyperirritability in infants; and depression and mental confusion in adults. Vitamin B_6 deficiency leads to the formation of xanthurenic acid, an abnormal metabolite of tryptophan, and the excretion of xanthurenic acid following a test dose of tryptophan shows a vitamin B_6 deficiency.

The recommended daily intake for vitamin B_6 is 2.0 mg per day for the adult female. Vitamin B_6 is widespread in foods, occurring in meats, cereals, lentils, nuts, and certain fruits and vegetables.

Folacin.   Folacin, a general name for folic acid and related compounds, plays a role in the formation of purines and pyrimidines from which nucleic acids are derived. It functions in the formation of red blood cells and also plays a role in certain amino acid interconversions and methylation reactions.

A folacin deficiency results in the accumulation of immature red blood cells (megaloblasts) in the bone marrow, leading to macrocytic anemia. Other deficiency symptoms include glossitis, gastrointestinal disturbances, and neurological damage.

The RDA for folacin for an adult woman is 400 mcg. Folacin is present in many foods, and those with a high content per unit of dry weight include yeast, liver, and other organ meats, green vegetables, and some fruits.

Vitamin B_{12}.   Vitamin B_{12}, or cobalamin, is required for normal red blood cell formation. It functions by incorporating purines and pyrimidines into nucleosides and nucleic acids. Vitamin B_{12} is also a cofactor in methyl donor reactions important in amino acid metabolism. It occurs only in foods of animal origin.

A deficiency of vitamin B_{12} results in pernicious anemia characterized by megaloblastic red blood cells and eventually extensive neurological damage. Vitamin B_{12} corrects the blood abnormalities of pernicious anemia and arrests the progress of nervous tissue damage. Folacin, given in the treatment of pernicious anemia, corrects blood abnormalities but does not have any effect on nerve damage. A deficiency of vitamin B_{12} is not normally caused by a dietary deficiency but is due to the lack of an intrinsic factor produced in the stomach and necessary for vitamin absorption.

The RDA for vitamin B_{12} for adult women is 3 mcg per day.

Pantothenic Acid. Pantothenic acid is a component of coenzyme A and is involved in the intermediary metabolism of carbohydrates, fats, and proteins. The symptoms of a dietary deficiency of this vitamin are not well defined. There is insufficient evidence on which to base an RDA, but safe and adequate daily dietary intakes are estimated to be in the range of 4–7 mg (**14**). Liver and other organ meats, egg yolk, and dry milk are good sources of pantothenic acid.

Biotin. Biotin functions as a coenzyme in the synthesis of fatty acids. It plays a role in carboxylation reactions and may also be involved in amino acid metabolism, as well as the metabolism of carbohydrates, fats, and protein. Deficiency symptoms can be produced by the consumption of extremely large amounts of raw egg white. Raw egg white contains a glycoprotein, avidin, that combines with biotin and prevents its absorption, but avidin is inactive in cooked egg white. No established RDA for biotin exists, but the daily safe intake is estimated to be between 100 and 200 mcg (**14**).

Vitamin C. Two hundred years ago physicians recognized that citrus fruit would cure scurvy. It was not until 1928, though, that vitamin C, ascorbic acid, was isolated and identified as the substance having antiscorbutic properties. Like the B-complex group, ascorbic acid is soluble in water.

Vitamin C plays a role in the synthesis of collagen, a protein that is part of the connective tissue which binds together and supports all the structures of the body. It is essential for maintaining the integrity of capillary walls; for proper growth and development of blood vessels, teeth, and bone; and for wound healing. It also plays a role in the metabolism of amino acids and is involved in the synthesis of epinephrine and anti-inflammatory steroids by the adrenal gland. Active in the transport of iron between the plasma and storage organs, it may also be important for iron absorption from the intestinal tract.

Early signs of vitamin C deficiency include weakness, irritability, bleeding gums, gingivitis, loosening of teeth, and a tendency to bruise easily. The onset of scurvy in adults can be detected 60 to 90 days after the beginning of a vitamin C deficiency. Symptoms of scurvy include spongy bleeding gums, weakness, loss of appetite, anemia, painful swollen joints, and a tendency to hemorrhage.

Many of these symptoms are a result of the breakdown of the collagenous structure of connective tissue, bone, and cartilage. Scurvy is not commonly seen in adults but does develop occasionally in infants fed exclusively on cow's milk.

Vitamin C is found chiefly in plant products. Citrus fruits and their juices— oranges, grapefruits, and lemons—as well as fresh strawberries are rich in this vitamin. Other important sources include tomatoes and tomato juice, broccoli, brussels sprouts, cabbage, canteloupe, cauliflower, green peppers, dark green leafy vegetables such as collards, kale, mustard greens, spinach, and turnip greens, potatoes and sweet potatoes, (especially when cooked in the jacket) and watermelons. Cereal grains contain almost no vitamin C.

The body has a limited capacity to store vitamin C; therefore adequate amounts must be consumed frequently. To prevent scurvy 10 mg of vitamin C per day is sufficient. The FNB lists the RDA for the adult female as 60 mg of vitamin C per day, an amount that replenishes the amount of ascorbic acid metabolized daily and maintains an adequate body pool.

Because of recent health claims made for vitamin C, many Americans now consume massive doses in vitamin supplements in the belief that they are deriving certain benefits. No acceptable scientific evidence exists now, though, that ascorbic acid will prevent or cure the common cold or other diseases. Very little is known about the adverse effects of long-term use of massive doses of vitamin C, although studies indicate that excessive doses of this vitamin could be dangerous. Excessive doses of vitamin C cause nausea and diarrhea in some persons, markedly enhance iron absorption, and mobilize minerals from bone. A continued excess of vitamin C can also result in a conditioned deficiency or a lack of response to normal doses of the vitamin, destroy substantial amounts of vitamin B_{12} in food, and lead to the development of kidney stones in certain persons who cannot adequately dispose of megadoses. Until further evidence is available, the safest course is to make certain that the daily diet provides the vitamin in the amounts recommended by the National Research Council.

Minerals

Twenty-six or more different minerals are found in varying amounts in the body, and about 15 of these are necessary for good nutrition. Although they make up only 4 percent of body tissue, minerals are necessary for vital body processes, playing an important part in building the bone framework. They also play a role in the regulation of many processes such as blood clotting, muscular contractions, nerve responses, oxygen transport, and various other chemical reactions. Certain minerals are required by the body in relatively large amounts and are referred to as macronutrients. These include calcium, phosphorus, sodium, chloride, potassium, and magnesium. Iron, manganese, copper, iodine, zinc, cobalt, fluorine, selenium, and chromium are trace or micronutrients and are required in smaller amounts.

Calcium.   Calcium is present in the body in greater amounts than any other mineral, and approximately 99 percent of body calcium is concentrated in the skeletal system. Throughout life calcium builds and shapes the framework of the body and gives strength to bones and teeth. The remaining 1 percent is distributed throughout the soft tissues. Calcium in the body fluids and soft tissues helps to regulate body processes, including the normal functioning of nerves, contraction of muscle tissue, and the clotting of blood.

The FNB (**14**) recommends that 800 mg of calcium be included in the daily diet of the adult female to maintain calcium equilibrium. Milk is an outstanding source of calcium, and a low dietary intake of calcium in the United States is generally associated with a low milk intake. Appreciable amounts of calcium are also found in cheese, ice cream, certain dark green leafy vegetables (collards, kale, mustard greens, turnip greens) and salmon and sardines, if the small bones are eaten. An insufficient supply of calcium may result in stunted growth, poor quality of teeth and bone, or other bone disorders. "Osteoporosis," a disorder of bone metabolism that occurs in middle and older age, is often attributed to low calcium intake. Other nutrients, however, such as vitamin D and fluoride, may also be involved.

A calcium deficiency of dietary origin is difficult to relate to these disorders, and hormonal changes may prove to be the underlying cause. Osteoporosis is a particular problem for the older woman, and most often appears after the childbearing years. Women over 50 are afflicted more than any other group. Estrogen therapy is beneficial in some cases, but dietary therapy does not appear to help (**29**).

Phosphorus.   Phosphorus is the second most abundant mineral in the body, with 70–80 percent being found in bone and teeth, where it occurs with calcium in a nearly constant ratio. The healthy human organism maintains a specific calcium : phosphorus ratio of 2.5 : 1 in bone tissue. Calcium combines with phosphorus in the bone in the form of calcium-phosphate salts. If either calcium or phosphorus is lacking, the other mineral becomes ineffective, since they must be incorporated into the bone together.

Phosphorus, present in the soft tissues and in the intra- and extracellular fluids, plays a role in almost every chemical reaction in the body. It is important in the utilization of carbohydrate, fat, and protein for growth, maintenance, and repair of cells and the production of energy. It is an essential part of nucleoproteins that are responsible for cell division and reproduction and the transfer of genetic traits from parent to offspring. Proper muscle contraction, kidney function, and transfer of nerve impulses also require phosphorus.

The intake of phosphorus in the average American diet is approximately 1.5 times that of calcium. In general, if calcium and protein needs are met by the diet, phosphorus requirements will also be met. A phosphorus deficiency appears in the human only in certain clinical conditions (**30**).

Sodium.   Sodium is divided approximately equally between bone and the body fluids, including blood plasma and the extracellular fluid. Sodium functions in the body to equalize the acid-base balance of the blood and to regulate water balance. It is also involved in muscle contraction and nerve stimulation.

No dietary requirement for sodium is established, but dietary deficiency probably does not occur in the human because the kidney efficiently conserves the needed amount of sodium. Excessive or prolonged sweating, severe vomiting, and diarrhea, however, can cause sodium depletion, especially if the water lost is replaced without replacing the lost sodium. The result may be nausea, apathy, exhaustion, and eventually, respiratory failure.

A high intake of sodium, primarily in the form of salt, is now recognized as a potential problem in the U.S. population (**21, 31**). Intakes of sodium by adults in the United States average about 2300—6900 mg per day or about 6—18 g of sodium chloride. The average requirement, however, is only about 250 mg per day (**31**). Safe and adequate daily intakes are estimated to be in the range of 1100—3300 mg of sodium (**14**). The high intakes result from salt added in the processing and preparation of foods and the addition of salt during actual consumption. Diets containing high amounts of salt contribute to the development of high blood pressure and excessive retention of fluid. The reduction of present intakes to about 5 g of salt daily was recently recommended (**21**). This figure has since been raised to 8 g per day (**32**).

Chloride.   Chloride is found in the extracellular fluid and is important in the maintenance of fluid balance in the body. It may also play a role in activating certain enzymes. It is essential for the formation of hydrochloric acid and is found in high concentrations in the gastric juice that is important for the digestion of food in the stomach.

Nearly all dietary chloride occurs as sodium chloride or table salt. There is no established RDA for chloride. Safe and adequate intakes are in the range of 1700—5100 mg per day (**14**). The daily turnover in adults (intake-output) ranges between 85 and 250 mEq. The same factors affecting sodium loss from the body tend to affect chloride loss. A deficiency of chloride would therefore occur under circumstances similar to those causing a deficiency of sodium.

Potassium.   Potassium is an essential nutrient found mainly in the intracellular fluid. With sodium it helps to regulate the water balance in the body. It also plays a role in the stimulation of nerve tissue and contraction of muscle tissue.

The FNB (**14**) has established a safe and adequate daily intake of 1875—5625 mg of potassium. This mineral is widely distributed in foods and occurs in large amounts in potatoes, carrots, oranges, bananas, and apricots. Minimal needs for the healthy adult are believed to be about 2.5 g per day, and intakes of potassium in the American adult average between 50 and 150 mEq per day (1 mEq = 39 mg).

Potassium deficiency is usually attributed to causes other than a dietary deficiency. Body potassium can be depleted by excessive excretion through the kidney because of kidney disease or high salt intake. Excessive vomiting, diarrhea, and stress following injury or surgery may also lead to a potassium deficiency. Symptoms of potassium deficiency include overall muscle weakness, weakness of respiratory and cardiac muscles, and eventually cardiac failure.

Magnesium.   Magnesium is found in all body tissues but principally in bone, where it occurs together with calcium and phosphorus. Thirty percent of body magnesium is found in soft tissues and body fluids. Magnesium is an essential part of many enzyme systems responsible for energy conversions in the body. It is also involved in bone growth and is necessary for proper functioning of nerve and muscle tissue.

The FNB (**14**) recommends a daily intake of 300 mg of magnesium for the adult female, but a high calcium or phosphorus intake can increase magnesium requirements. The amounts of protein and vitamin D in the diet also influence the magnesium requirement. Magnesium is found in goodly amounts in nuts, whole grain products, dry beans, dry peas, and dark green vegetables.

A magnesium deficiency is not common in the healthy individual who eats a variety of foods, but it has been seen in postsurgical patients and people with diabetes, kidney malfunction, or severe malabsorption caused by chronic diarrhea or vomiting. Symptoms of magnesium deficiency include muscle tremors and mental confusion.

Iron. The best-known micronutrient is probably iron, and two-thirds of the iron in the body is present in the blood, mainly as a component of "hemoglobin." *Hemoglobin* is the pigment in red blood cells that carries oxygen from the lungs to the tissues, where it is needed for basic life functions. The remainder of body iron is in the form of storage iron found in the liver, spleen, bone marrow, and muscle.

The primary function of iron is to enable hemoglobin, an essential component of red blood cells, to carry oxygen needed for cellular respiration. Iron serves as a mediator of the oxidative process. Iron-containing heme compounds carry oxygen to tissue cells and move hydrogen along the electron transport chain. In addition, a small amount of body iron is incorporated into certain enzymes, and iron also plays a role in the synthesis of collagen.

Dietary intakes for iron are ten times greater than actual needs, because the percentage of food iron absorbed by the body is as low as 10 percent of the amount actually consumed. The average American adult diet supplies about 15 mg of iron per day, but the need for iron in the adult female is larger because of menstrual losses. The FNB (**14**) establishes the daily recommended iron allowance for women at 18 mg. This allowance may not be met by ordinary diets, and supplements may be necessary. Only a few foods contain much iron, but liver is a particularly good source. Lean meats, heart, kidney, shellfish, dry beans, dry peas, dark green vegetables, dried fruit, egg yolk, and molasses are also good sources of iron. Whole grain and enriched breads and cereals contain smaller amounts of iron but when eaten frequently become important sources.

Iron-deficiency anemia is probably the most widespread nutritional deficiency in the United States today. This is because iron consumption can easily be low unless there is a conscious effort to include iron-rich foods in the diet. The enrichment of cereal grain products with iron has been practiced since 1943, but in 1973 concern about the incidence of anemia led the FDA to examine its fortification standards. The proposed changes would essentially triple the amount of iron presently in bread and cereal products. Controversy and confusion still exist, though, about the benefits and risks of the recommended increases in fortification levels, largely because a toxic level of iron (a condition known as "hemosiderosis") can occur in some individuals. This is due to a genetic error of metabolism in which excessive iron is absorbed. The FDA decided, therefore, not to approve increased iron enrichment (**33**).

Manganese.   Manganese is a trace mineral essential for the development of normal tendon and bone structure, reproduction, and normal function of the central nervous system. It also plays a role in the activation of numerous enzymes. The average adult intake varies from 2 to 9 mg per day. In view of the remarkably steady tissue concentrations of manganese in the U.S. population and of the low toxicity of dietary manganese, an occasional intake of 10 mg per day can be considered safe. But to include an extra margin of safety, a safe and adequate daily intake for manganese has been set at 2.5−5.0 mg over long periods of time (**14**).

Copper.   Copper is required in the body to incorporate dietary iron into hemoglobin, develop bone and connective tissue, and to assure normal functioning of the central nervous system. In the adult female 2 mg of copper per day will maintain copper balance. Safe and adequate daily dietary intakes are set at 2−3 mg per day (**14**).

A dietary deficiency of copper is extremely unlikely, since adequate amounts of copper are in the normal mixed diet. A copper deficiency can result, though, from a defect in the formation of "ceruloplasmin," the copper-carrying protein in blood. Wilson's disease, characterized by nerve degeneration and liver changes, is due to an accumulation of excessive copper in the tissues, caused by the genetic absence of a liver enzyme.

Iodine.   The only known function for the trace mineral iodine is its role in the production of thyroid hormones, those that regulate the rate of body metabolism. The human requirement for iodine is small, and the FNB (**14**) recommends a daily intake of 150 mcg for the adult female.

An iodine deficiency will lead to enlargement of the thyroid gland, a condition known as "goiter." Cretinism is often found in children born to mothers who had a limited intake of iodine during adolescence and pregnancy. These children are physically dwarfed and mentally retarded. Iodine deficiency can occur in areas isolated from the ocean and where the soil and water, and thus the food crops, are low in iodine.

The high incidence of goiter led to the introduction of iodized salt in 1924. To a large extent, this eliminated the problem. However, goiter still occurs in the United States, because iodination of salt is not mandatory. The FDA has requested federal legislation to require the addition of iodine to salt. Regular use of iodized salt, and the consumption of seafood, especially during growth and pregnancy, is recommended to insure an adequate iodine intake (**14**).

Zinc.   Zinc is a constituent of at least 25 enzymes involved in digestion and metabolism. It is essential in nucleic acid synthesis. It is also necessary for growth and proper development of the reproductive organs, plays a role in wound healing, and is important in taste acuity.

The FNB (**14**) recommends a daily dietary intake of 15 mg of zinc for the adult female. The average zinc content of a mixed diet consumed by an American adult is 10−15 mg. Although this appears to be adequate, recent studies on the loss of a sense of taste and on delayed wound healing indicate that a zinc deficiency may exist in some persons in the United States.

Cobalt.   Cobalt is an essential part of vitamin B_{12} or cobalamin that plays a role in the prevention of pernicious anemia. Vegetarians who do not eat meat, eggs, or dairy products can become vitamin B_{12} deficient, since they get only trace amounts from plants.

Fluoride.   Fluoride contributes to sound tooth formation and results in a decrease in the incidence of dental caries, especially in children. Studies suggest that fluoride also plays a role in strengthening bone and that an adequate fluoride intake may be important as a protection against osteoporosis. Less osteoporosis seems to exist in areas where the fluoride content of water is adequate. A deficiency of fluoride in infancy and childhood can also result in incomplete calcification of the teeth, leaving them relatively unprotected from decay.

Fluoride is found in small and varying amounts in water, soil, plants, and animals. To a large extent, the amount of fluoride in foods is dependent on the content of the soil in which they were grown. A major source of fluoride, however, may be in the water supply. In areas where the drinking water does not contain fluoride the addition of the mineral to the public water supply, raising it to what is considered a desirable level (fluoridation), can be an important public health measure. The most generally accepted level of fluoridation is one part per million (ppm) in the public water supply.

Intakes of fluoride of 1.5−4.0 mg per day are considered to be safe and adequate (**14**). Most adults have intakes of between 0.5 and 4.0 mg daily.

Selenium.   Selenium functions in the body as an antioxidant, protecting the membrane of red blood cells and hemoglobin against oxidative changes. Recent research (**34**) demonstrates that selenium is a component of an enzyme in the red blood cell that functions to degrade peroxides. Biochemically, selenium resembles sulfur and can replace it in the sulfur-containing amino acids methionine, cystine, and cysteine. It also plays a protective role against mercury and cadmium toxicity.

Very little is known about the human requirement for selenium. Selenium intakes in the range of 50−200 mcg per day can be obtained easily from a varied diet. This intake can be considered to be safe and adequate (**14**).

Chromium.   Chromium was first recognized by the FNB as an essential element for human beings in 1974. It functions to maintain normal glucose metabolism, and glucose utilization has responded to chromium supplements in persons suspected of having marginal intakes (**35**).

There is no established recommendation for daily chromium intakes, but a chromium intake of 50−200 mcg per day is tentatively recommended for adults (**14**). Good sources of chromium are meats and whole grain products. Chromium nutriture may be a problem in the elderly and in the pregnant woman, but much more research is needed to elucidate the role of this element.

Water

Water is the most critical and most abundant nutrient found in the body, accounting for one-half to three-fourths of body weight. The concentration of water in body tissues varies, being 72 percent in muscle, 20−35 percent in fat tissue, and 10 percent in bone. Every cell in the body contains water, and two-thirds of total body water is found in the intracellular compartment. The remaining one-third is found in the extracellular compartment, where it exists in circulatory fluids, blood and lymph, and in interstitial fluid that is found outside the vascular system and within tissue spaces (Figure 1.2). The exchange of fluid between the intracellular and extracellular compartments is regulated by several factors, including the relative concentrations of protein, sodium, and potassium in each compartment.

Water acts as a solvent and a medium of transport for all body solutes. It carries nutrients and hormones to individual cells as they are needed. It also carries waste products from the cells, where they are produced, to the lungs, skin, or kidney for excretion.

Water forms the intracellular medium in which chemical reactions can occur. In the cell, water acts as a medium for many biological reactions and transports nutrients from one organelle to another.

Water acts as a lubricant in certain transcellular fluids, including saliva and the synovial fluid of joints. Water from the digestive juices in the stomach enters into a variety of hydrolytic reactions involved in nutrient breakdown, for example, splitting of peptide bonds. In the cerebrospinal fluid, water acts as a cushion for the nervous system. In the ear, water transports sound. In the eye, it serves to transmit light.

Water also plays a role in regulating and maintaining body temperature, since the high conductivity properties of water allow for an even distribution of

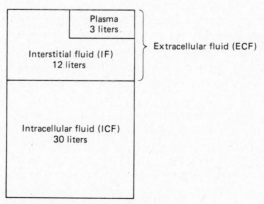

Figure 1.2 *Body fluid compartments.*

heat in the body. Evaporation of water from the body surface removes excess heat produced in the metabolism of carbohydrate, fat, and protein from the body.

The major source of body water is from fluids consumed in beverages. This amount varies from 900 to 1500 ml per day in the adult, with an average intake of 1100 ml. Water is also supplied in food in amounts varying from almost none to 96 percent. A 2000 kcal diet of mixed foods provides 500 to 800 ml of water. Water is one of the end products of metabolism of carbohydrate, fat, and protein, and this is known as "metabolic water." One hundred grams of carbohydrate yields 56 g of water; 100 g of protein, 37 g of water; and 100 g of fat, 107 g of water. About 15 percent of the daily water need is provided as metabolic water. In an average diet providing 2000 kcal per day and consisting of 50 percent carbohydrate, 35 percent fat, and 15 percent protein, the water of metabolism would be approximately 264 ml.

Water losses from the body occur through the kidneys, lungs, and skin. Urine volume per day is 1–2 liters, and 97 percent of this volume is water. Water loss through the lungs is approximately 300–400 ml per day. In colder climates the loss of water by evaporation from the skin is approximately 500–600 ml per day. About 200 ml of water per day is lost through the feces. One thousand ml of water should be consumed for every 1000 kcal in the adult diet to compensate for water loss in the urine and feces and through the skin and lungs. Two-thirds of this amount should be supplied by beverages. The remainder can be supplied by food. The following summary represents a typical water intake and loss for an adult (Table 1.8).

Body fluid content is regulated by the kidney that acts to preserve the normal chemical composition of the blood plasma and extracellular fluid. If the sodium concentration of blood rises as little as 1 percent because of a decrease in blood volume, the thirst regulating mechanism in the brain is stimulated, causing a desire for and consequent increase in water intake. At the same time, the secretion of antidiuretic hormone stimulates the kidney to retain more fluid, causing the blood volume to return to its normal level.

Electrolytes as well as water are lost under certain conditions in which large amounts of body fluid are lost through excessive perspiration, vomiting, or diarrhea. Water intoxication can develop if water is replaced without a simultaneous replacement of electrolytes. As the sodium concentration in the extracellular fluid decreases, water moves into the cell, causing a decrease in extracellular fluid volume. This eventually leads to a decrease in blood pressure and general

TABLE 1.8 TYPICAL DAILY WATER BALANCE FOR AN ADULT

Fluids	1500	Urine	1500
Foods	800	Skin	600
Metabolism	300	Lungs	400
		Feces	100
Total	2600	Total	2600

weakness. Symptoms of dehydration appear when body fluids are reduced as much as 10 percent, and a reduction of 20 percent can be fatal. On the other hand, an abnormal retention of water to levels above 10 percent causes edema.

PLANNING FOOD INTAKE
FOR THE PRECONCEPTIONAL FEMALE

So far we have discussed why good nutrition is important for women of childbearing age and what nutrients are essential and in what amounts. It is not enough to know what one should eat to be healthy, however. Guidelines for food selection and the application of the principles of good nutrition to everyday living must be available and acceptable to the woman of childbearing age. We all select food to suit our personal tastes. The choices we make are influenced by availability, cost, color, flavor, texture, and temperature of the food. The degree of hunger we feel enters into the choices made—as well as food habits; the desire to lose, gain, or maintain weight; and the circumstances or traditions we associate with any particular meal.

Of all the factors involved in food selection, the nutritional value of food is often of least concern. Yet nutrition must certainly be a prime consideration when making food selections. Health professionals, using their knowledge of nutrition, can help young women translate their nutrient needs into an acceptable, appealing, nutritious diet. They can guide this audience of potential mothers toward an understanding of why the food they eat affects not only their health but also the health and well-being of their future children.

We have discussed nutritional requirements in terms of RDAs. It is difficult, however, for the average individual to evaluate meals each day to determine if they are providing all the essential nutrients. A relatively simple method to help plan a healthy diet is based on the Daily Food Guide or, more commonly, the Basic Four of the USDA (Table 1.9). The Basic Four evolved in 1955 as a simplification of an earlier guide to food selection, the Basic Seven. The Basic Four concept has been increasingly criticized, though, on the basis that with the most recent knowledge of nutrient requirements an individual can no longer follow the Basic Four guide and select a diet adequate in all nutrients (**36**). It is also suggested that the Basic Four concept has been overemphasized to young people and that this group may no longer be interested in hearing about it. A more accurate but equally simple guide has not been developed, however. Although they are divided in their opinions regarding the need for a new food guide, many nutritionists feel that the current guide is acceptable. They view the guide as a valuable tool as long as its limitations are recognized, and they believe that less dissatisfaction will be encountered if the guide is used as such and not as an absolute. The guidelines offered today are based on present knowledge and may well change in the future as new understandings are developed of the relationship between nutrition and health.

Recently, the USDA added a fifth group of foods to the original four (**37**). The fifth group, Fats-Sweets-Alcohol, provides mainly calories and little in the way of nutrients (Table 1.9.).

Nutritionists have divided foods containing similar nutrients into four groups to help young women make wise selections from the numerous foods available to them. These groups are meat and meat alternates, milk and milk products, fruits and vegetables, and breads and cereals. The fifth group, mentioned earlier, consisting of fats, sweets, and alcohol, was added only recently.

Selecting a variety of foods from this Daily Food Guide is a step toward providing the essential nutrients described earlier. The health professional must emphasize to the young woman seeking dietary counseling that no one food and no one food group can supply all the essentials; an excess dietary intake of one nutrient will not compensate for the lack of another. The Daily Food Guide in Table 1.9 explains the food groups in greater detail. Using this as a guide, young women can plan meals and snacks of infinite variety to suit their needs and preferences. The suggested numbers of servings in the Guide provide approximately 1200 calories for the adult female, adequate protein, and most of the vitamins and minerals needed daily. Each day's food intake can be built around this foundation to insure a nutritious diet. Young women need to keep in mind that the Guide gives only the basics. With a knowledge of their own food habits (their likes and dislikes) and the help of a health professional they can choose foods to meet their unique needs. Income, health, and activity levels are other factors that will enter into meal planning. A sample menu pattern is shown (Table 1.10) and can be compared with the other sample menus provided (Table 1.11). The sample menu pattern or menus will obviously not fit into everybody's lifestyle, but the food choices can be rearranged to suit an individual's work, study, recreational, social, and leisure schedules. No one, of course, should become tied to a stereotyped menu pattern.

Food from one food group can be combined with those from another food group. Examples are shown in Table 1.12. Women, too, should be encouraged to make use of new recipes and food service ideas. Numerous sources of food selection and preparation information are available, including the food columns in many magazines and newspapers. Many food companies also distribute booklets of tested recipes, and government agencies publish bulletins related to food, nutrition, meal planning, food preparation, buying, preservation, and production. Such bulletins are available at county or state Extension offices, from the U.S. Department of Agriculture or from the Government Printing Office in Washington, D.C.

Good nutrition, then, is not eating foods you do not like because they are good for you. There is no one essential food to eat or dietary pattern to follow. Preferred foods can be selected from the tremendous amount available. Good nutrition does depend on making an intelligent selection based on some knowledge of foods and their nutritive value and the ways in which they can be chosen to best meet individual nutrient requirements and lifestyles.

TABLE 1.9 DAILY FOOD GUIDE

Food group	Nutrients supplied	Serving size	Basic servings/day
Meat and meat alternates (meat, poultry, fish, dry beans or peas, soybeans, lentils, eggs, seeds, nuts, peanut butter)	Protein, phosphorus, vitamins B_6, B_{12} (animal sources), iron, other vitamins and minerals	2–3 oz cooked lean meat. The following are equivalent to 1 oz of meat: 1 egg; ½–¾ cup cooked dry beans, peas, soybeans, or lentils; 2 tablespoons peanut butter; ¼–½ cup nuts or seeds	2
Milk and milk products (milk in any form, yogurt, ice cream, ice milk, cheese)	Calcium, riboflavin, protein, vitamins A, B_6, B_{12}, and D when fortified)	One 8 oz cup of milk; common portions of some dairy products and their milk equivalents are 1 cup plain yogurt = 1 cup milk 1 oz Cheddar or Swiss cheese = ¾ cup milk 1 in. cube Cheddar or Swiss cheese = ½ cup milk 1 oz process cheese food = ½ cup milk ½ cup ice cream or ice milk = ⅓ cup milk ½ cup cottage cheese = ¼ cup milk	Teens 4 Adults 2 Pregnant women 3 Nursing mothers 4

32

TABLE 1.9 (Continued)

Food group	Nutrients supplied	Serving size	Basic serving/day
Fruits and vegetables (all fruits and vegetables)	Vitamin A (dark green and deep yellow fruits and vegetables); vitamin C (dark green vegetables, citrus fruits, melons, berries, tomatoes); calcium (greens—collards, kale, mustard, turnip, and dandelion); riboflavin; folacin; iron; magnesium; fiber	½ cup or a typical portion—one orange, one-half grapefruit or canteloupe, one medium potato, and so on	4 (a vitamin C source each day; a vitamin A source every second day)
Breads and cereals (all products made with whole grains and enriched or fortified flour or meal: bread, biscuits, muffins, waffles, pancakes, cooked or ready-to-eat cereals, flour, grits, macaroni, spaghetti, noodles, rice, and so on	B-vitamins, iron, protein, magnesium, folacin, fiber	1 slice bread; ½–¾ cup cooked cereal, cornmeal, grits, macaroni, noodles, rice, spaghetti, 1 oz ready-to-eat cereal	4
Fats, sweets, and alcohol (butter, margarine, mayonnaise, salad dressings, candy, sugar, jams, jellies, soft drinks, alcoholic beverages, refined but unenriched breads, pastries, and flour products)	Mainly calories in the form of fat and sugar; low in protein, vitamins, and minerals in proportion to calories	No specified serving size	No suggested number of servings

TABLE 1.10 SAMPLE MENU PATTERN

BREAKFAST

1 serving Fruit-Vegetable Group

1 or more servings Bread-Cereal Group (or 1 serving Meat Group, plus 1 serving Bread-Cereal Group)

1 serving Milk Group

1 or more servings Fats-Sweets-Alcohol Group

LUNCH

1 serving Meat Group

1 or more servings Fruit-Vegetable Group

1 serving Bread-Cereal Group

1 serving Milk Group

1 serving Fats-Sweets-Alcohol Group

DINNER

1 serving Meat Group

2 or more servings Fruit-Vegetable Group

1 serving Bread-Cereal Group

1 serving Milk Group

1 serving Fats-Sweets-Alcohol Group

SNACKS

1 serving Bread-Cereal Group

or

1 serving Fruit-Vegetable Group

or

1 serving Fats-Sweets-Alcohol Group

TABLE 1.11   SAMPLE MENUS

BREAKFAST

1/2 cup orange juice	**or**	1/2 grapefruit
1 scrambled egg		cereal (iron-fortified with milk)
2 slices toast		1 ounce Cheddar cheese on 1/2 toasted English muffin
1 cup of milk		
1 tsp. butter		1 tsp. butter
jelly		

LUNCH

vegetable soup	**or**	Chicken sandwich: 2 ounces chicken, 2 slices whole wheat bread, lettuce,
Chef's salad: 1 ounce ham, 1 hard-cooked egg, 1 ounce cheese, lettuce and tomatoes, French dressing		butter or mayonnaise
		1 cup hot chocolate
1 hard roll		honeydew melon (1/8 medium-sized)
butter		
baked custard		
iced tea		

DINNER

3 oz roast beef	**or**	3 oz baked flounder
½ cup buttered green beans		1 baked potato
½ cup summer squash		½ cup buttered asparagus
popover		carrot sticks
butter		1 glass of milk
½ cup ice cream with blueberries		apple pie (1/6 of 9 in.) with 1 oz Cheddar cheese
coffee		

SNACKS

2 graham crackers with
1 oz Swiss cheese
or
1 medium tangerine
or
1 glass lemonade

TABLE 1.12   FOODS CAN BE A COMBINATION OF FOOD GROUPS

Food	Food group
Beef taco	Meat = ground beef Milk = shredded cheese Fruit-Vegetable = shredded lettuce and tomato Bread-Cereal = taco shell
Sausage and cheese pizza	Meat = sausage Milk = cheese Fruit-Vegetable = tomato sauce, vegetable garnish Bread-Cereal = crust
Cheeseburger	Meat = hamburger Milk = cheese Fruit-Vegetable = tomato, lettuce Bread-Cereal = bun
Rhubarb crisp	Fruit-Vegetable = rhubarb Bread-Cereal = pastry Fats-Sweet-Alcohol = butter, sugar
Custard	Meat = eggs Milk = milk
Macaroni, ground beef, and tomato casserole	Meat = ground beef Fruit-Vegetable = tomato Bread-Cereal = macaroni

DIETARY COUNSELING FOR THE YOUNG WOMAN

The young woman, prior to pregnancy, represents an ideal audience for a nutrition education that can have benefits extending far beyond her present circumstances. The learning and application of these sound nutrition principles can have a lasting influence on a young woman, and through her, on her family. An assessment of a woman's present nutritional status and nutrition education and the supervision of her nutrient intake are all important components of dietary counseling.

Dietary counseling is a process of mutual exchange. The nutritionist, or other health professional who does the counseling, will want to learn as much as possible about the woman's present dietary habits. To this end, a 24-hour dietary recall would be useful to a degree, the counselee writing down all the food and the amounts she consumes in a 24-hour period. A calculation of the total nutrient intake from the day's supply of food can then be made. More information can be gathered by asking additional questions. What is the woman's primary source of nutrition information? Does the woman know what the basic four food groups are? Does the woman consciously consider her food choice each day in relation to the basic food groups or another food guide? Has the woman ever tried a fad diet? What were the results of the diet? Would the woman try such a diet again? Why or why not? What does the term "health food" mean to her? Can the woman trace any of her attitudes toward food back to her parents' or grandparents' attitudes toward food? What are her favorite foods? Does she enjoy a wide variety of foods or only a few? Was she considered to be a "good eater" as a child? Why or why not? How have her eating habits changed since childhood?

These and similar questions will provide some basis for determining a woman's food habits and nutrient intake. If inadequacies are found, some necessary dietary changes can be suggested. Sound and appropriate dietary patterns that emerge should be encouraged and reinforced. Any advice given should be specific, rather than general, with respect to types of foods, portion sizes, and frequency of consumption.

Some young women may need information on food assistance programs. In general, each State Health Department has a nutrition division that may be contacted for information about nutrition services in the state. The American Dietetic Association can also provide information about nutrition services. Several food assistance programs of the USDA serve low-income groups and other target populations. Such programs are discussed in greater detail in Chapter 12.

Written and pictorial material can be of great value in dietary counseling. This can include publications to reinforce verbal nutritional advice, graphs, charts, and videotapes for independent use by the patient.

Any educational aids used, however, should never replace direct personal contact between the young woman and the nutrition counselor. An important factor in persuading a woman to establish sound nutritional habits is continued personal encouragement by the counselor. A young woman, motivated by concern for her future children, will welcome nutrition information if it is adapted to her own situation or if it is presented in the context of personal experience.

The health professional must consider cultural and environmental factors that may influence dietary habits. Where is the young woman being fed—at home, the local fast food restaurant, or the office cafeteria? Who decides what the young woman eats—the young woman, friends or a physician? Who has the most influence on her food practices—the young woman, school peers, husband? The nutritionist must explore the basics of sound nutrition with every potential mother in the light of the emotional and cultural factors affecting her food choices. In this type of supportive atmosphere the nutritionist can guide young women to investigate the role of nutrition in human development from before conception through adolescence.

Some of the questions about why young people eat as they do must be answered and some of the related problems corrected; otherwise, it can be expected that many young women in the future will continue to enter their first pregnancies with a significant nutritional risk. Failure to deal with nutrition-related concerns of the young will compound the high human and economic costs borne by mothers, their children, and society in general. By improving the preconceptional nutritional status of women, health professionals have the opportunity to help guide superior pregnancies as well as to improve the general long-term health of the women involved (**38**).

SUMMARY

The state of the mother's nutrition prior to pregnancy is all important for a successful pregnancy and the future health of her infant. The conditions in the uterus at the time of conception determine whether the fertilized egg will successfully implant itself in the uterine wall and begin normal development. The best provision for the well-being of both mother and child during pregnancy is for the mother to arrive at the point of pregnancy in good nutritional and physiological condition, since the well-nourished mother nourishes her fetus well. In turn, the infant who is healthy at birth has reserves to provide for healthy growth and development throughout childhood. The best insurance, then, for a healthy infant is a mother who is healthy and well nourished throughout her entire life, as well as during the pregnancy itself.

Dietary counseling can result in dietary improvement for young women who are at nutritional risk. Frequently, potential mothers can be motivated to adopt sound nutritional practices when they realize that good nutrition affects not only their health but also the health of future generations.

Pregnancy wastage and neonatal mortality are greater when the nutriture of the mother is habitually poor. Therefore, a lifetime of good nutrition should help insure successful pregnancies, maternal health, and vigorous infants.

STUDY QUESTIONS AND TOPICS FOR INDIVIDUAL INVESTIGATION

1. Interview one of your female classmates. Try to determine the woman's eating habits. What is the woman's favorite food and meal? Would the woman consider herself a good eater? Why or why not? Does she select foods from the Basic Four food guide in planning her dietary intake? Does she ever consider how her eating habits and health before pregnancy could influence the health of the next generation?

2. Using the list of Basic Four foods that follows create a day's menus (three balanced meals plus nutritious snacks) for an 18-year-old female.

MEAT	BREAD AND CEREAL	FRUIT AND VEGETABLE	MILK
Egg	Rice	Strawberries	Yogurt
Peanut butter	Cereals	Carrots	Cheese
Liver	Spaghetti	Spinach	Ice cream
Shrimp	Waffles	Pineapple	Milk
Baked chicken	Bread	Squash	
	Pasta	Canteloupe	

3. "Food," a publication on food and nutrition developed by the U.S. Department of Agriculture, has up-to-date, reliable information about food and nutrition issues and suggestions on how to apply this information to food decisions. The Daily Food Guide is discussed and ways of choosing food for their nutritional value are outlined. Breakfast, snacking, sugar in the diet, fiber, and nutrition labeling are some issues covered. Recipes and practical guidelines are offered to help consumers plan nutritious appetizing meals. You may want to obtain a copy of this book for your own use. Write to Superintendent of Documents, U.S. Government Printing Office, Washington, D.C. 20402, and ask for "Food—Home and Garden Bulletin No. 228."

4. Poor nutrition may be a way of life for many young women. These women may not realize that nutrition affects the health of future children. Discuss in class reasons young women may not eat well. Make a list of reasons, and compare it with a list of reasons for establishing sound dietary habits. What could you, as a nutrition educator, do to help young women switch from poor to good eating behavior?

REASONS FOR POOR EATING BEHAVIOR	REASONS FOR GOOD EATING BEHAVIOR
Apathy	Appearance
Stress	Athletic ability
Habit	Health
Others	Others

Swift and Company, Chicago, Illinois, and the National Foundation, March of Dimes, White Plains, N.Y., have developed nutrition education materials in a comic book format to reach young people. You may want to order some of these materials to see how you might use such a format to reach the preconceptional female with nutrition information.

5. Using the RDAs and a table of food composition, evaluate a 24-hour food intake record of a young adult female. Are there deficiencies in the intake of certain nutrients? (Generally, a value of two-thirds of the RDA can be considered to be adequate.) How would you help this young woman improve her dietary intake if the need exists? How can you encourage the young woman to continue good food habits if her dietary intake looks good?

REFERENCES

1. Winick, M., ed. *Nutritional Disorders of American Women.* Wiley, New York, 1977.
2. Moghissi, K., and T. Evans, eds. *Nutritional Impacts on Women Throughout Life with Emphasis on Reproduction.* Harper & Row, New York, 1977.
3. Wishik, S. The implications of undernutrition during pubescence and adolescence on fertility. In: *Nutritional Impacts on Women Throughout Life with Emphasis on Reproduction,* eds. K. Moghissi and T. Evans. Harper & Row, New York, 1977.
4. McGanity, W. J. Nutrition in the adolescent. In: *Nutritional Impacts on Women Throughout Life with Emphasis on Reproduction,* eds. K. Moghissi and T. Evans. Harper & Row, New York, 1977.
5. Carruth, B. R. Nutrition and teenage pregnancies. In: *Nutrition Update: Accent on Youth.* Proceedings of the 1978 Nutrition Education Workshop, ed. B. Tanis, American Home Economics Association, New Orleans, 1978.
6. Sabry, Z., J. Campbell, M. Campbell, and A. Forbes. Nutrition Canada. *Nutrition Today,* 9:5, 1974.
7. Lowenstein, F. W. Major nutrition-related risk factors in American Women. In: *Nutritional Disorders of American Women,* ed. M. Winick. Wiley, New York, 1977.
8. Preliminary Findings of the First Health and Nutrition Examination Survey, United States, 1971–1972: Dietary Intake and Biochemical Findings, Public Health Service (PHS), Department of Health, Education and Welfare (DHEW) Publication No. (HRA) 74–1219–1, 1974.
9. Preliminary Findings of the First Health and Nutrition Examination Survey, United States, 1971–1972: Anthropometric and Clinical Findings. Public Health Service (PHS), Department of Health, Education and Welfare (DHEW) Publication No: (HRA) 75–1229, 1975.

10. Roe, D. A. Nutrition and the contraceptive pill. In: *Nutritional Disorders of American Women,* ed. M. Winick. Wiley, New York, 1977.

11. Rose, D. P. The Pill and Nutrition: A Most Intimate Relationship. In: The *Professional Nutritionist.* Foremost Foods Co., San Francisco, Summer 1977.

12. Prasad, A., K. Moghissi, K. Lei, D. Oberleas, and J. Stryker. Effect of oral contraceptives on micronutrients and changes in trace elements due to pregnancy. In: *Nutritional Impacts on Women Throughout Life with Emphasis on Reproduction,* eds. K. Moghissi and T. Evans. Harper & Row, New York, 1977.

13. Belsey, M. Hormonal contraception and nutrition. In: *Nutritional Impacts on Women Throughout Life with Emphasis on Reproduction,* eds. K. Moghissi and T. Evans. Harper & Row, New York, 1977.

14. Food and Nutrition Board. *Recommended Dietary Allowances,* 9th ed. National Academy of Sciences, Washington, D.C., 1980.

15. Dwyer, J. *Dietary Goals of the United States,* 2nd ed. Select Committee on Nutrition and Human Needs, U.S. Senate, Washington, D.C., 1977, p. 9.

16. Heald, F. P. The natural history of obesity. *Advances in Psychosomatics,* 7:102, 1977.

17. Oscanova, K. Trends of dietary intake and prevalence of obesity in Czechoslovakia. In: *Recent Advances in Obesity Research,* ed. H. Newman. Publ. Ltd., 1973.

18. Mayer, T. *Overweight: Causes, Cost, and Control.* Prentice-Hall, Englewood Cliffs, N.J., 1968.

19. Grande, F. Assessment of body fat in man. In: *Obesity in Perspective,* Vol. 2, ed. G. Bray. DHEW Publication No. 75–708. U.S. Government Printing Office, Washington, D.C., 1975.

20. D'Angelli, A., and H. Smicklas-Wright. The case for primary prevention of overweight through the family. *Journal of Nutrition Education,* 10:76, 1978.

21. Select Committee on Nutrition and Human Needs, U.S. Senate. *Dietary Goals for the United States,* 2nd ed. Washington, D.C., 1977.

22. Calloway, D. H. Dietary components that yield energy. *Environmental Biology and Medicine,* 1:175, 1971.

23. Friend, B. Nutritional review. In: National Food Situation No. 142. U.S. Department of Agriculture, Hyattsville, Md., 1972, p. 25.

24. Mendeloff, A. I. Dietary fiber. In: *Present Knowledge in Nutrition.* Nutrition Foundation, New York, 1976, p. 392.

25 U.S. Department of Agriculture. Handbook of Agriculture Charts. Agricultural Handbook No. 504, USDA, 1976.

26. McGill, H. C., and G. E. Mott. Diet and coronary heart disease. In: *Present Knowledge in Nutrition.* Nutrition Foundation, New York. 1976, p. 376.

27. Turpeinen, O. Future trends in nutrition: Fats and oils. In: *Future Trends in Nutrition and Dietetics.* S. Karger, New York, 1975.

28. Anderson, H. C., E. S. Cho, P. A. Krouse, K. C. Hanson, G. F. Krouse, and R. C. Wixom. Effects of dietary histidine and arginine on nitrogen retention of men. *Journal of Nutrition,* 107:2067, 1977.

29. Avioli, L. V. The Osteoporosis problem. In: *Nutritional Disorders of American Women,* ed. M. Winick. Wiley, New York, 1977.

30. Harrison, H. E. Phosphorus. In: *Present Knowledge in Nutrition.* Nutrition Foundation, New York, 1976, p. 241.

31. Meneely, G. R., and H. D. Battarbec. Sodium and potassium. In: *Present Knowledge in Nutrition.* Nutrition Foundation, New York, 1976, p. 259.

32. McGovern, G. The nutrition gazette. *Nutrition Today,* 14(2):5, 1979.

33. Anonymous. Anatomy of a Decision. *Nutrition Today,* 13(1):6, 1978.

34. Rotruck, J. T., A. L. Pope, H. E. Ganther, A. B. Swanson, D. G. Hateman, and W. G. Hoekstra. Selenium: Biochemical role as a component of glutathione peroxidase. *Science,* 179:588, 1973.

35. Mertz, W. Effects and metabolism of glucose tolerance factor. In: *Present Knowledge in Nutrition.* Nutrition Foundation, New York, 1976, p. 365.

36. King, J., S. Cohenour, C. Corruccin, and P. Schneeman. Evaluation and modification of the basic four food guide. *Journal of Nutrition Education,* 10(1):27, 1978.

37. U.S. Department of Agriculture. *Food—Home and Garden Bulletin No. 228.* Science and Education Administration, Washington, D.C., 1979.

38. Chapman, N. Incorporating nutrition into family planning services. *Journal of Nutrition Education,* 10(3):129, 1978.

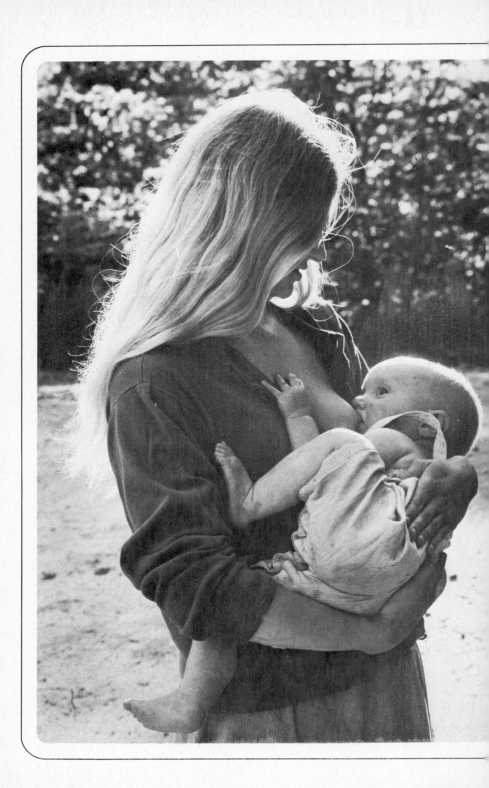

CHAPTER 2

PREGNANCY AND LACTATION

Human growth and development begin with conception and continue until maturity. This development must be adequately supported in the fetus, infant, growing child, and adolescent. Good nutrition provides the basis for both satisfactory growth and health in all four. Serious consequences can result from inadequate nutrition at any stage of the entire process of growth and development but may be most severe during the very earliest stages of life, during pregnancy or gestation.

The relationship between the mother and fetus, the functions of the placenta, and the increasing nutritional needs of the mother are all involved in this development process. A clear comprehension of the physiological changes that occur during pregnancy, therefore, provides the basis for understanding the nutritional needs of the mother and fetus.

Pregnancy causes many changes in the physical and emotional health of the woman, and the normal woman easily recognizes these changes. Breathing may be difficult, and the pregnant woman's heart beats faster. Urine excretion occurs more frequently. She seems hungry and is ill at times. The shape of her body changes, so clothes must be altered, and new ones bought. She becomes concerned about the health of her expected baby and, perhaps for the first time, about her own health. As she embarks on this new and exciting phase of her own life she is bombarded with well-intentioned but often conflicting, misleading, and erroneous advice from family, friends, and associates.

What does being pregnant mean? Who knows the answers to questions about pregnancy, growth of the fetus, and the mother's nutritional needs? Professionals in nutrition, dietetics, child development, family relations, health education, home economics, and allied health areas have many of the answers and can be a source of sound advice. This chapter, too, addresses these questions with basic information about pregnancy, the changes that occur in the maternal system, and the woman's nutritional needs during this time.

THE FEMALE REPRODUCTIVE SYSTEM

The female reproductive system is comprised of several anatomical parts (Figure 2.1).

The ovaries, which are in the lower abdominal cavity, have two primary functions: (1) the production of ova or eggs and (2) the secretion of the primary female sex hormones, estrogens and progesterone. Ova are normally released during the menstrual cycle from menarche, or the onset of puberty, to the onset of menopause. This time in a woman's life is often referred to as the "childbearing years," and it is during this span that the nutritional needs of the female may be different from those of the male and of the female prior to or following the childbearing period.

The released ova pass through the fallopian tubes or oviducts into the uterus, usually on the thirteenth or fourteenth day after the onset of the previous menstruation. Ovulation does not occur during pregnancy. Oral contraceptives prevent ovulation through hormonal control and thus prevent conception. This is why the effect of oral contraceptives may be referred to as "pseudo" or false pregnancy.

The cervix is a muscular ring between the uterus and the vagina. The vagina extends to the exterior of the body, receives sperm from the male during sexual intercourse, and serves as the birth canal at the end of pregnancy. The sequence of events that join sperm and ovum to form a fertilized egg requires about one week (Figure 2.2).

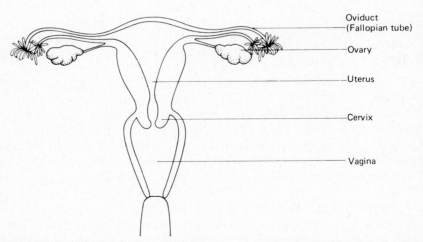

Figure 2.1 *The female reproductive system.* (*Source:* Reprinted with permission from *Biology of Sex,* by C. J. Avers. Copyright © 1974 by John Wiley & Sons, Inc., New York.)

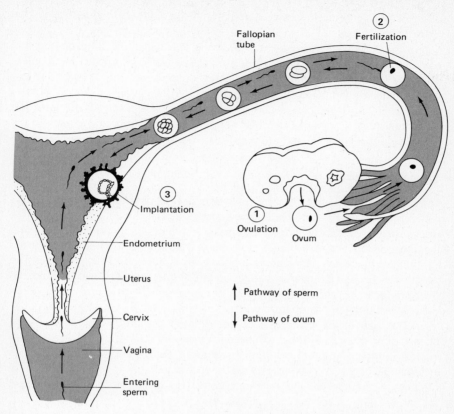

Figure 2.2 *Pathways of sperm, ovum and the fertilized egg during ovulation, fertilization and implantation. (Source: Reprinted with permission from Biology of Sex, by C. J. Avers. Copyright © 1974 by John Wiley & Sons, Inc., New York.)*

PHYSIOLOGICAL DEVELOPMENT AND CHANGES DURING PREGNANCY

The physiological and biochemical development of the egg begins after fertilization or conception. Cell division begins in the fertilized egg or zygote while it moves down the fallopian tubes, and by the time the fertilized egg reaches the uterus the cluster of cells has been transformed into a hollow mass known as a "blastocyst." The transit time through the tubes is from three to four days, and during this time the number of cells increases from 2 to approximately 100. Nutrients and oxygen for this growing cellular mass are supplied by secretions of the uterus.

The fetus and the placenta begin to emerge from the blastocyst about the seventh day as the process of differentiation begins. Implantation begins approximately seven days after fertilization, with the blastocyst adhering to, and later being embedded in, the wall of the uterus. When fertilization occurs, the ovary enlarges and is filled with fatty materials. The entire structure that develops in the ovary is the "corpus luteum" that persists throughout pregnancy and functions during the implantation process by secreting the hormones progesterone and estradiol. Both of these hormones act to establish an appropriate environment within the uterus for implantation. Implantation does not occur if the corpus luteum fails to function, and the process then ceases.

Continued development and differentiation of the placenta and fetus are rapid, however, if implantation does happen. These events occur early in the development of the fetus and are outlined in Table 2.1.

THE PLACENTA

The placenta is developed fully by the twelfth week of pregnancy or by the end of the first trimester and is a unique and complex tissue. It functions as the lungs, kidney, and gastrointestinal tract for the developing fetus. In addition to serving the transport function for the fetus, the placenta has several biochemical functions important to the maintenance of pregnancy and the development of the fetus. The various functions of the placenta are important to the health and well-being of the developing fetus, and these aspects of the placental role are examined in subsequent parts of this chapter.

The size of the placenta increases throughout pregnancy. In the early phases of pregnancy, the placenta exceeds the fetus in weight. The two are equal in size at about the fourth month of pregnancy. Thereafter, the fetus becomes increasingly larger in weight relative to the placenta. At the termination of pregnancy placental weights will range from 10 to 20 percent of the fetal weight with an average of about 15 percent (**3, 4**).

Amniotic Sac

The embryo develops within the amniotic sac that includes the placenta, umbilical cord, amniotic cavity, "bag of waters," and other tissues (Figure 2.3). The embryo

TABLE 2.1 DEVELOPMENT OF THE FETUS FOLLOWING FERTILIZATION

Age	Development event
1–3 days	Cleavage of zygote in fallopian tube
4–7 days	Blastocyst develops in the uterus
7–13 days	Implantation
3 weeks	Embryo is three-layered row; heartbeat begins
4 weeks	Organs rapidly developing
5 weeks	Umbilical cord organized
6 weeks	Thyroids and parathyroids present; hemopoiesis begins in the liver
10 weeks	Kidney begins secretion
12 weeks	First islets in pancreas

Source: Adapted and reprinted with permission from D. B. Villee, *New England Journal of Medicine, 281,* 473, 1969. Copyright © 1969 by the New England Journal of Medicine, Boston, Massachusetts.

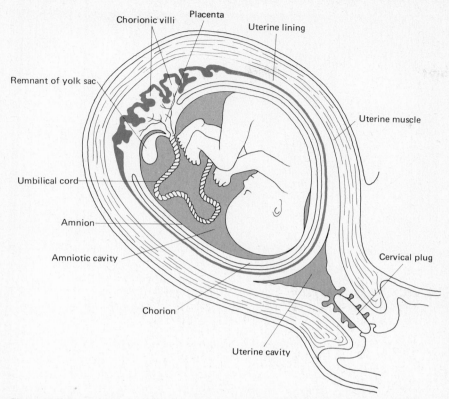

Figure 2.3 The fetal-maternal tissues of the placenta. *(Source:* Reprinted with permission from *Biology of Sex,* by C. J. Avers. Copyright © 1974 by John Wiley & Sons, Inc., New York.)

almost fills the sac in the early part of pregnancy, but as pregnancy progresses the sac becomes proportionally larger, allowing the fetus to move freely (Figure 2.4).

Period of Intrauterine Growth

The development of the embryo and fetus is much more rapid in the early phases of pregnancy than in the latter part, and the initial organ development is completed by the end of the second month. After that, development is primarily an increase in size and in the elaboration of the cellular patterns. The developing and growing organism may be referred to by various terms that are indicative of the stage of development or the length of time following fertilization. Common terms are (1) "zygote" or "fertilized ovum," used during the first two weeks after fertilization or until implantation is completed; (2) "embryo," used during the period from two to eight weeks when major differentiation of organs and tissues occurs; (3) "fetus," used for the period from eight weeks until birth or through the remainder of intrauterine life; and (4) "infant," applied to the newborn who is

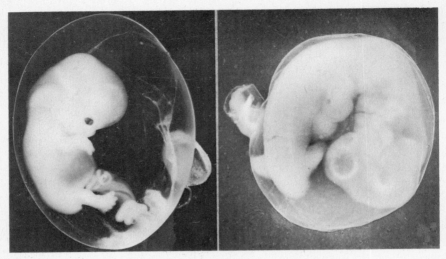

Figure 2.4 *Relative size of the amniotic sac and the fetus at gestation time of five weeks* (right) *and eight weeks* (left). (*Source:* Reprinted by permission from *Pathology of the Fetus and the Infant,* 3rd edition, by E. L. Potter and J. M. Craig. Copyright © 1975 by Year Book Medical Publishers, Inc., Chicago.)

completely outside the body of the mother and separated from the maternal system.

The following provides some idea of the change in weight and length of a fetus based on information from one source (**5**) (Table 2.2). The reader should recognize that there will be considerable individual variation.

TABLE 2.2 AVERAGE WEIGHTS AND LENGTHS FROM 8 TO 26 WEEKS

Gestation week	Weight (g)	Length (cm) (crown-heel)
8	10	—
9	11	—
10	14	—
12	25	7
14	38	10
16	73	14
18	161	19
20	227	23
22	348	25
24	361	25
26	394	27

Source: Adapted from Potter and Craig (**5**). Reproduced with permission from *Pathology of the Fetus and the Infant,* 3rd edition, by E. L. Potter and J. M. Craig. Copyright © 1975 by Year Book Medical Publishers, Inc., Chicago.

HORMONAL ASPECTS OF PREGNANCY

The development and maintenance of the reproductive systems of both males and females generally are controlled by a variety of hormones. Since pregnancy and fetal development in the female system are governed by a series of hormones it is important to understand the nature and function of the two.

Two hormones, known generally as the "female sex hormones," play a basic role throughout the childbearing years. Estrogen is responsible for the development of the entire female reproductive tract, including the uterus, oviducts, vagina, glands in the reproductive tract, external genitalia, breasts, and pelvis. This hormone is even responsible for secondary sex characteristics, such as growth of hair and fat and muscle distribution throughout the body. The second hormone, progesterone, acts primarily on the endometrium, or lining of the uterus, during the menstrual cycle, but it does have effects on the breast and the smooth muscle of the uterus during pregnancy.

The key role of the corpus luteum during implantation has been mentioned previously in this chapter. The hormones from the corpus luteum maintain the endometrium of the uterus in readiness for implantation of the fertilized egg.

The placenta also functions as an endocrine organ. That is, it can synthesize hormones. The placenta produces several hormones, including estrogens, progesterone, chorionic gonadotrophin (HCG), chorionic somatomammotrophin (HCS), and possibly others.

IMMUNOLOGICAL FUNCTIONS OF THE PLACENTA

A clear separation exists between the fetus and mother during pregnancy despite the obvious intimacy of the two. The placenta separates the two circulatory systems throughout gestation. The barrier, however, permits a limited passage of materials such as the cellular elements of the blood and certain large molecules.

Five major classes of immunoglobulins are found in the human: IgG, IgA, IgM, IgD, and IgE. Only one of these, IgG, is transferred from the maternal system to the fetal system; the other substances involved in immunity do not seem to transfer.

From an immunological view, the human placenta has two functions (**6**). First, it protects the fetus from invading microorganisms by selecting appropriate immunoglobulins from the mother. Second, the placenta protects the fetus from an attack of maternal immunological substances by controlling the passage of potentially destructive materials.

TRANSPORT OF MATERIALS ACROSS THE PLACENTA

The placenta transports or transfers materials between the maternal and fetal systems and serves as an effective but selective barrier between the two systems (**7**). It severely restricts the movement of certain materials, such as blood cells, functioning as a "placental barrier" for particulate matter. Yet the transfer of the essential nutrients is actually enhanced by transporting mechanisms in the placenta.

Transport of Gases

The placenta was described earlier as the "fetal lung." Gases cross the placenta by simple diffusion, the primary force being the concentration of the gas on either side of the membrane or the partial pressures of physically dissolved gas in the circulating blood of the maternal and fetal systems.

The transport of oxygen to the fetal system is complicated by several factors. These include the needs of the placenta itself for oxygen, diffusion resistance of the membranes, and "shunts" that represent blood lows not exposed to the membrane for gas exchange purposes. The amount of oxygen delivered is dependent primarily on the circulatory factors. These are the differences in the concentrations of oxygen and the flow rates of blood in the maternal and fetal circulations that determine the uptake of oxygen by the fetus.

Carbon dioxide is transferred from the fetal to the maternal circulatory system to rid the fetus of this end product of metabolism. The membrane exhibits little resistance to this movement of carbon dioxide. Carbon dioxide in the blood is present as hemoglobin bound (30 percent of the total), as bicarbonate (62 percent), and as dissolved carbon dioxide (8 percent). An equilibrium exists between the three forms, but carbon dioxide release from hemoglobin in the fetus is enhanced by the uptake of oxygen (O_2). The following figure (Figure 2.5) shows the exchange of gases across the placenta.

Water

Water crosses the placental barrier in apparent response to two different physiological phenomena. First, water moves across the placenta to maintain osmotic equilibrium between the maternal and fetal systems (**8**). Second, the fetus

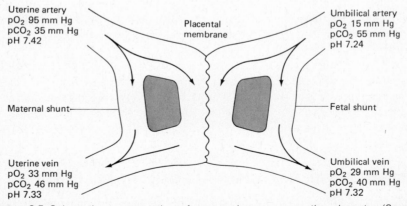

Figure 2.5 *Schematic representation of gas exchange across the placenta.* (*Source:* Reproduced with permission from J. Dancis and H. Schneider in *The Placenta*, ed. P. Gruenwald. Copyright © 1975 by MTP Press Limited, Lancaster, England.)

accumulates water, electrolytes, and other molecules as new tissues form and increase in size. Water is also retained to create physiological osmotic forces (**7**).

Electrolytes

A simple diffusion mechanism does not account for the movement of most of the electrolytes, including those generally regarded as effective in maintaining osmotic forces and relations across membranes: sodium, potassium, and chloride. Sodium seems to move freely across the placental barrier, and the accumulation of sodium, the major cation in the extracellular fluid, is essential to the well-being of the fetus. Sodium may also be involved in the transport of nutrients such as amino acids and glucose to the fetus. Chloride, the major anion, generally seems to follow the movement of sodium as it does in most cells and membranes. The movement of potassium, the major cation of the intracellular fluid, across the placenta is controlled by physiological forces other than simple diffusion.

The concentrations of these three ions are approximately equal in the mother and fetus (Table 2.3). Movement across the placental barrier, particularly for sodium and chloride, is a two-directional mechanism: the electrolytes moving from mother to fetus and returning to the maternal system.

TABLE 2.3   RELATIVE LEVELS OF SOME CONSTITUENTS OF MATERNAL AND FETAL BLOOD

	About equal	Lower in fetus	Higher in fetus
Amino acids			+
Urea	+		
Uric acid	+		
Creatinine	+		
Inorganic P			+
Free fatty acids		+	
Cholesterol		+	
Glucose		+	
Lactic acid			+
Calcium			+
Magnesium	+		
Chloride	+		
Sodium	+		
Potassium	+		
Iron			+
Vitamins			
Fat soluble		+	
Water soluble			+
Chorionic gonadotrophin (HCG)		+	
Placental lactagen		+	
Growth hormone			+

Source: From Dancis and Schneider (**7**). Reproduced by permission from J. Dancis and H. Schneider in *The Placenta,* ed. P. Gruenwald. Copyright © 1975 by MTP Press Limited, Lancaster, England.

Minerals

Essential elements, such as calcium, phosphorus, magnesium, iron, zinc, and iodine, move across the placenta against a concentration gradient, since concentrations in the fetus tend to be higher than in the maternal blood (Table 2.3). Movement against a concentration gradient indicates an active transport mechanism for these ions (**7**).

Glucose

Although the concentration of glucose is higher in the maternal blood (approximately 96 mg per 100 ml) than the fetal blood (about 75 mg per 100 ml), the rate of movement by simple diffusion would not meet the fetal needs for glucose. Indications are that an active transport system is involved in this movement.

Amino Acids

The mechanism for the movement of amino acids into the fetus also seems to involve an active transport mechanism, and the rate of transport differs for each (**9**). This passage of amino acids to the fetus is against a concentration gradient (Table 2.3). Amino acids may contribute, along with glucose, to the energy needs of the fetus as well as being utilized in the synthesis of protein for the developing tissues.

Proteins

Several plasma proteins, in spite of their large molecular size, are transported to the fetus, but at a slower rate than the amino acids. The transfer of IgG is important for survival of the fetus as indicated in the section on immunological aspects of the placenta.

Lipids

Free fatty acids pass through the placenta at a relatively slow rate but in sufficient amounts to meet fetal needs for the synthesis of adipose tissue. Toward the end of gestation the fetus can produce fat from its own resources (**10**). Higher molecular size lipids—such as cholesterol, phospholipids and neutral triglycerides—are transported in small amounts to the fetus.

Fat-Soluble Vitamins

Vitamins A, D, E, and K are probably transported across the placenta by simple diffusion, although the mechanism is not clear. In any event, the concentrations of these vitamins are lower in the fetus than in the mother (Table 2.3).

Water-Soluble Vitamins

An active mechanism also is probably involved in transporting the water-soluble vitamins, since higher levels of vitamin C, thiamin, riboflavin, vitamin B_6, vitamin B_{12}, and folic acid are found in the fetal blood than in the maternal circulation.

Fetal Metabolic End Products

The placenta is sometimes described as the kidney for the fetus. This implies that metabolic end products, such as urea, uric acid, creatinine, and bilirubin, move from the fetus to the maternal system. Bilirubin is transported by a mechanism similar to that involved in estrogen transfer. Urea seems to move by a simple diffusion (**7**).

CHANGES IN THE MATERNAL SYSTEM DURING PREGNANCY

The nutritional needs of the combined maternal-fetal system must be viewed in terms of the changes that occur within the maternal system during a normal pregnancy, as well as the nutrient requirements of the growing and developing fetus. These changes in the physiological system of the mother should be viewed as normal and progressive rather than as abnormal (**11**).

Blood Volume and Composition

Changes in the components of the blood are summarized in Table 2.4.

Plasma volume and the total blood volume begin to rise at the third month, reaching a maximum amount at about two weeks prior to term. Plasma volume then drops about 200 ml during the last two weeks of gestation.

Red cell volume also increases during gestation, but the rise is proportionally less than the plasma volume, resulting in a decreased concentration of hemoglobin and hematocrit. The change in hemoglobin is referred to as the "physiological anemia of pregnancy," since the concentration of hemoglobin drops by approximately 2 g per 100 ml at this time. Hemoglobin levels of 13.5−14.0 g in the nonpregnant woman may drop to 11.0 to 12.0 g in pregnancy. Clinicians differ in their opinions about whether this hemoglobin drop constitutes a true iron-deficiency anemia.

TABLE 2.4 PLASMA VOLUME, RED CELL VOLUME, TOTAL BLOOD VOLUME AND HEMATOCRIT[1] IN PREGNANCY

		Weeks of pregnancy		
	Nonpregnancy	20	30	40
Volume (ml)				
Plasma	2600	3150	3750	3600
Red cell	1400	1450	1550	1650
Total blood	4000	4600	5200	5250
Hematocrit (percentage)				
Body	35.0	31.5	29.5	31.5
Venous	39.8	35.8	34.0	35.8

Source: Reprinted with permission from F. E. Hytten and A. M. Thomson in *Biology of Gestation,* Vol. 1, ed. N. S. Assali. Copyright © 1968 by Academic Press, New York.
[1]Assuming hematocrit ratio of 0.88.

The composition of the blood plasma also changes during pregnancy (**11**), with the concentration of total protein dropping from approximately 7 g per 100 ml of plasma to a level of 5.5−6 g during the first trimester. Not all protein fractions follow this change, however. In fact, the decline in total protein is a reflection of the significant decrease in albumin level that drops from approximately 4 to 2.5 g to 3 g per 100 ml. The globulins actually rise in concentration, and the fibrinogen rises significantly throughout pregnancy. Most lipids, including cholesterol, phospholipids, and free fatty acids, increase in concentration during pregnancy. Cholesterol rises from 200 to 250−300 mg per 100 ml. Fatty acids increase from about 800 mEq per l to around 1330 mEq per l. Phospholipids rise to maintain the prepregnancy ratio between cholesterol and phospholipids.

Changes in the Cardiovascular System
Important differences are readily apparent in the cardiovascular system if comparisons are made between the nonpregnant and pregnant conditions. Cardiac output rises during pregnancy by approximately 1.5 l per minute above the normal range of 4.5−5.0 l per minute. This change occurs during the first half of pregnancy when both the heart rate and the stroke volume are increased to provide for the more rapid movement of blood. Pulse rate rises throughout pregnancy, increasing to about 15 beats per minute above the normal rate, and the blood flows more rapidly to the kidney and skin, both sites of the elimination of metabolic end products.

Changes in the Respiratory System
Anatomical changes occur in the chest even prior to significant growth of the fetus and placenta. The rate of ventilation changes from about 7 l to 10 l per minute, and this is the result of an increase in the volume of air rather than in the rate of breathing. Considerable overbreathing also occurs, even in early pregnancy.

Changes in the Kidney Function
During pregnancy the entire renal tract is dilated and relatively atonic and thus has a larger capacity for urine. Renal blood flow increases from about 500 ml to above 700 ml per minute, and the glomerular filtration rate rises. Waste products (urea, creatinine, and uric acid) and nutrients (amino acids, folate, iodine, and sugar) are thus readily excreted from the body.

Changes in the Alimentary Function
The changes here are contradictory in nature. Although the body's use of food materials becomes more efficient, the pregnant woman is often bothered by nausea, constipation, and heartburn—all general indications of an impaired function. She also usually has an increased appetite and an increased saliva flow but reduced gastric function and reduced motility. The liver function is not altered, but the gall bladder follows the general slowdown of the gastrointestinal tract.

Changes in Weight and Water Retention

The amount of total body water increases during pregnancy, and except for women with edema, this gain can be attributed to increased blood volume and water in the fetus, placenta, and other products of conception.

Careful investigation shows that fat is the major material stored in the maternal system. The total weight gain, though, can be accounted for by the products of pregnancy: the expanded maternal blood volume, an increase in the reproductive organs, and gain in fat by the mother. The components of the weight gain and the rate of gain of each component are illustrated in Figure 2.6.

Wide variations are seen in both the total amount of weight gained and in the components of gain. The distribution of weight gained by 746 healthy women during their first pregnancy is shown in Figure 2.7. The average gain was 12.5 kg.

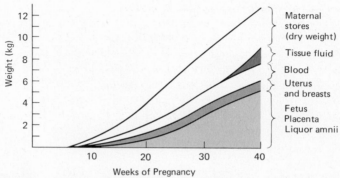

Figure 2.6 *The components of weight gain in normal pregnancy.* (*Source:* Reproduced with permission from F. E. Hytten and A. M. Thomson in *Biology of Gestation,* Vol. 1, ed. N. S. Assali. Copyright © 1968 by Academic Press, New York.)

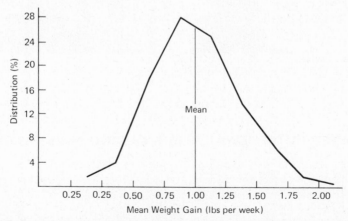

Figure 2.7 *Distribution of the mean rate of weight gain between 20 weeks and delivery for a selected group of healthy young primigravidas.* (*Source:* Reproduced with permission from *The Physiology of Human Pregnancy,* 2nd edition, by F. E. Hytten and I. Leitch. Copyright © 1971 by Blackwell Scientific Publications Ltd., Oxford, England.)

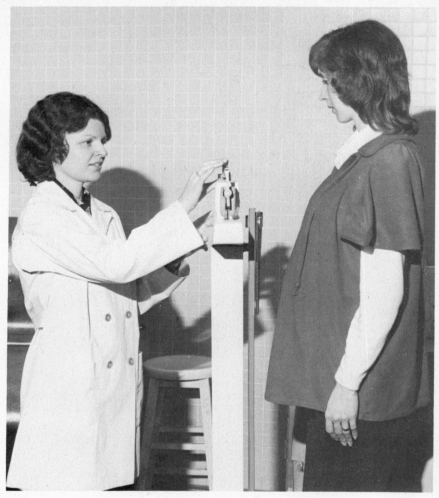

Sound health care and nutritional advice during pregnancy is essential for normal fetal development.

INCREASED NUTRITIONAL NEEDS DURING PREGNANCY

During pregnancy the body increases its needs for most nutrients to provide for the building of new tissues for the fetus and placenta and for the mother (**14**). The recommended allowances for the adult female were discussed in Chapter 1, and additional attention is given to certain nutrients in later sections of this book. A brief discussion, though, of the increased nutritional needs seems appropriate at this point. The extra needs for nutrients during pregnancy, as suggested by the FNB, National Research Council are summarized in Table 2.5 (**14**).

TABLE 2.5 COMPARISON OF RECOMMENDED
DAILY ALLOWANCE FOR THE
NONPREGNANT AND PREGNANT ADULT FEMALE

	Nonpregnant	Pregnant	Lactating
Energy (kcal)	2100	2400	
Protein (g)	44	74	64
Vitamin A (mcg R.E.)[1]	800	1000	1200
Vitamin D (mcg)[2]	5	10	10
Vitamin E (mg α T.E.)[3]	8	10	11
Vitamin C (mg)	60	80	100
Folacin (mcg)	400	800	500
Niacin (mg N.E.)[4]	13	15	18
Riboflavin (mg)	1.2	1.5	1.7
Thiamin (mg)	1.0	1.4	1.5
Vitamin B_6 (mg)	2.0	2.6	2.5
Vitamin B_{12} (mcg)	3.0	4.0	4.0
Calcium (mg)	800	1200	1200
Phosphorus (mg)	800	1200	1200
Iodine (mcg)	150	175	200
Iron (mg)	18	18+[5]	18+[5]
Magnesium (mg)	300	450	450
Zinc (mg)	15	20	25

Source: Food and Nutrition Board, *Recommended Dietary Allowances,* 9th edition. National Academy of Sciences, Washington, 1980 (**14**).

[1] 1 Retinol equivalent (R.E.) = 1 mcg retinol or 6 mcg β-carotene.
[2] As cholecalciferol. 10 mcg cholecalciferol = 400 IU vitamin D.
[3] α-tocopherol equivalents. 1 mg D-α-tocopherol = 1 α-T.E.
[4] One niacin equivalent (N.E.) = 1 mg niacin or 60 mg dietary tryptophan.
[5] The increased requirement during pregnancy cannot be met by the iron content of habitual American diets or by the existing iron stores of many women; therefore, the use of 30–60 mg of supplemental iron is recommended. Continued supplementation of lactating mothers for two to three months after parturition is advisable to replenish stores depleted by pregnancy.

Energy
The metabolic rate of women increases with pregnancy. Therefore, an increased energy supply is needed to accommodate their larger energy needs with no decrease in physical activity. An extra allowance of 300 kcal per day, or a total of 80,000 kcal throughout gestation is suggested (**14**).

Protein
Approximately 925 g of protein is deposited in the fetus and other tissues associated with the developing fetus during pregnancy. This protein is deposited at estimated rates of 0.6, 1.8, 4.8, and 6.1 g per day during the four successive quarters of pregnancy. Studies suggest that considerable protein also is stored in the maternal tissues (**15**).

Vitamins A, D, and E
An increased allowance or intake is suggested to reflect the amounts stored in the fetus.

Thiamin, Riboflavin, and Niacin
The higher recommended allowances are suggested to assist in the metabolism of the required increased energy intake. The estimates are based on urinary excretion studies, a commonly used index of water-soluble vitamin sufficiency. The daily levels of thiamin intake are 0.5−0.6 mg per 1000 kcal. The increased needs for riboflavin are estimated to be 0.3 mg per day; those for niacin are estimated to be 2 mg per day.

Folacin
The need for folacin increases markedly during pregnancy. The increased need is from 200 to 400 mcg per day to meet the needs of the fetus and mother.

Vitamin B_6
The increased allowance of 0.6 mg per day is sufficient to maintain serum levels and normal metabolic function. The placenta concentrates vitamin B_6 and provides the fetus with an ample supply of this vitamin.

Vitamin B_{12}
The FNB recommends an increased allowance of 4 mcg per day of vitamin B_{12} during pregnancy, although research suggests the need for approximately 0.3 mcg per day in addition to that amount.

Calcium, Phosphorus, and Magnesium
These macro minerals are deposited in relatively large quantities in the fetus. Approximately 25 g of calcium are found in the infant at birth, and most of that is deposited during the last trimester of pregnancy. Phosphorus follows the same pattern as calcium.

Sodium and Potassium
An increased amount of sodium of about 25 g is required during pregnancy or about 4 mEq per day. The restriction of sodium during pregnancy was recommended for many years, but this practice was found to be damaging; maternal weight gain was reduced, and babies were correspondingly smaller (**16**). No additional requirements for potassium seem to exist during pregnancy since the normal diet usually provides sufficient amounts.

Iron
Large amounts of iron are stored in the fetus and large amounts enter the maternal circulation system. Estimates of the extra iron stored during pregnancy suggest about 370 mg in the fetus and other tissues and 290 mg in the maternal blood. The

FNB suggests supplements of 30−60 mg of iron daily to compensate for these iron stores.

Iodine
The approximate need for iodine is 1 mcg per kg of body weight, with slightly higher levels during pregnancy. Intakes of approximately 150 mcg are suggested for the nonpregnant adult female, with a recommended intake of 175 mcg during pregnancy.

Zinc
The recommendation for zinc rises from 15 mg for the nonpregnant adult female to 20 mg during pregnancy.

SOURCES OF NUTRIENTS DURING PREGNANCY

Pregnant women can obtain most of the nutrients they need in adequate amounts from normal food consumption. Iron may be the key exception to this generalization, and the doctor may recommend iron supplements. In the case of other nutrients, an increased food intake to provide for the energy needs of the pregnant woman will be sufficient if the woman consumes a variety of foods. The pregnant woman should place a high priority on foods with a high nutrient density and avoid high-energy, low-nutrient foods. For example, potato chips, pastries, and other snacks offer incomplete nourishment. However, most are so filling that they leave less room for the necessary foods. The pregnant woman need only eat a little more than usual if her eating habits have always been good (Table 2.6).

An expectant mother needs three 8 oz cups of whole or skim milk each day for the first three months of pregnancy and four cups daily for the next six months to meet calcium requirements for herself and the baby. Milk is also a source of protein, certain vitamins, zinc, magnesium, and phosphorus for the pregnant

TABLE 2.6 SUMMARY OF FOODS NEEDED DURING PREGNANCY[1]

Food group	Servings per Day	
	First trimester	Second-third trimesters
Milk (8 oz cup)	3	4
Meat, eggs, fish (2−3 oz servings)	3	4
Whole grains and breads	3−4	3−4
Fruits and vegetables		
Total servings	4	4
Vitamin C source	1	1
Vitamin A source	1	1

[1]See appropriate textual discussion for foods that apply to each of these groups.

woman. Part of the milk requirement can be met by adding milk to cream soups, cocoa, custards, or puddings. Milk that has been fortified with vitamin D should be used.

Cheese or other milk products can also be substituted for part of the milk requirement. A 1½ oz piece of hard or semisoft cheese is equivalent to 1 glass of milk. The pregnant woman may prefer 1 cup of yogurt or 1½ cups of creamed cottage cheese or ice cream instead of 1 cup of milk. She must remember, though, that while ice cream provides the same nutrients as milk, it provides more fat and sugar. Some women may not be able to tolerate milk or may simply not like it. The doctor, dietitian, or nutritionist can plan a diet for these women using milk substitutes. For example, many women who can't drink milk can digest homemade yogurt. Green leafy vegetables are also a good alternative source of calcium for anyone who can't drink milk.

Three 2–3 oz servings of protein-rich foods are required daily during the first trimester of pregnancy. Four are needed each day thereafter. Meat, poultry, fish, and eggs are animal foods that supply complete protein in the diet. They also provide important vitamins, iron, and other necessary minerals. Vegetable protein foods such as dried beans, peas, and nuts are incomplete sources of protein and when eaten alone cannot build body tissue in the same way that complete protein can. Vegetable protein foods need to be combined with other complementary protein foods or with a small amount of animal protein to improve the overall protein quality.

Cereal grains are excellent sources of the B-vitamins, minerals, and a certain amount of incomplete protein. At least three to four servings of whole grain or enriched breads and cereals are needed each day throughout pregnancy. Any of the following make up one serving from the bread and cereal group: one slice of bread; one-half cup of whole grain brown rice, enriched white rice, whole grain or enriched cereal, or cooked pasta; two corn tortillas, one muffin, one biscuit, one dumpling, one pancake, one 2 in. square of cornbread, one hot dog roll or hamburger bun, or ¾ cup of ready-to-eat cereal.

The pregnant woman should eat one serving of fruits or vegetable supplying vitamin C, one serving supplying vitamin A, and at least two other servings per day. The day's requirement for vitamin C can be supplied by 1 orange, ½ grapefruit, 4 oz of orange or grapefruit juice, 12 oz of tomato or pineapple juice, ¾ cup of green peppers or chili peppers, or 2 tomatoes. Other good sources are cantaloupe, mangoes, fresh strawberries, blackberries, raspberries, cabbage, brussels sprouts, broccoli, and cauliflower.

One cup of raw or one-half cup of cooked green leafy vegetables supplies vitamin A as well as other vitamins, iron, and magnesium. The pregnant woman can choose from asparagus, broccoli, cabbage, endive, escarole, romaine, beet greens, collards, kale, spinach, and Swiss chard. Other excellent sources of vitamin A are the dark orange and yellow fruits and vegetables such as apricots, carrots, sweet potatoes, and winter squash.

Two servings of other fruits and vegetables should be eaten daily in addition to those just mentioned. Nutrient values vary among fruits and vegetables, so it is a good idea to choose from a wide variety. Peaches, apples, bananas, pears, grapes, watermelons, potatoes, peas, corn, eggplants, onions, and many others are all good choices.

The number of servings from each food group mentioned here provides the minimum recommended nutrients for a pregnant woman. She can obtain extra energy from additional servings and from butter, margarine, salad oils, and other fats used in cooking. In addition, she should drink six to eight glasses of water or other fluids daily.

Some women experience nausea early in pregnancy. It is important for the baby's sake for the pregnant woman to eat correctly even during this difficult time when she may not have an appetite. Eating small amounts of food throughout the day or eating something before getting out of bed in the morning can be helpful. Medicine, however, to alleviate nausea should not be taken without a doctor's advice. The pregnant woman will probably be more comfortable during the last trimester if she does not overload the stomach at one meal. Several smaller meals eaten throughout the day should solve this problem. These minimeals should be planned to provide the required number of servings of the basic foods mentioned before.

The nutritional health and well-being of the fetus is, therefore, inherently related to the functions of the maternal system and placenta, as well as to nutrient intake of the mother. The maternal-fetal system operates in a manner that first meets the needs of the fetus. That is, the fetus derives more than its proportional share of the nutrients available, even when these nutrients are limited or are in short supply. The fetus, because of its rapid growth and development, receives more nutrition per unit weight than the mother. Thus a nutritionally adequate diet for the pregnant woman is extremely important for her own health as well as that of her baby. The partition of nutrients is represented schematically in Figure 2.8.

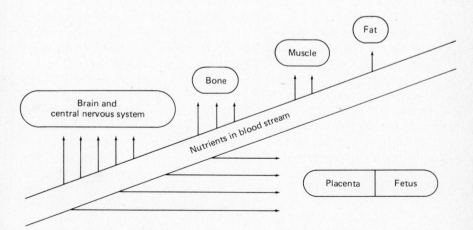

Figure 2.8 Schematic representation of partition of nutrients according to metabolic activity. (*Source:* Reprinted with permission from *Farm Animals,* 3rd edition, by J. Hammond, Jr. Copyright © 1960 by Edward Arnold (Publishers) Ltd., London, England.)

THE LACTATING MOTHER

A renewed interest in the practice of breast-feeding appeared in the United States during the 1970s, but despite this trend, less than one-half of all new mothers in this country breast-feed their babies today (**18**). On a percentage basis more women in western states breast-feed than do those in the eastern states (**19**). In addition, babies are being breast-fed longer. However, only one infant in five is breast-fed for as long as six months (**18**).

As in pregnancy, it is difficult to make accurate physiologic observations during lactation, and the knowledge we have of the metabolic and functional changes associated with lactation progresses slowly. Much less is known about the physiological adjustments during lactation than during pregnancy. According to Thomson and Hytten there is no reason to suppose that lactation is accompanied by large-scale metabolic adjustment in the maternal organism (**20**). Both mother and baby are now physiologically independent individuals. Changes in the maternal system, therefore, are related to the return of the woman's metabolism to a nonpregnant condition. Of course, certain modifications necessary for the production and secretion of milk will be superimposed on these changes.

MAMMARY SYSTEM

The mammary gland consists of glandular epithelium and a duct system embedded in interstitial tissue and fat. The nipple, elevated above the breast, contains 15−20 lactiferous ducts. These ducts extend radially from the nipple toward the chest wall to form the sinuses where milk is stored. The ducts terminate in epithelial masses that form lobules and tubules. The terminal tubules and glandular structures are generally most numerous during the childbearing years. The mammary gland of the nonpregnant woman is inadequately prepared for secretory activity. During pregnancy and lactation, however, the breast structures achieve a full physiological development so that milk production and secretion are possible. Ovarianlike hormones, including HCS, secreted by the placenta in large quantities, appear to stimulate rapid growth and development of the breasts in pregnant women. Following birth, the infant's sucking stimulates a hypothalamic response that causes the anterior pituitary to produce the hormone prolactin. This hormone acts on cells in the mammary tissue to promote continued milk production and release. The "milk ejection" or "let-down" reflex is a neurohormonal mechanism regulated partially by the central nervous system. The primary stimulus, again, is sucking on the nipple that triggers the release of the hormone oxytocin from the posterior pituitary. Oxytocin acts on the smooth muscles surrounding the alveoli of the nipples, causing them to contract and permit the release of milk. Medicinal or "food galactogogues," substances believed to stimulate lactation, have evolved in most cultures. These include garlic, cottonseed, candy, beer, ale, and large quantities of milk (**18**).

EARLY STAGES OF BREAST-FEEDING

The decision to breast-feed is generally made early in pregnancy. Once the decision to breast-feed is made the woman's success in doing so will depend on several factors. These include the woman's own health and nutritional status and her basic attitude toward breast-feeding and understanding of the process of lactation and the support and encouragement she receives from medical personnel and members of her family (**18**). At least 99 percent of the women who attempt breast-feeding their infants are successful (**21**).

Full lactation does not begin at birth. A small amount of colostrum is secreted from the breasts during the first two or three days after birth, followed by an increase in milk secretion. Lactation is generally well established by the end of the first week when the daily milk output usually reaches 500 ml. Lactation, however, may not be fully established until the third week or even later in primiparas. The continuation of milk secretion requires the hormonal factors from the pituitary already mentioned. The pituitary release of these essential hormones will cease, and milk secretion will slow down or stop altogether if sucking is discontinued during the lactation period. For this reason, formula feedings should be avoided during the first two weeks after birth, since they may adversely affect the establishment of the milk supply. An occasional bottle after this period will not significantly affect the supply, especially if the milk from a skipped feeding is expressed manually into a sterile container and kept for the next bottle feeding

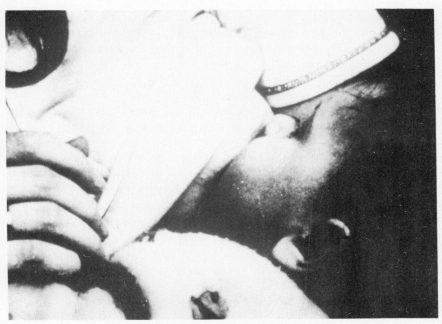

Successful breast feeding promotes sound growth and development in the infant.

(**18**). It is a good idea to introduce the breast-fed baby to an occasional bottle at least by the end of the second month of life, simply because the nursing mother will sometimes need to be away from her infant during a normal feeding time.

INCREASED NUTRIENT NEEDS DURING LACTATION

Certain nutritional recommendations must be followed during the postpartum period for breast-feeding to be successful for the mother and infant both physiologically and psychologically. As in pregnancy, the maternal diet plays a significant role in supplying nutrient requirements for both mother and child. The best basis for successful breast-feeding is an adequate diet during pregnancy that develops the necessary nutrient reserves. Then a good diet is necessary during lactation to maintain maternal tissues and to replenish the nutrient stores (**22**). In addition, a nutritious diet aids in the production of sufficient amounts of high-quality breast milk to help promote proper growth and development of the infant.

An inadequate diet during lactation can have adverse consequences. Poor maternal nutriture during lactation may result in a failure of the mother to return to acceptable health, in a decreased volume of breast milk, and, in some cases, in a reduction in the nutrient content of the milk (**22, 23**). The latter two factors can cause the infant to have health problems.

The RDAs for lactation are shown in Table 2.5. These values are based on even less quantitative data than are the RDAs for pregnancy. Several factors, including a lack of clearly defined information on the nutrient composition of breast milk, the volume of milk production, and the efficiency of that milk production, make it difficult to establish standards (**18**). But according to most research, the nutrient intake levels suggested here will support an average milk production of 850 ml per day.

Energy

Contrary to popular belief, the diet of the lactating mother must contain an even higher number of calories than that of the pregnant woman. The energy required to provide for the needs of lactation is proportional to the amount of milk produced and will vary considerably from one woman to another. In general, approximately 900 kcal of energy are required to produce 1 l of milk in the adult female. Therefore, the woman who secretes an average of 850 ml of breast milk daily over a six-month lactation period requires an additional 750 kcal per day. Of this amount, 150 kcal are required for the synthesis and secretion of milk. The remaining 600 kcal represent the energy content of the milk itself.

The pregnant woman who adds 11−12.5 k of weight will store approximately 2−4 k of this in her body as fat. This fat store can be used to supply a part of the additional energy the woman will require for lactation. Storage fat will provide 200−300 kcal per day during a three-month lactation period. The remaining energy needs should come from an additional 500 kcal in the daily diet during the first three months of lactation. The daily extra energy allowance should be increased accordingly if lactation continues beyond the initial three months or if maternal weight falls below the ideal for the mother's height. Moderate to severe restriction of caloric intake during lactation can lessen a woman's ability to produce breast milk and should be discouraged by health professionals.

Protein

Along with the recommended energy increment, a 20 g increase in daily protein is advised for lactating women. The additional protein needs are dependent on the amount of milk protein being produced. The average daily milk yield is 850 ml, but it can range as high as 1200 ml. Assuming a protein content of 1.2 percent, the secretion of the average 850 ml of milk requires about 10 g of protein. The secretion of the maximum 1200 ml requires 15 g of protein. The RDA is now set at 20 g above normal needs to allow for the consumption of protein that is not always of high biological value and assumes a 70 percent efficiency of protein utilization.

Calcium

The calcium content of human milk indicates that approximately 250 mg of calcium daily are required for normal milk production during early lactation. Approximately 300 mg are required after three months of lactation. No evidence exists that the calcium composition of human milk is influenced by dietary calcium intake. However, it is well known that dietary calcium deficiency results from the use of maternal bone calcium to maintain milk calcium levels (**24**). Therefore, an allowance of 1200 mg of calcium, or 400 mg above normal, is recommended during lactation.

Trace Minerals

The iron, copper, and fluoride content of human milk does not appear to be altered by the administration of these trace elements to lactating women (**19**). Also, the total fluoride content of milk from mothers drinking fluoridated water does not differ essentially from that of mothers using nonfluoridated water (**25**). The selenium content of breast milk appears to be higher in lactating women who reside in areas where forage crops are high in selenium. However, the general information on the subject is far from conclusive (**26**). As a whole, the total mineral content of human milk is fairly constant. Specific amounts may vary considerably with variations in the maternal diet and the stage of lactation but not to the extent that certain vitamins vary.

Fat-Soluble Vitamins

The fat-soluble vitamins, especially D, E, and K, do not appear to move easily from blood to milk. The vitamin A concentration in breast milk, however, is strongly influenced by the quality and quantity of the nursing mother's diet.

Water-Soluble Vitamins

Ascorbic acid, riboflavin, and thiamin are the vitamins whose content in the maternal diet is most greatly reflected in breast milk composition.

Extra servings of citrus fruit or juice can provide the 100 mg of ascorbic acid needed by the lactating mother. It is assumed that the additional amount of riboflavin needed during lactation is equal to the amount secreted by breast milk. Based on a mean riboflavin content in human milk of approximately 40 mcg per 100 ml, the increased requirement would be 0.34 mg. Also assuming a utilization of the additional riboflavin at approximately 70 percent, the additional daily intake is set at 0.5 mg.

A thiamin deficiency in the mother's diet is reflected directly in a deficiency in her breast milk. Therefore, an intake of 0.5 mg per 1000 kcal is recommended to produce milk with adequate thiamin levels.

SOURCES OF NUTRIENTS DURING LACTATION

The nutritive demands of the lactating mother exceed those she experienced during pregnancy, with the most significant demands being in protein and energy. Therefore, careful daily diet planning is of utmost importance to insure successful lactation and the maintenance of the woman's health. Although nutrient needs increase during lactation, these increased needs can be provided by a well-balanced diet. Ethnic, social, and economic factors will, as discussed in Chapter 1, influence the mother's dietary intake, and these factors must be considered by the health professionals who counsel the nursing mother.

The nursing mother will find guides available to help her plan an adequate diet (**22**). The number of servings and the types of food needed to meet the RDAs for lactating women are shown in Table 2.7. For the most part, though, the quantities and kinds of food needed during lactation are similar to those required during pregnancy. These recommended nutrient increases can be satisfied by the equivalent of an additional meal of approximately 500 kcal of protective foods each day. Increased amounts of protein-rich foods, green and yellow fruits or

TABLE 2.7 SERVINGS AND TYPES OF FOODS
NEEDED TO MEET THE RDAs FOR LACTATING WOMEN

Type of food	Examples	Number of servings
Meat and meat alternates	Red meat, poultry, fish, eggs, peanut butter, dried beans, dried peas	2
Milk and milk products	Milk, cheese, yogurt	4+
Breads and cereals	Bread, pasta, rice, cereal	4
Fruits and vegetables		
Vitamin C rich	Citrus fruits, tomatoes, greens, green peppers, strawberries, cantaloupes	1
Vitamin A rich	Broccoli, spinach, kale, sweet potatoes, carrots, apricots	1 every second day
Others	Apples, pears, bananas, corn, celery, potatoes, beets, squash, eggplant, peas	2-3

vegetables, citrus fruits, and the equivalent of two to three cups of whole milk over and above a normal well-balanced diet should supply the additional nutrients needed during lactation. As during pregnancy, some women may find it difficult to incorporate the extra food into three regular meals. In such cases five to six smaller meals each day may be effective.

Fluid

The nursing mother should consume two to three quarts of liquid daily to provide the liquid volume essential for the production of adequate breast milk. Nutritionists have not established the relationship between fluid intake and the volume of breast milk. However, milk production appears to be limited only when the total fluid intake is less than the volume of milk usually produced. A liberal fluid intake is also necessary to preclude the formation of a highly concentrated urine in compensation for a lack of fluid.

Foods to Avoid

Most foods that are well tolerated during pregnancy will be well tolerated by the mother and infant during lactation. No basis exists for the breast-feeding mother to avoid garlic, curry, sulfur-containing vegetables, or other foods. A food, however, that consistently seems to bother the mother or child can be omitted to see if relief occurs.

Nutrient Supplements

In general, the increased nutrient needs associated with lactation can be provided by a well-balanced diet, so nutrient supplements are generally unnecessary. In certain cases, though, carefully selected vitamin and mineral supplements may be beneficial for some women. The use of such supplements does not minimize the importance of a varied and balanced diet for the mother.

During lactation there may be a need to supplement the maternal diet with certain nutrients. Since relatively little iron is transferred to the infant through milk, the need for iron in the maternal diet does not increase above that needed during pregnancy. The RDAs for nursing mothers do not require any increases in dietary iron over the nonpregnant state. But, as in pregnancy, a supplement of 30 – 60 mg of elemental iron should be taken daily during lactation (**24**). This supplement should be continued for at least two to three months postpartum to replenish maternal iron stores that were reduced during pregnancy.

In the past vitamin and mineral supplements were prescribed for lactating women to prevent nutrient depletion. Few studies evaluated the actual dietary intake of lactating women to determine the need, if any, for such supplements (**27**). Recent studies indicate that neither the nutrient status of the mother nor the nutrient content of breast milk suffers in women receiving no vitamin and mineral supplements, provided the women were healthy and were eating an adequate diet (**27, 28**). Vitamin and mineral supplements, however, may be indicated in the case of less well nourished women.

Drugs

The effect of drugs on the composition of mother's milk and on the infant is not understood fully. It is, however, known that drugs can be transmitted through breast milk to the infant (**29**–**31**). Therefore, as pointed out in Chapter 4, the use of any drug during lactation must be seriously evaluated. The infants of nursing mothers who use oral contraceptives, for instance, show a slower growth rate than the infants of nursing mothers who do not use oral contraceptives (**32**). If oral contraceptives are taken sooner than six weeks postpartum, the amount of breast milk can be diminished (**33**–**35**). The estrogen and progesterone in these preparations reduce milk production, and the low growth rate seen in some infants has been attributed to a low milk supply. Other studies report a decrease in the amount of certain nutrients in the breast milk of women who take oral contraceptives (**36**).

SUMMARY

The normal growth and development of the fetus must be supported by an adequate nutrient supply. Several major physiological changes occur during pregnancy that affect the nutritional requirements of the pregnant woman and developing fetus. To provide the pregnant woman with sound nutritional advice, students of nutrition, dietetics, child development, and other health-related fields need an understanding of the physiological changes that take place during pregnancy. They need to know the ways these changes affect nutritional requirements in the mother and fetus and, ultimately, the growth and development of the infant.

Physiological and biochemical development of the embryo begins immediately following conception. In the very early stages nutrients and oxygen for the growing cellular mass are supplied from the uterine secretions. By the twelfth week of pregnancy the placenta is developed fully. This unique and complex tissue has several biochemical functions important to the maintenance of pregnancy and normal development of the fetus. Despite the obvious closeness of the fetus and mother during pregnancy, there is a clear separation of the two. The placenta acts as a barrier separating the two circulatory systems throughout gestation. It does, however, permit the passage of materials necessary for normal growth and development of the fetus.

The human placenta functions in an immunological capacity to protect the fetus from invading microorganisms by selecting appropriate immunoglobulins from the mother. Proteins, carbohydrates, lipids, vitamins, minerals, and water also cross the placenta either by simple diffusion or with the aid of some active transport mechanism.

Fetal development is accompanied by significant changes in the physiology and metabolism of the maternal system. Blood volume and composition change throughout pregnancy, and the cardiac output rises. Heart rate and stroke volume increase to provide for the more rapid movement of blood. Changes in the renal and gastrointestinal systems can also be observed in the pregnant woman. An increase in water retention because of the increased blood volume and water content of the fetus, placenta, and other products of conception and an increase in tissue deposition contribute to a weight gain of approximately 12.5 kg during pregnancy.

Pregnancy results in an increased need for most nutrients to provide for the laying down of new tissues in the fetus and placenta and for increased needs of the mother. The increased requirements for most nutrients, with the exception of iron, can be met through the consumption of a balanced diet including a wide variety of foods. The pregnant woman must be careful to choose foods that offer a high nutrient return for calorie content. The nutritional health and well-being of the fetus are linked inherently to the functions of the maternal system and placenta as well as to the nutrient intake of the mother.

Similarly, the nutritional health and well-being of the nursing mother and her infant depend to a large extent on the mother's diet, and these nutritional demands generally exceed those of pregnancy. The most significant nutrient increases are for protein and energy. In general, the increased nutritional needs associated with lactation can be provided by a well-balanced diet. Health professionals, though, need to increase their efforts to determine and understand the factors influencing lactation in a quantitative and qualitative sense so that they can evaluate more fully the role of lactation in society today.

STUDY QUESTIONS AND
TOPICS FOR INDIVIDUAL INVESTIGATION

1. The placenta is fully developed by the twelfth week of pregnancy. It performs several biochemical functions important to the maintenance of pregnancy and development of the fetus. Discuss and evaluate the unique and varied functions of this tissue.

2. *Great Expectations*—a film on nutrition for nursing and pregnant mothers—can be ordered from the Society for Nutrition Education, 2140 Shattuck Avenue, Suite 1110, Berkeley, California 94704. The film discusses the importance of wise daily food selection and offers possible solutions to common diet-related problems of pregnancy and nutrients of special concern to pregnant mothers. Why not view the film as a class? Discuss ways in which the film could be used in different settings, Special Supplemental Food Program for Women, Infants, and Children (WIC) centers, Extension classes, parent education groups, high schools, community colleges, and the like, to teach pregnant women about the importance of good nutrition during pregnancy.

3. It takes three to four 8 oz glasses of milk or milk products daily to provide the calcium the pregnant woman and her baby need. If she does not like or cannot drink milk, what other sources of calcium might you suggest to the pregnant woman? Plan three daily menus designed to meet the nutritional needs of this individual.

4. Discuss the increased need for the following nutrients during pregnancy: (a) sodium, (b) iron, (c) vitamin B_{12}, (d) protein. How are the increased needs related to changes in the maternal system? How are the increased needs related to fetal growth and development?

5. How can you, as a future health professional, best educate a woman about the process of growth and development and nutritional needs during pregnancy? How would you convey the material presented in this chapter to an individual concerned about the physiological changes taking place in her body during pregnancy and about the nutritional needs of herself and her unborn child? Several nutrition education aids may be helpful. These include the following:

   (a) "Straight Talk"—a slide series developed by the National Foundation-March of Dimes in cooperation with the Extension Service, U.S. Department of Agriculture—reflects not only the latest medical knowledge but also the basic concerns many women have about pregnancy. The objectives of this educational material are to present facts on pregnancy and help the viewer realize the importance of good health care and practices during the development of the child from conception to birth.

   (b) "Be Good to Your Baby Before It Is Born"—a pamphlet developed by the National Foundation-March of Dimes—is directed to parents and stresses health care during pregnancy.

   (c) *Nutrition in Maternal Health Care*—a pamphlet developed by the American

College of Obstetricians and Gynecologists—is designed as a guide to the nutritional component of maternal health services and deals with nutritional care as an essential aspect of complete maternity care.

6. You are a dietitian or nutritionist working in a clinic setting. A 25-year-old woman who has been using oral contraceptives for four years comes to the clinic. She now wants to become pregnant. How can she prepare adequately for this pregnancy? How will you use the material presented in this chapter to discuss this concern with the woman? What are her current nutritional habits? Does she follow a well-balanced eating pattern? Does she go on fad diets? Is her diet deficient in any nutrients? Could her diet be improved? How motivated is she to make any changes? How much money does she have to spend on food? Is she aware of what good nutrition really is? What other information might you need before giving this woman nutritional advice to meet the needs of her particular situation? Finally, what advice, suggestions, techniques, and so on, will you share with her to help her prepare best for this pregnancy?

7. Following the format outlined in question 6 what nutritional problems and other factors will you consider in developing sound nutritional advice to aid the following individuals?

   (a) A young woman will have her first child in six months and wants to breast-feed. She is intelligent and has an adequate income. She is very concerned with slimness and returning to her prepregnancy weight soon after the baby is born.

   (b) A young pregnant woman and her husband are college students and follow a vegetarian lifestyle. She feels that they do not have extra income to spend on meat.

   (c) An obese pregnant woman feels that if she could gain less weight during this pregnancy than during her previous two she could end the pregnancy a few pounds lighter than she entered. The woman's husband has not worked for four months, and the family qualifies for food stamps.

REFERENCES

1. Avers, C. J. *Biology of Sex.* Wiley, New York, 1974.
2. Villee, D. B. Development of endocrine function in the human placenta and fetus. *New England Journal of Medicine,* 281:473, 1969.
3. Hepner, R. The placenta and the fetus. *Journal of the American Medical Association,* 172:81, 1960.
4. Lowrey, G. H. *Growth and Development of Children,* 6th ed. Year Book Medical Publishers, Chicago, 1973.

5. Potter, E. L., and J. M. Craig. *Pathology of the Fetus and the Infant,* 3rd ed. Year Book Medical Publishers, Chicago, 1975.

6. Lanman, J. T. Immunological functions of the placenta. In: *The Placenta,* ed. P. Gruenwald. University Park Press, Baltimore, Md., 1975.

7. Dancis, J., and H. Schneider. Physiology: transfer and barrier function. In: *The Placenta,* ed. P. Gruenwald. University Park Press, Baltimore, Md., 1975.

8. Bruns, P. D., A. E. Hellegers, A. E. Seeds, Jr., R. E. Behrman and F. C. Battaglia. Effects of osmotic gradients across the primate placenta upon fetal and placental water contents. *Pediatrics,* 34:407, 1964.

9. Ghadimi, H., and P. Pecora. Free amino acids of cord plasma as compared with maternal plasma during pregnancy. *Pediatrics,* 33:60, 1964.

10. Dancis, J., V. Jansen, H. J. Kayden, H. Schneider, and M. Levitz. Transfer across perfused human placenta. II. Free fatty acids. *Pediatric Research,* 7:192, 1973.

11. Committee on Maternal Nutrition/Food and Nutrition Board. *Maternal Nutrition and the Course of Pregnancy.* National Academy of Sciences, Washington, D.C., 1970.

12. Hytten, F. E., and A. M. Thompson. Maternal physiological adjustments. In: *Maternal Nutrition and the Course of Pregnancy.* National Academy of Sciences, Washington, D.C., 1970.

13. Hytten, F. E., and I. Leitch. *The Physiology of Human Pregnancy.* Blackwell, Oxford, England, 1964.

14. Food and Nutrition Board/National Research Council. *Recommended Dietary Allowances,* 9th ed. National Academy of Sciences, Washington, D.C., 1980.

15. King, J. C., D. H. Calloway, and S. Margen. Nitrogen retention, total body ^{40}K and weight gain in teenage pregnant girls. *Journal of Nutrition,* 103:772, 1973.

16. Khokhar, S. A., and R. L. Pike. Aldosterone producing capacity of adrenal glands of sodium-restricted pregnant rats. *Journal of Nutrition,* 103:1126, 1973.

17. Hammond, J. *Farm Animals,* 3rd ed. Edward Arnold Publishers, London, 1960.

18. Guthrie, H. A. *Introductory Nutrition,* Mosby, St. Louis, 1979.

19. Filer, L. Relationship of Nutrition to Lactation and Newborn Development. In: *Nutritional Impacts on Women Throughout Life with Emphasis on Reproduction,* eds. K. Moghissi and T. Evans. Harper & Row, New York, 1977.

20. Thomson, A., and F. Hytten. Physiologic Basis of Nutritional Needs During Pregnancy and Lactation. In: *Nutritional Impacts on Women Throughout Life with Emphasis on Reproduction,* eds. K. Moghissi and T. Evans. Harper & Row, New York, 1977.

21. Worthington, B. S. Lactation, Human Milk, and Nutritional Considerations. In: *Nutrition in Pregnancy and Lactation,* by B. S. Worthington. Mosby, St. Louis, 1977.

22. California Department of Health. *Nutrition During Pregnancy and Lactation.* Maternal and Child Health Unit, California Department of Health. California Association for Maternal and Child Health, 1975.

23. Fomon, S. J. *Infant Nutrition.* Saunders, Philadelphia, 1974.
24. Atkinson, P. J., and R. R. West. Loss of Skeletal Calcium in Lactating Women. *Journal of Obstetrics and Gynaecology of the British Commonwealth,* 77:555, 1970.
25. Dirks, O., J. Jongeling-Eijndhoven, T. Flissebaalje, and I. Gedalia. Total and free ionic fluoride in human and cow's milk as determined by gas-liquid chromatography and the fluoride electrode. *Caries Research,* 8:181, 1974.
26. Shearer, T., and D. Hadjimarkos. Geographic distribution of selenium in human milk. *Archives of Environmental Health,* 30:230, 1975.
27. Thomas, M. R., and J. Kawamoto. Dietary evaluation of lactating women with or without vitamin and mineral supplementation. *Journal of the American Dietetic Association,* 74:669, 1979.
28. Thomas, R., J. Kawamoto, S. Sneed, and R. Eakin. The effects of vitamin C, vitamin B_6, and vitamin B_{12} supplementation on the breast milk and maternal status of well-nourished women. *American Journal of Clinical Nutrition,* 32:1679, 1979.
29. Kesaniemi, Y. Ethanol and acetaldehyde in the milk and peripheral blood of lactating women after ethanol administration. *Journal of Obstetrics and Gynaecology of the British Commonwealth,* 81:84, 1974.
30. Knowles, J. A. Excretion of drugs in milk—a review. *Journal of Pediatrics,* 80:401, 1972.
31. O'Brien, T. E. Excretion of drugs in human milk. *American Journal of Hospital Pharmacy,* 31:844, 1974.
32. Filer, L. J. Maternal nutrition in lactation. *Clinical Perinatology,* 2:353, 1975.
33. Miller, G. H., and L. R. Hughes. Lactation and genital involution effects of a new low-dose oral contraceptive on breast-feeding mothers and their infants. *Obstetrics and Gynecology,* 35:44, 1970.
34. Kaetsawang, S., P. Bhiraleus, and T. Chiemprojert. Effects of oral contraceptives on lactation. *Fertility and Sterility,* 23:24, 1972.
35. Chopra, J. G. Effect of steroid contraceptives on lactation. *American Journal of Clinical Nutrition,* 25:1202, 1972.
36. Barsivala, V. M., and K. D. Virkar. The effect of oral contraceptives on concentrations of various compounds in human milk. *Contraception,* 7:307, 1973.

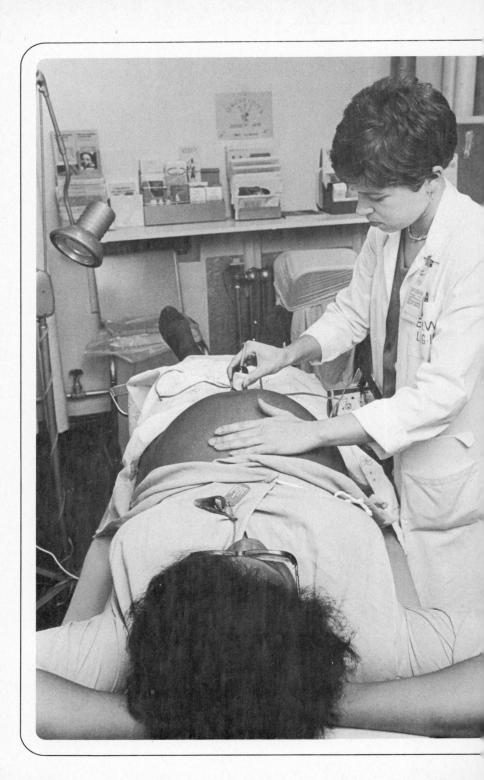

CHAPTER 3

PHYSIOLOGICAL DEVELOPMENT OF THE FETUS AND INFANT

Many physiological and biochemical developments occur during the 280-day fetal period, each aimed at helping the infant function as a distinct entity at birth. Nutrition of the mother and young child, therefore, is an important factor in the development of essential metabolic pathways. Moreover, understanding the body's physiological responses to foods and its use of nutrients will provide a sound basis for the comprehension of the nutrition needs of the fetus and young child. This chapter focuses on the cellular, tissue, and metabolic development of the fetus and infant.

Fetal development is characterized by a series of morphological, physiological, and biochemical changes. These changes occur in an orderly sequence, but the rate of change and timing of events differ in different organisms. Also, two physiological processes—growth and differentiation—are involved in the development of the organism.

Differentiation is the process in which groups of cells take on special characteristics permitting them to operate in a more highly organized and functional state. *Growth* is defined as a quantitative increase in total size because of an increase in both the number and size of cells.

Tissues and organs progress toward final physiological maturity at different rates during gestation and in the years after birth. The maturation of each system is influenced by both environmental and hereditary factors. Of these environmental influences nutrition is probably the major one affecting the entire process of growth and development.

CELLULAR GROWTH OF THE FETUS

An increase in the deoxyribonucleic acid (DNA) content in any tissue or organ represents a corresponding increase in the number of cells. The amount of DNA is constant in each diploid nucleus for any particular organism. Therefore, the total number of cells in an organ or tissue can be determined by measuring total DNA content and dividing by the DNA content per diploid nucleus (**1**). The ratio of protein to DNA can be used as an index of cell size in an organ or tissue, so an increase in this ratio would represent an increase in the mass of each cell.

Cellular growth of an organ or tissue is the result of three distinct phases: (1) a period of rapid increase in DNA content indicative of active cell division. This period is known as "hyperplasia" and results in an increase in cell number, (2) a transitional phase characterized by an increase in the size of cells, or "hypertrophy," occurring simultaneously with hyperplasia, and (3) a phase of hypertrophy alone in which cell division has essentially ceased. The transition from one phase of cellular growth to another depends on the slowing down and finally the cessation of DNA synthesis. The time when this occurs varies from organ to organ but is specific to each one. When net DNA synthesis stops, all growth is by hypertrophy (**2, 3**) or an increase in cell size.

By determining the protein and DNA content of growing organs and tissues one can establish a major investigative tool to identify the type of growth occurring at any given time. Hyperplasia is reflected by a proportionately greater increase in DNA than in protein content. A proportionately greater increase in protein content with little or no increase in DNA is indicative of hypertrophy.

Cellular growth patterns have been studied in several organs and tissues during normal development of the human fetus (**4**). Cell number in the spleen, thyroid, thymus, esophagus, stomach, large and small intestines, tongue, brain, lungs, adrenal gland, and diaphragm, determined by measuring total organ DNA content, increases from 13 weeks of gestation to term. Cell size, determined by measuring either weight/DNA or the protein/DNA ratio, does not change throughout gestation in the spleen, thyroid, thymus, esophagus, stomach, large and small intestines, and tongue. From the beginning of the seventh month of gestation to term, cell size increases slowly in the brain, lungs, adrenal gland, and diaphragm (Table 3.1). DNA and protein/DNA ratios have also been determined in kidney, heart, liver, and gastrocnemius muscle of fetuses and newborn infants of 13–42 weeks of gestational age. In these four systems the total amount of DNA doubles every week from the thirteenth to the twenty-fifth weeks of gestation (**1**). From then on the rate of increase in cell number is slower. Before 30 weeks of gestation, some increase in cell si..e is noted in the kidney, heart, and gastrocnemius muscle. During the last 10 weeks of intrauterine life a rapid increase in cell size occurs in all four systems. At term, the cell number in the kidney, heart, and liver is less than 20 percent of the adult value, yet cell size in the kidney and liver is almost equal to adult cell size. In the heart, however, cell size is only one-half of the mature cell size. The cytoplasm associated with each nucleus in muscle tissue is 60 percent of the adult value.

A limited amount of data is available on cellular growth during the first year

TABLE 3.1 DNA CONTENT OF VARIOUS ORGANS IN NORMAL HUMAN FETUSES (mg)

Weeks of gestation	13	17	23	25	27	31	33	34	39	40
Fetal weight (gm)	31.7	163	320	580	610	1080	1525	1720	3300	4040
Brain	25	85	134	251	240	285	385	—	620	685
Heart	0.51	2.8	8.1	15.4	17.3	18.2	38.6	40.2	54.7	55.6
Liver	16.5	50	53.9	97.3	105.1	175	203	247	328	329
Kidney	0.72	6.8	—	38.7	59.6	—	73	79	107	128
Spleen	0.41	1.2	2.5	7.7	9.8	15.3	—	64.4	84.6	90.9
Thyroid	0.02	0.10	—	0.84	0.97	2.7	—	4.5	5.8	6.9
Adrenal	0.24	0.71	1.31	1.87	2.14	5.84	6.97	8.04	10.2	12.6
Right lung	3.0	23.6	50.9	64	—	66.4	68.5	—	148.7	166.8
Left lung	2.5	18.7	37.5	41.8	—	55.6	59.4	—	126	132
Thymus	0.39	3.99	10.96	21.8	26.5	47.3	105.4	160.6	249	303
Esophagus	0.17	0.60	0.64	0.78	0.80	1.38	3.69	4.21	6.1	6.9
Stomach	0.53	2.3	3.6	5.0	5.7	6.8	22.3	26.8	32.7	40.7
Small intestine	3.8	6.1	16.2	26.3	32.8	48.7	157	179	512	529
Large intestine	0.37	2.97	5.8	10.0	11.2	26.3	47.2	525	129.6	137.2
Diaphragm	0.38	2.1	5.2	6.8	7.2	18.7	24.7	31.7	38.5	45.3
Tongue	0.39	1.21	2.4	3.5	3.7	4.9	—	—	—	—

Source: Reprinted with permission from M. Winick, J. A. Brasel, and P. Rosso in *Nutrition and Development*, Vol. I, ed. M. Winick (**1**). Copyright © 1972 by John Wiley & Sons Inc., New York.

79

TABLE 3.2 DNA CONTENT OF
VARIOUS ORGANS IN NORMAL INFANTS (mg)

	Months after birth				
	2	3	5	10	12
Brain	—	858	890	917	1000
Heart	72.8	88	152	—	—
Liver	360.0	662	848	1130	1200
Kidney	191.84	342	768	—	—
Spleen	108.15	127	156	224	260

Source: Reprinted with permission from M.
Winick, J. A. Brasel, and P. Rosso in *Nutrition and
Development,* Vol. I, ed. M. Winick (**1**). Copy-
right © 1972 by John Wiley & Sons Inc., New
York.

of life (**1**). These data show that cell number continues to increase rapidly in heart, liver, kidney, and spleen during this period. The size of cells in the heart begins to increase after the third month. Cell size does not appear to change during the first year of life in the kidney, liver, and spleen (Table 3.2).

STRUCTURAL AND FUNCTIONAL DIFFERENTIATION DURING THE FETAL PERIOD

"Organogenesis," or the establishment of organs, proceeds rapidly during the embryonic period of prenatal life. Development throughout the subsequent fetal period, from eight weeks of gestation to birth, continues the growth and maturation of tissues and organs that began to develop in the embryo. The differentiation of systems during the fetal period involves the elaboration of their structure and the development of early functional activity (**5, 6**).

BODY GROWTH

The human infant grows at the most rapid rate of its entire lifetime during the fetal stage (Figure 3.1). This fetal growth rate follows a general S-shaped curve characteristic of postnatal growth with growth rate accelerating during the third and fourth months of pregnancy. The most rapid growth occurs during the last trimester (Figure 3.2). Birth weight, traditionally, is an important index of the quality of fetal development. The human fetus increases in weight from 6 g at two months of gestation to about 3500 g at term. Between 21 and 25 weeks of gestation the fetus begins to increase in weight substantially and, although still lean, appears better proportioned. By the twenty-ninth week subcutaneous fat has been laid down and the fetus is less wrinkled. Under favorable conditions weight increases in a linear fashion from mid-gestation to approximately 37 weeks when the curve begins to flatten (Figure 3.3).

Maturation proceeds from the head to the foot and from the central axis of

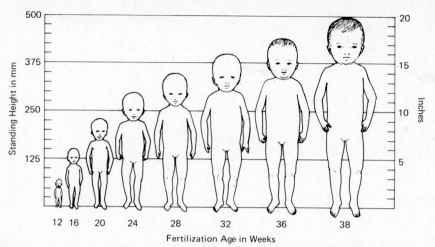

Figure 3.1 Diagram illustrating the changes in size of the human fetus when drawn to scale. (*Source*: Reproduced with permission from *Development and Growth of the External Dimensions of the Human Body in the Fetal Period*, by R. E. Scammon and E. L. Calkins. Copyright © 1929 by the University of Minnesota Press, Minneapolis.)

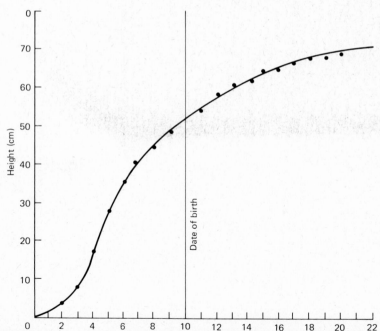

Figure 3.2 Human growth curve during prenatal and early postnatal development. (*Source:* Reproduced with permission from *On Growth and Form*, 2nd edition, by D. A. W. Thompson. Copyright © 1948 by Cambridge University Press, New York.)

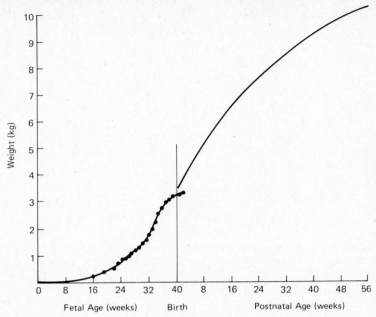

Figure 3.3 *Growth of human fetus and infant.* (*Source:* Reproduced with permission from E. M. Widdowson in *Biology of Gestation,* Vol. 2, ed. N. S. Assali. Copyright © 1968 by Academic Press, New York.)

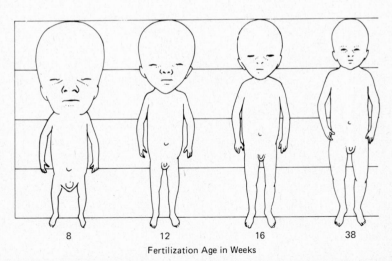

Fertilization Age in Weeks

Figure 3.4 *Diagram illustrating the changing proportion of the body during the fetal period; cell stages are drawn to the same total height.* (*Source:* Reproduced with permission from *Development and Growth of the External Dimensions of the Human Body in the Fetal Period,* by R. E. Scammon and E. L. Calkins. Copyright © 1929 by the University of Minnesota Press, Minneapolis.)

the body outward toward the extremities. At the beginning of the fetal period the head makes up almost half of the fetal body (Figure 3.4). At this point the growth rate of the head slows considerably in relation to the rest of the body. By the end of the twelfth week the upper limbs have reached their final relative lengths. The lower limbs are still short and small, compared with their final length. At 16 weeks the fetal head is relatively small, compared with that of the 12-week fetus and the legs have lengthened. Between the seventeenth and twentieth week of gestation the rate of growth slows. The fetus continues to increase in length until the lower limbs reach their final relative proportions. At about five months of gestation the fetus reaches its peak in height gain. From this point and continuing into the postnatal period the growth rate declines. At birth, the length and weight of the human infant are relatively proportional (**10**).

DEVELOPMENT OF THE FETAL RESPIRATORY SYSTEM

The respiratory system includes nostrils, the nasal cavity and paranasal sinuses, part of the pharynx, the larynx, trachea, and bronchi, as well as the lungs and associated nerves and vessels (**11**). In the embryo the respiratory system begins to develop at 24 days. By the beginning of the fetal period most of the structure of the respiratory system is established.

Lung development occurs in four principal stages. First, the bronchial or pseudoglandular stage covers approximately the initial eight weeks of fetal life. Growth and subdivision during this period result in the formation of 75 percent of the total final number of bronchial tubules in the developing lung. By the sixteenth week of gestation the structural lung is essentially complete, except for those elements involved with aeration. Second, the respiratory portion begins to form about the sixteenth week. The bronchi and bronchioles enlarge, and the lung becomes highly vascularized. By the twenty-fourth week, the alveolar ducts are lined with a respiratory membrane capable of supporting gas exchange. Third, the terminal sac stage encompasses the period from 24 weeks of gestation to birth. During this period the alveolar ducts give rise to terminal air sacs or alveoli. Fourth, the alveolar stage begins late in gestation and extends into postnatal life. The alveoli increase in number, and further vascularization of the lung tissue occurs. At birth one-eighth to one-sixteenth of the adult number of alveoli is present. The adult number is achieved by the eighth year.

The development of the alveoli is accompanied by the formation of a "surfactant" (**12**). The surfactant is responsible for reducing surface tension forces at the air-fluid interface in the alveoli of the postnatal lung. This reduction of surface tension forces is necessary to maintain air breathing. Surface tension would otherwise increase upon expiration when the alveoli are at their minimum size and cause their collapse. Failure by the fetal lung to produce adequate amounts of surfactant is a predisposing factor in the development of respiratory distress or hyaline membrane disease in the newborn (**13**).

The fetal lung usually matures between the thirty-third and thirty-seventh weeks of gestation (**14**). A 25-week-old fetus, born prematurely, usually dies within a few days because of respiratory problems. But premature infants between 26 and 29 weeks can survive because the central nervous system has matured to a stage at which it can direct rhythmic breathing movements (**15**). Mortality rates are still high, though, and the infant has a better chance of survival if born between 29 and 36 weeks, when more adequate amounts of surfactant are present. Before birth, the respiratory system has no immediate contact with the true environment of the organism and until that time does not function in a respiratory capacity.

DEVELOPMENT OF THE FETAL KIDNEY

Primitive glomeruli and secretory tubules or nephrons (the functional units of the kidney) can be distinguished in the embryo at six weeks and appear to be functional from around the ninth week. An increase in the number of nephrons formed begins at seven to eight weeks of gestation and continues until 32 to 34 weeks. Progressively larger numbers of nephrons are associated with increasing the functional capacity of the developing kidney (**16**). Twenty percent of the nephrons are relatively mature at 11 to 13 weeks of gestation, and 30 percent are mature by 16 to 20 weeks of gestation. The total number of nephrons in each kidney increases from 350,000 at 20 weeks of gestation to 820,000 at 40 weeks. From 100 days of gestation to term the growth of the kidneys forms a higher proportion of body weight than in later life (**17, 18**).

Urine formation begins at ten weeks and continues to increase in volume until term, the fetus passing the urine into the amniotic fluid. This fetal urine is "hypotonic," containing a much lower concentration of sodium, chloride, and urea than the mother's urine that is formed at the same time. Sixteen to forty-four milliliters of urine are present in the bladder at birth (**18**).

Apparently, the role of the fetal kidney in regulating acid-base balance in the fetus is of little importance. The mature kidney is the major route by which excess acid or base is eliminated from the body. In the fetus, however, there is no essential need for the kidney to function in this manner, since short-term adjustment in the acid-base balance can be regulated by the maternal lungs and kidneys by way of the placenta (**18**).

The infant acquires renal processes and regulatory functions of the kidney gradually until it is 2 years old. No new nephrons develop after birth, but the existing nephrons complete their differentiation during infancy and continue to increase in size to adulthood. In the neonate the kidney is also characterized by a low glomerular filtration rate. The normal adult pattern is established in 30 percent of the glomeruli by the fifth month of gestation, and glomeruli continue to increase in diameter from 100 millimeters (mm) at birth to an adult diameter of 200 mm by the twentieth year (**17, 18**).

DEVELOPMENT OF THE FETAL LIVER

The human liver is formed at an early stage of embryonic development, and the major structural elements of the liver can be distinguished in the 31-day-old

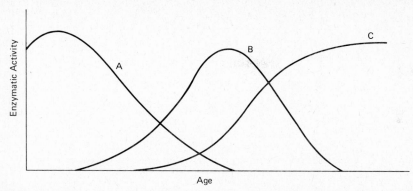

Figure 3.5 *Changes in enzymatic activity during development (A) Enzymes concerned mainly with growth. (B) Enzymes related primarily to functional development. (C) Enzymes concerned with the process of maturation. (Source:* Reproduced with permission from D. Richter, *British Medical Bulletin 17,* 121, 1961. Copyright © 1961 by the British Medical Bulletin, London, England.)

embryo (**19**). The fetal liver at 100 days of gestation weighs 1 g, about 10 percent of the total fetal weight. It increases in weight from that time, following a growth curve similar to that of the body as a whole so that liver weight remains relatively constant as a proportion of body weight. In late pregnancy the relative liver weight of the human fetus is 5.2 g per 100 g of body weight.

During prenatal life, the liver differs from the adult liver in structure and function and in the response it has to environmental factors (**19**). The fetal liver functions in the formation of erythrocytes, or red blood cells, and hemoglobin. Throughout the fetal period, the liver serves to store nutrients such as iron, copper, and zinc.

Essential to growth and cell reproduction, enzymes, whose activity relates specifically to organ function, are active early in fetal life. They increase in activity in late gestation and continue to develop functionally after birth (Figure 3.5). Although many of the morphological characteristics of liver cells are relatively mature during gestation, most enzymes concerned with homeostatic functions of the liver show negligible activity at term.

DEVELOPMENT OF THE FETAL HEART

The human heart differentiates early and the development of the heart as a functional organ is virtually complete by 31 days of gestation. By the sixth week of embryonic life the heart has acquired its characteristic shape (**19, 21**). The heart's size in relation to the embryonal body, however, is nine times that of the adult. During the fetal period the heart grows at a similar rate to the total body, increasing in size by a factor of 100. As a proportion of total body weight, it remains constant from 100 days of gestation to term.

Whereas the composition of the heart changes little during the fetal period (Table 3.3), a decrease in the concentration of potassium and an increase in the concentration of sodium in the heart can be observed between 20 weeks and

TABLE 3.3   COMPOSITION OF FETAL HEART[1]

Constituent	Fetus (20−22 weeks)	Term
Weight of heart (g)	1.6	17
Water (g)	860	841
Total N (g)	14.0	19.6
Nonprotein N[2] (g)	1.5	1.7
Collagen N (g)	0.8	2.0
Cellular protein N, by difference (g)	11.7	15.9
Sodium (mEq)	46.1	64.2
Potassium (mEq)	81.1	54.3
Chlorine (mEq)	41.0	45.2
Phosphorus (mmoles)[3]	49.7	47.0

Source: Reproduced by permission from E. M. Widdowson and J. W. T. Dickerson in *Mineral Metabolism,* Vol. 2, Part A, eds. C. L. Comar and F. Bronner (**22**). Copyright © 1964 by Academic Press Inc., New York.
[1]Per kilogram of fresh fat-free weight.
[2]N = Nitrogen.
[3]Millimoles.

term. This is related to the decrease in interstitial fluid. The heart, thus, acquires a mature chemical composition earlier than does skeletal muscle that does not function until after birth (**22**).

DEVELOPMENT OF THE FETAL BRAIN

The brain develops from the neural plate, and by three weeks of gestation the future brain region has enlarged locally to form the three principal brain components: forebrain, midbrain, and hindbrain (Figure 3.6). Relatively large throughout the fetal period and up to the thirtieth week of gestation, brain weight follows a sigmoid curve. The brain of a full-term newborn infant is one-quarter the weight of the adult brain, compared to a proportion of about one-twentieth for other organs. All neurons are present by seven to eight months. The subsequent fourfold growth of the brain is mainly because of an increase in the number of glial cells, deposition of myelin, elaboration of the dendritic processes, and a considerable increase in the amount of vascular tissue present. The weight of the brain, therefore, and its gross appearance can be used as a reliable indicator of gestational age.

Brain growth in the human seems to be linear prenatally but the rate of growth slows after birth and attains maximum size by 8−12 months (Figure 3.7) (**23**).

The functional development of the human brain has been studied by measuring electroencephalographic (EEG) and reflex activity. This maturation of the brain has been divided into four major phases including (1) neuronal division up to the last trimester; (2) growth of neurons, division and growth of glial cells, and development of dendritic processes during the last trimester; (3) rapid myelination of nerve cells from the sixth month of gestation and continuing to the

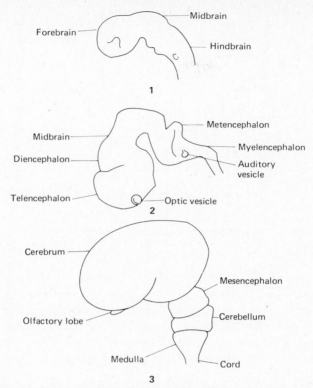

Figure 3.6 *Development of the fetal brain shown by stages: Stage 1, Regions easily seen; 3 weeks of age. Stage 2, at 7 weeks, five major areas are present. Stage 3, at 11 weeks, definite form of the brain has evolved. (Source:* Reproduced with permission from *Growth and Development of Children,* 7th edition, by G. H. Lowrey. Copyright © 1978 by Year Book Medical Publishers, Inc., Chicago [Modified from *Human Embryology,* 3rd edition, by B. M. Patten. McGraw-Hill, New York, 1968.].)

third postnatal month; and (4) slow final completion of myelination and differentiation continuing up to 13–25 years postnatal life.

Early in prenatal life, at around 43 days of gestation, a spontaneous electrical activity can be detected in the human brain. This EEG pattern is essentially one of slow frequency and low voltage until mid-gestation. Signs of maturation in the EEG pattern appear by the seventh to eighth month of gestation. Sleep-wake patterns have been differentiated, and reactivity to auditory and visual stimuli can be detected. The mature EEG pattern is generally established by the thirteenth year. From birth until that time spontaneous electrical activity continues to increase in voltage (**19, 25**).

DEVELOPMENT OF THE FETAL GASTROINTESTINAL TRACT

During fetal life the placenta assumes the function of exchanging nutrients and waste between the developing fetus and its environment. Thus the demands on

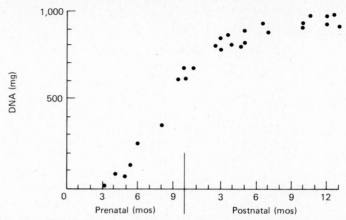

Figure 3.7 *Total DNA content of the human brain determined from fetuses and infants who died from a variety of causes.* (*Source:* Reprinted with permission from M. Winick, *Federation Proceedings 29,*1510–1515, 1970.)

the alimentary tract are minimal and final gastrointestinal development occurs relatively late in the gestational period. The period immediately before birth is one of extensive and rapid differentiation of specialized structures so that the majority of the biochemical and physiological functions of the gastrointestinal system are established by that time. Functions continue to mature during the early neonatal period (**6, 19**).

By the fourth week of embryonic life, the stomach is recognizable and the intestine is visible as a single tube beginning in the stomach. Subdividing into small and large segments, the intestine elongates at a faster rate than the total body and by the sixth week can no longer be contained in the abdomen. It moves into the umbilical cord, where it remains until the tenth week, when it reenters the abdominal cavity. Between the fifth week of gestation and birth, the intestine increases its total length 1000 times, with the length of the small intestine becoming 6 times that of the large one.

The secretory cells of the digestive tract are mature and potentially functional at birth. These are the cells that secrete hormones, mucus, and digestive enzymes. Digestive enzymes, such as the peptidases, maltase, lactase, and sucrase are present early in the fetal system. The transport and absorptive capacity of the intestine is well developed at term (**6**).

At birth, the gastrointestinal system is theoretically capable of digesting solid foods. Tissues associated with the mechanical processes of digestion, however, are limited, and the neonate lacks teeth, and the masticatory muscles are still weak. Since the growth of jaw muscles involved in the sucking and then the chewing process proceeds with general muscle growth after birth, the mechanical functioning level of the infant gastrointestinal system is suited to a predominantly liquid diet. Hormonal and nerve regulation of the gastrointestinal system is also not fully established in the neonatal infant (**6, 19**).

ACCUMULATION OF NUTRIENTS BY THE FETUS

The rate of growth before birth depends primarily on the nutrient supply available to the fetus and on the ability of the fetus to utilize those nutrients. From very early in gestation the placenta responds to insure that all substances needed for growth and development reach the fetus in sufficient amounts and to return nutrient surpluses and waste products to the mother's circulation. Thus the nutrient supply and the growth rate of the fetus throughout gestation involve a close dependence on maternal reserves, maternal diet, and the normal functional capability of the placental-fetal complex (26).

Within three weeks of implantation the beginnings of placental circulation are established, forming an exchange center between the maternal and embryonic blood through a system of two vascular networks: fetal and maternal in intimate contact. Once the placental circulation is fully established at the twelfth week of gestation, all nutrients required by the fetus reach it through its umbilical blood vessels. Nutrients from the maternal blood stream are delivered to the fetus through the two umbilical arteries, and waste products are returned by the umbilical vein. The nutrient supply available to the fetus depends primarily on the quantity of maternal blood reaching the fetus and to a lesser extent on the concentration of nutrients in the maternal plasma.

A wide variety of nutrients in adequate amounts and proper equilibrium are required for maintenance, differentiation, and growth of the fetus. The nutrient requirements of the fetus also vary during the different phases of development. For instance, nutrient requirements for maintenance are smaller than those for differentiation, that in turn are smaller than those for growth. As growth progresses, absolute requirements increase. Quantitative data on minimal nutrient requirements of the fetus during the various stages of growth are limited. Knowledge of such requirements results from studies of the chemical composition of the fetus, levels of nutrients in the maternal blood needed to promote normal fetal growth (Table 3.4), and data collected from the study of nutrient requirements in premature infants. Essentially, information comes from observations of various defects caused by deficiencies in the maternal diet.

TABLE 3.4 CALCULATED REQUIREMENTS OF THE HUMAN FETUS FOR CALCIUM, PHOSPHORUS, AND MAGNESIUM IN TERMS OF THE AMOUNTS IN THE MOTHER'S PLASMA

Constituent	Calcium	Phosphorus	Magnesium
Total amount required by fetus during last three months of gestation (g)	28	16	0.7
Amount required by fetus per hour (mg)	13	7.4	0.32
Total amount of mother's plasma (mg), assuming a volume of 2.5 l	250	75	50
Fetal requirement per hour as a percentage of the amount in mother's plasma	5	10	0.6

Source: Reproduced by permission from E. Widdowson in *Biology of Gestation*, Vol. 2, ed. N. S. Assali (9). Copyright © 1968 by Academic Press Inc., New York.

METABOLISM AND THE USE OF NUTRIENTS

In the mature human, nutrients are made use of through digestion and absorption, and these essential systems are developed in the fetus and during early childhood. The proper functioning of the entire gastrointestinal tract is necessary for the functioning of the other parts of the physiological system. The development of the digestive system seems to be primarily in response to the diet.

Swallowing begins in the fetus between the third and fifth month when amniotic fluid is swallowed (**27**). The movement of this fluid through the stomach and intestines begins early in the fetus. Spontaneous movement of the small intestine, in fact, has been observed as early as six to seven weeks, and peristaltic movements appear at approximately three to five months. After birth the propulsive motility of most of the gastrointestinal tract accelerates with age (**28**). Passage, however, through the large intestine declines with age. The emptying of the large intestine is most rapid in the premature infant, less in the full-term infant, and slows with further growth and development of the infant (**28**). The general sites of absorption of nutrients are shown in Figure 3.8.

Digestion, metabolism, and the use of nutrients are covered in great detail in other readily available books and references. This section does not attempt to provide that information but gives a brief account of those aspects of nutrient metabolism that are unique to the fetus and infant.

Carbohydrate

The plasma concentration of glucose in the fetus is lower than in the mother. Glucose crosses the placenta by facilitated diffusion. Fructose is not transported, although the molecular weight is the same as glucose. Thus there is a specific mechanism for glucose (**30**). Glucose is used at a high rate and seems to be the major source of energy for the fetus. There is an active transport of hexoses during gestation that appears to begin the mature absorption process (**31**). This absorption is influenced by the state of maturity, and glucose absorption is slower in the premature infant than in the full-term baby (**32**).

Glycogen, the storage form of carbohydrate in the body, is formed from glucose in the placenta during the first months of pregnancy and is in a state of continuous exchange between maternal and fetal glucose. During the last trimester the fetus begins to synthesize its own glycogen, and the concentration of carbohydrate rises in the liver and skeletal muscles of the fetus. A high concentration of glycogen is also present in cardiac muscle at term. Fetal glycogen stored in the placenta, liver, and muscle serves as a possible source of fetal glucose. The main sources of glucose during the last trimester, therefore, include maternal blood glucose and maternal and fetal glycogen stores (**33**).

Liver glycogen values begin to rise at the thirty-sixth week of gestation (Figure 3.9), but a rapid fall in liver glycogen occurs during the first 24 hours after birth. The carbohydrate that accumulated in the fetal body is the major food reserve of the infant at birth. The oxidation of carbohydrate provides the calories the body needs during the first hours after birth and before sufficient nutrients are available from milk (**34**).

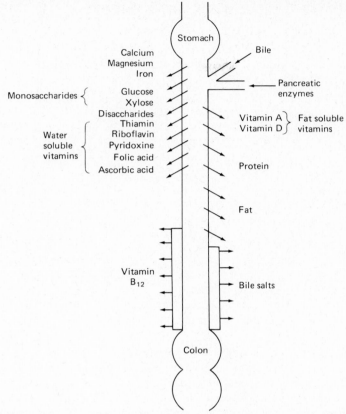

Figure 3.8 *Known sites of absorption in the small intestine.* (*Source:* Reproduced with permission from C. C. Booth in *Handbook of Physiology,* Section 6, Vol. III, ed. C. F. Code. Copyright © 1968 by the American Physiological Society, Bethesda, Md.)

Several disaccharidases that are active in the human appear prenatally. Lactase is found prior to birth and actually is more active at that time. The activity of this enzyme decreases after birth. Lactase is present in higher amounts in the mucosa of the small intestine of the newborn than in the adult (**33**). Animal studies show, in fact, that lactase is active the entire length of the small intestine in early life but exists only in the upper small intestine in the adult. Other disaccharidases, maltase and sucrase, attain maximum activity between six and eight months of gestation. The activity of these enzymes, however, is the same in the newborn as in the adult (**33**).

Lipid

The major site of lipid digestion is the duodenum, and the pancreatic secretion is the source of the lipolytic or fat-splitting enzymes. The rate at which fat enters the small intestine from the stomach seems to be dependent on the capability of lipolytic enzymes from the pancreas to digest this fat.

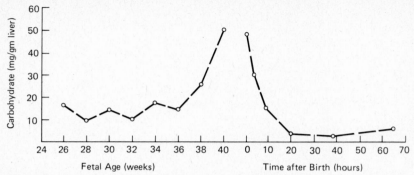

Figure 3.9 *Glycogen in human liver before and after birth.* (*Source:* Reproduced with permission from H. J. Shelley and G. A. Neligan, *British Medical Bulletin, 22,* 34, 1966. Copyright © 1966 by British Medical Bulletin, London, England.)

Pancreatic lipase acts on triglyceride molecules to cleave the 1,3-fatty acids from glycerol, leaving two free fatty acids and a monoglycerol. In the intestinal lumen, micelles are formed under the influence of bile salts. The monoglycerols are trapped by the micelles, and the free fatty acids are dissolved as are cholesterol and the fat-soluble vitamins. This mixture, with the bile salts acting almost as detergents, is brought into contact with the intestinal mucosa (Figure 3.10).

Both pancreatic lipase and bile salts are present in the duodenum shortly after birth. The premature infant, however, exhibits lower concentrations of both than the fully developed infant. Fatty acids, up to 85 percent of the intake, are absorbed well in the fully developed infant, and the infant seems to retain more fat from breast milk than from any other food. Retention of 85 to 90 percent of fat from breast milk is common, compared to a retention of about 70 percent of fat from cow's milk (**37**).

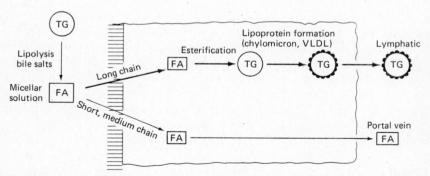

Figure 3.10 *Scheme showing the major steps in lipid intake by the mucosal cell; the metabolism of lipid and its exit into the lymph as chylomicra or short-chain fatty acids.* (*Source:* Reproduced with permission from K. J. Isselbacher and R. M. Glickman in *Transport Across the Intestine,* eds. W. L. Burland and P. M. Samuel. Copyright © 1972 by Churchill Livingstone, Longman Group Ltd., London, England.)

The fetus synthesizes fat from glucose, essential fatty acids, and precursors, such as acetate, that cross the placenta rapidly. In the early stages of gestation the developing organism lays down no fat other than the essential lipids in the nervous system and phospholipids in cell membranes. The human fetus contains only 0.5 percent fat in the body until mid-gestation. Then the rate of fat synthesis increases steadily until term. At 140 days of gestation approximately 6 kcal of energy per day is stored as fat. Near term the rate increases to 100 kcal per day. At 28 weeks of gestation, when the fetus weighs approximately 1.2 kg, the percentage of fat in the fetal body is 3.5 percent. This value increases to 7.5 percent at 34 weeks and a weight of 2.2 kg. At term, with an infant weighing 3.5 kg, 16 percent of the body weight is fat (Figure 3.11). The time during which large amounts of fat are deposited corresponds with the fetus' most rapid growth period. This rapid weight gain is not simply caused by the deposition of fat, however. It is also the result of an accelerated gain in lean body tissue (**9**).

Lipids are stored in the adult and to a lesser extent, in the fetus in the form of triglycerides in the adipose tissue. This storage provides a readily available source of energy, primarily in the form of free fatty acids. During its early growth, the fetus' energy needs are derived almost exclusively from glucose. The continuous supply of glucose to the fetus, however, exceeds the immediate needs for energy, and the excess is stored as triglycerides in the adipose tissue. This adipose tissue develops during the latter part of pregnancy and apparently serves the same purpose in the adult (**38**).

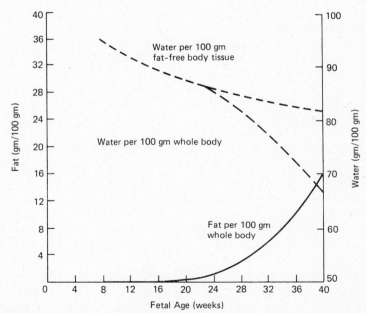

Figure 3.11 *Percentage of water and fat in the human fetus in relation to fetal age.* (*Source:* Reproduced with permission from E. M. Widdowson in *Biology of Gestation,* Vol. 2, ed. N. S. Assali. Copyright © 1968 by Academic Press, New York.)

In the newborn infant, triglycerides are hydrolyzed and fatty acids are mobilized as a source of energy. This occasions a rapid rise in the concentration of free fatty acids, ketones, and glycerol in the blood and a rapid drop in the respiratory quotient (RQ) (**39**). These events indicate a shift from carbohydrate as the major source of energy to that of fat. The body fat of the newborn, thus, is the major source of energy until a normal feeding pattern is established. Soon after birth the incorporation of fatty acids into triglycerides decreases. The human fetus seems capable of oxidizing fatty acids but likely does not, except in cases of chronic placental insufficiency (**40**). The accumulation of fat as an energy source, though, serves a real purpose during the initial days after birth.

Types of Adipose Tissue

Two distinct types of adipose tissue form in the fetus. One is normal white adipose tissue that is responsible for the storage and release of lipids. The second type, brown adipose tissue, functions as it does in other mammals, but data are not available about the development of brown adipose tissue in the human. Brown adipose tissue's presence is demonstrated morphologically and by skin temperature measurements, and the tissue disappears gradually after birth. This brown adipose tissue is related to heat production and serves to maintain body temperature, warming the blood on its route to the brain and heart (**41**). The maintenance of body temperature in the early phase of newborn life by the use of brown adipose tissue is referred to as the mechanism of "nonshivering thermogenesis."

Protein and Amino Acids

Proteins are very large and complicated structures that must be degraded to component units for use by the body. This degradation occurs as a result of proteolytic activity in the stomach and small intestine of the human, appearing as early as the sixteenth week of the gestation period. Digestion of protein in the fetus and infant during this early postnatal period seems to be confined to the duodenum. The digestion of protein is minimal in the stomach of the young infant. (**37**).

Amino acids, the products of the digestion process, are absorbed rapidly. The young mammal does absorb intact proteins. This mechanism ceases as the infant begins to ingest food and is absent generally in the adult. Absorbing intact protein serves the useful purpose of allowing the infant to obtain antibodies and passive immunity from the mother (**42**). The ingestion of milk protein causes the intestinal mucosa to lose its capacity to absorb intact protein, but by this time, the gamma globulin concentration in the young is equal to adult levels.

Protein deposition is most rapid in the fetus before it achieves a body weight of 1 kg, with the maximum protein deposition rate occurring between approximately 220 and 260 days of gestation. At this time 8 g per day are deposited. From this point the rate of deposition declines slowly. At eight weeks of fetal age the proportion of nitrogen in the fat-free tissue is 0.8 percent. This percentage increases continuously to term when the value reaches 2.4 percent of fat-free body tissue (Figure 3.12), approximately two-thirds the nitrogen value in the fat-free tissue of the adult human (**22**).

The distribution of nitrogen in the body of the fetus is different from that occurring later in the adult body. Normal growth during the last half of gestation and early postnatal life reveals specific patterns of amino acids at different times for each tissue and organ.

Vitamin Absorption

The water-soluble vitamins, with the exception of vitamin B_{12}, are readily absorbed by the body. This absorption mechanism has been generally assumed to be simple diffusion, but it is now being seen that an active transport mechanism is involved with these essential nutrients.

The fat-soluble vitamins are absorbed by specific mechanisms, many of which are still under study. Absorption of these vitamins, though, is usually associated with the transport of lipids.

Mineral Absorption

Absorption of the inorganic nutrients is controlled by many different physiological states. This absorption does not occur by a simple process; both rate and degree are influenced by specific carriers and controls. Research in this area, particularly

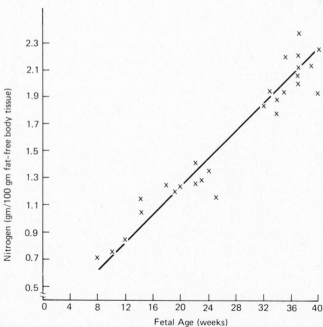

Figure 3.12 Concentration of nitrogen in the fat-free tissue of the fetus. (*Source:* Reproduced with permission from E. M. Widdowson in *Biology of Gestation,* Vol. 2, ed. N. S. Assali. Copyright © 1968 by Academic Press, New York.)

for calcium and iron, has been active in recent years, and attention is now being focused on certain of the trace elements, such as zinc and copper.

NUTRIENT TRANSPORT

As they are transferred across the intestinal wall, nutrients and other materials become available for use by the body. The blood plasma serves as the transportation medium for these nutrients, permitting their movement to the cells and also the removal of waste or excretory products from the cell. A continuous interchange exists between the plasma and cells to maintain homeostasis and the continued well-being of the entire physiological system. The entire cycle from the ingestion of food to the excretion of metabolic products is outlined in Figure 3.13.

HORMONAL DEVELOPMENT AND CONTROL

Hormones, although produced in very minute amounts by various endocrine glands, regulate most of the physiological activities in the body (**44**). This hormonal stimulation and release is controlled in a hierarchical manner (Figure 3.14). The hypothalamus located at the base of the brain receives a neural input and releases a small quantity of specific releasing factors. These factors then function through the anterior pituitary to trigger the release of a specific hormone. The hormones pass through the blood to specific target glands and those glands then produce characteristic hormones to act on final target tissues. Certain

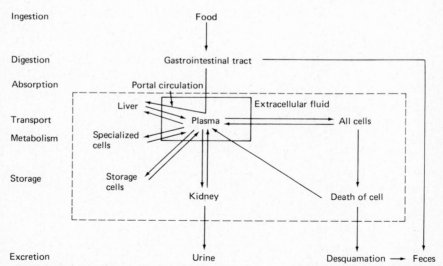

Figure 3.13 *The pathways through which the nutrients in food become available and are transported to the individual cells. (Source: Reproduced with permission from Nutrition: An Integrated Approach, 2nd edition, by R. L. Pike and M. L. Brown. Copyright © 1975 by John Wiley & Sons, Inc., New York.)*

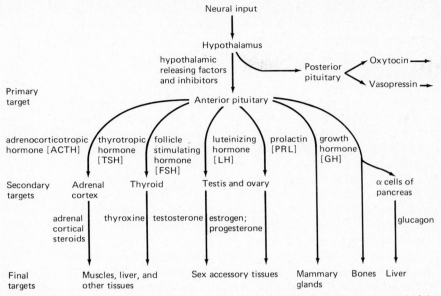

Figure 3.14 *The hierarchical organization of endocrine regulation under the control of the hypothalamus. (Source:* Reproduced with permission from *Biochemistry,* 2nd edition, by A. L. Lehninger. Copyright © 1975 by Worth Publishers, Inc., New York.)

hormones are under less control by the pituitary, including calcitonin, parathyroid hormone, insulin, glucagon, epinephrine and norepinephrine.

In the adult, hormones may act by (1) transferring information from one cell to another, (2) limiting the concentration of metabolites or nutrients, and (3) through feedback controls.

Although metabolic processes within the physiological system are under hormonal control, the role of hormones in the development of the enzymatic system is questionable. There is also evidence that at certain stages of development some organs respond differently to hormones than during adult life.

The processes of cellular development and hormonal control may have a common function, since each may cause the production of specific enzymes. Hormones can regulate cellular activities by altering the permeability of the cell membrane or the membranes around subcellular parts. The concentrations of substrates may be altered through this action, and the patterns of metabolism can be changed in the cell. In addition, hormones may cause protein molecules to attain enzymatic activity by changing the conformation of the molecule.

Certain enzymes that are present in low concentrations during fetal development rise markedly soon after birth. Some enzymes change in response to food intake; others change in response to specific substrates, and others appear to increase activity in simple response to the new environment.

Studying the significant influence and control of hormones is exhaustive in itself and far beyond the intent of this text. The effects and influences of specific hormones appear in other sections of this book, but those sections focus on the nutrition and development of the human rather than on the more fundamental aspects of endocrinology.

SUMMARY

Many physiological, morphological, and biochemical developments occur during the fetal period that allow the infant to function as a distinct and independent entity at the moment of birth. Such development is influenced by various environmental and hereditary factors, nutrition being a major environmental influence affecting the entire process of early growth and development.

Cellular growth of each organ and tissue in the body is the result of hyperplasia or an increase in cell number and hypertrophy, an increase in cell size. Cellular growth patterns, differentiation, and maturation differ in individual organs and tissues, depending on the stage of development in both the fetal and newborn organism.

The embryonic respiratory system begins to develop at twenty-four days, and the fetal lung generally matures between the thirty-third and thirty-seventh weeks of gestation. The respiratory system does not come into contact with the true air environment of the infant until birth and does not function in a respiratory capacity until that time.

A primitive kidney can be distinguished in the embryo at the sixth week of development, and renal structure and regulatory functions are gradually acquired from that time until 2 years of age. The major structural elements of the embryonic liver can be observed at 31 days. The fetal liver differs from the adult liver in structure, function, and response to environmental factors. The human heart differentiates very early and as a functional organ is virtually complete by 31 days of gestation. Brain growth in the human begins in the embryo and continues until 13–25 years postnatal life. The demands on the alimentary tract of the fetus are minimal, and final gastrointestinal development occurs relatively late in the gestational period.

The rate of development in the fetus depends primarily on the nutrient supply available to the fetus and its ability to use that supply. The maintenance, differentiation, and growth of the fetus, therefore, require a wide variety of nutrients in adequate amounts and proper equilibrium. These requirements vary with the stage of development. The fetal nutrient supply and, therefore, normal growth and development involve a close dependence on maternal reserves, maternal diet, and the normal functional capability of the placental-fetal complex.

STUDY QUESTIONS AND
TOPICS FOR INDIVIDUAL INVESTIGATION

1. Tissues and organs progress toward final physiological maturity at different rates during gestation and in the years after birth. Trace and compare the changes in several organs or tissues (for example, the liver, heart, and intestine). Discuss both cellular and functional changes from conception to maturity.
2. The maturation of each system is influenced by environmental and hereditary factors. Choose one tissue or organ (for example, the intestine, kidney, and lung). Discuss the functional maturation in terms of the fetal and infant demands or requirements, nature of the immediate physical environment, and adequacy of the nutrient supply.
3. Discuss energy requirements in the fetus and newborn infant. How does fetal development progress to meet those requirements? The discussion should include nutrient deposition, storage, and metabolism in the fetus and newborn infant.
4. Certain enzymes that are present in low concentrations during fetal development rise markedly soon after birth (for example, pancreatic lipase). Others are present in higher concentrations and are more active prior to birth, with the amount and activity decreasing from the moment of birth until adulthood (for example, lactase). Enzyme activity changes in response to changes in the environment, including nutrient intake. A detailed discussion of enzyme development is beyond the scope of this chapter, but you may be interested in pursuing further the changes that do occur in fetal and newborn enzymatic development in response to changes in the nutritional environment.

REFERENCES

1. Winick, M., J. A. Brasel, and P. Rosso. Nutrition and cell growth. In: *Nutrition and Development,* ed. M. Winick. Wiley, New York, 1972.
2. Enesco, M., and C. P. Leblond. Increase in cell number as a factor in the growth of the organs and tissues of the young male rat. *Journal of Embryology and Experimental Morphology,* 10:530, 1962.
3. Winick, M., and A. Noble. Quantitative changes in DNA, RNA and protein during prenatal and postnatal growth in the rat. *Development Biology,* 12:451, 1965.
4. Cheek, D. M. *Fetal and Postnatal Cellular Growth.* Wiley, New York, 1975.
5. Arey, L. B. *Developmental Anatomy: A Textbook and Laboratory Manual of Embryology,* 5th ed. Saunders, Philadelphia, 1947.

6. Lowrey, G. H. *Growth and Development of Children,* 6th ed. Year Book Medical Publishers, Chicago, 1973.
7. Scammon, R. E., and L. A. Calkins. *The Development and Growth of the External Dimensions of the Human Body in the Fetal Period.* University of Minnesota Press, Minneapolis, 1929.
8. Thompson, D. A. W. *On Growth and Form,* 2nd ed. Cambridge University Press, New York, 1942.
9. Widdowson, E. M. Growth and Composition of the fetus and newborn. In: *Biology of Gestation,* Vol. 2, ed. N. S. Assali. Academic Press, New York, 1968.
10. Timiras, P. S., and T. Valcana. Body growth. In: *Developmental Physiology and Aging,* ed. P. S. Timiras. Macmillan, New York, 1972.
11. Towers, B. The fetal and neonatal lung. In: *Biology of Gestation,* Vol. 2, ed. N. S. Assali. Academic Press, New York, 1968.
12. Clements, J. A., J. Nellenbogen, and H. J. Trahan. Pulmonary surfactant and evolution of the lungs. *Science,* 169:603, 1970.
13. Avery, M. E., and J. Mead. Surface properties in relation to atelectasis and hyaline membrane disease. *American Journal of Diseases of Children,* 97:517, 1959.
14. Boyden, E. Development of the human lung. In: *Practice of Pediatrics,* Vol. 4, ed. J. Brennemann. W. F. Prior Co., Hagerstown, Md., 1971.
15. Boyden, E. The pattern of terminal air-spaces in a premature infant of 30 to 32 weeks that lived nineteen and a quarter hours. *American Journal of Anatomy,* 126:31, 1969.
16. Vernier, R. L., and A. Birch-Anderson. Studies of the human fetal kidney. I. Development of the glomerulus. *Journal of Pediatrics,* 60:754, 1962.
17. Valcana, T. Development of kidney function. In: *Developmental Physiology and Aging,* ed. P. S. Timiras. New York, 1972.
18. Vernier, R. L., and F. G. Smith, Jr. Fetal and neonatal kidney. In: *Biology of Gestation,* Vol. 2, ed. N. S. Assali. Academic Press, New York, 1968.
19. Timiras, P. S. *Developmental Physiology and Aging.* Macmillan, New York, 1972.
20. Richter, D. Enzymatic activity during early development. *British Medical Bulletin,* 17:121, 1961.
21. Assali, N. S., G. A. Bekey, and L. W. Morrison. Fetal and neonatal circulation. In: *Biology of Gestation,* Vol. 2, ed. N. S. Assali. Academic Press, New York, 1968.
22. Widdowson, E. M., and J. W. T. Dickerson. Chemical composition of the body. In: *Mineral Metabolism, An Advanced Treatise,* eds. C. L. Comar and F. Bronner. Academic Press, New York, 1964.
23. Patten, B. M. *Human Embryology.* Blakiston, Philadelphia, 1946.
24. Winick, M. Nutrition and nerve cell growth. *Federation Proceedings,* 29:1510, 1970.
25. Timiras, P. S., A. Vernadakis, and N. M. Sherwood. Development and plasticity of the nervous system. In: *Biology of Gestation,* Vol. 2, ed. N. S. Assali. Academic Press, New York, 1968.

26. Committee on Maternal Nutrition/Food and Nutrition Board. Maternal nutrition and the course of pregnancy. National Academy of Sciences, Washington, D.C., 1970.

27. Mistilis, S. D., and P. Mearrick. Absorption and excretion of radio copper in neonatal rats: A model for study of Wilson's disease. *Gastroenterology,* 58:286, 1970.

28. Smith, C. A. *The Physiology of the Newborn Infant,* 2nd ed. Thomas, Springfield, Ill., 1953.

29. Booth, C. C. *Handbook of Physiology,* Vol. 3. American Physiological Society, Washington, D.C., 1968.

30. Widdas, W. F. Inability of diffusion to account for placental glucose transfer in the sheep and consideration of the kinetics of a possible carrier transfer. *Journal of Physiology,* 118:23, 1952.

31. Jacobson, E. D. The circulation of the stomach. *Gastroenterology,* 48:85, 1965.

32. Borgstrom, B., B. Lindquist, and G. Lundh. Enzymes concentration and absorption of protein and glucose in duodenum of premature infants. *American Journal of the Diseases of Children,* 99:338, 1960.

33. Auricchio, S., A. Rubino, and G. Murcot. Intestinal glycosidase activities in the human embryo, fetus and newborn. *Pediatrics,* 35:944, 1965.

34. Shelley, H. J. Glycogen reserves and their changes at birth and in anoxia. *British Medical Bulletin,* 17:137, 1961.

35. Shelley, H. J., and G. A. Neligan. Neonatal hypoglycemia. *British Medical Bulletin,* 22:34, 1966.

36. Isselbacher, K. J., and R. M. Glickman. *Transport Across the Intestine,* eds. W. L. Burland, and P. D. Samuel. Churchill Livingstone, Edinburgh and London, 1972.

37. Koldovsky, O. Hormonal and dietary factors in the development of digestion and absorption. In: *Nutrition and Development,* ed. M. Winick. Wiley, New York, 1972.

38. Van Duyne, C. M., and R. J. Havel. Plasma unesterified fatty acid concentration in fetal and neonatal life. *Proceedings, Society for Experimental Biology and Medicine,* 102:599, 1959.

39. Van Duyne, C. M. Free fatty acid metabolism during perinatal life. *Biology of the Neonate,* 9:115, 1965.

40. Harding, P. G. R. Chronic placental insufficiency; an experimental model. *American Journal of Obstetrics and Gynecology,* 106:857, 1970.

41. Dawkins, M. J. R., and D. Hull. Brown adipose tissue and the response of newborn rabbits to cold. *Journal of Physiology (London),* 172:216, 1964.

42. Branbell, F. W. R. *The Transition of Passive Immunity from Mother to Young.* Elsevier, New York, 1970.

43. Pike, R. L., and M. L. Brown. *Nutrition: An Integrated Approach,* 2nd ed. Wiley, New York, 1975.

44. Jonxix, J. H. P., H. K. A. Visser, and J. A. Troelstra. *Metabolic Processes in the Fetus and Newborn Infant.* Williams and Wilkins, Baltimore, Md., 1971.

45. Lehninger, A. L. *Biochemistry,* 2nd ed. Worth Publishers, New York, 1975.

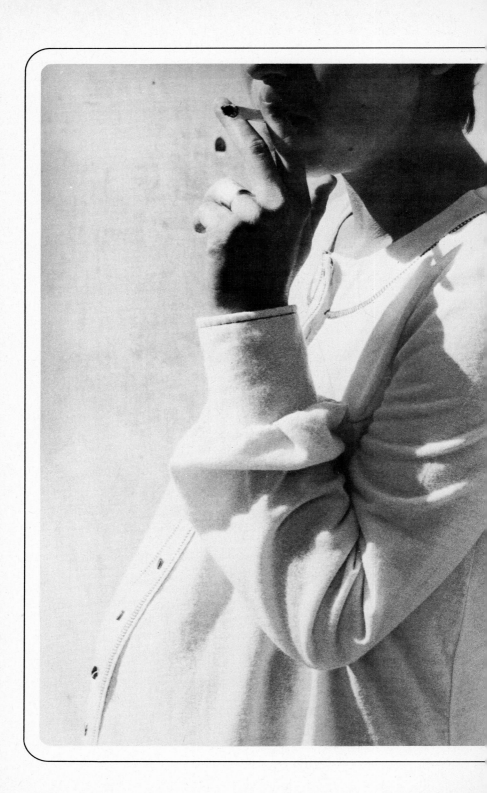

CHAPTER 4

NUTRITIONAL COMPLICATIONS OF PREGNANCY

The importance of maternal nutrition before and during pregnancy has been stressed because it influences not only the immediate outcome of pregnancy but also affects the child's lifelong physical and mental development. A major development in the field of nutrition within the past few years has been the demonstration that malnutrition during prenatal life may retard physical and mental development and lead to the permanent stunting of physical stature and mental capacity.

Growth of the normal human fetus is regulated by the interaction of numerous factors: genetic and metabolic potential of the fetus; placental size and function; and various maternal factors, including nutrition. Nutritional disturbances can and do influence all stages of prenatal growth and development. The majority of stillbirths, premature births, neonatal deaths, low birth weights, functional limitations, and congenital defects occur among infants born to mothers with poor to very poor prenatal diets that are representative of long-term poor eating habits (**1**). Considerable speculation exists about how maternal nutritional deprivation influences fetal growth (**2**), but the present methods of assessment are not adequate to answer all the questions raised. It is known that improving the maternal diet at any point in pregnancy increases the infant's chances for survival during the fetal stage and for a healthy life after birth (**3**). The ideal situation, though, is for the mother to maintain an excellent nutritional status from her own birth throughout life. The unfavorable outcome of some pregnancies can thus be reduced through the establishment of effective programs for nutritional counseling and food supplementation for pregnant women. These programs will enable the mother to provide her unborn child with the uterine environment most conducive to healthy growth (**1, 4**). This chapter reviews the subject of malnutrition and fetal development, emphasizing the influence of maternal diet and nutritional status.

MALNUTRITION AND PHYSICAL GROWTH

Fetal malnutrition implies a reduction in the nutrient supply from the mother of enough magnitude and duration to retard fetal growth significantly below its full genetic potential. Fetal malnutrition is characterized by small body size for gestational age as well as other biochemical and pathophysiological features associated with undernutrition.

The failure of an infant to thrive *in utero* is related to several factors, including biological immaturity of the mother, low prepregnancy weight for height, low total weight gain during pregnancy, infection, and poor nutritional status of the mother prior to and during pregnancy. The relative role played by any single factor is difficult to assess. However, many reports show that a major contributing factor in fetal malnutrition is poor nutrition by the mother before and during pregnancy (**1, 2**). Malnutrition, particularly in the United States, has only recently become a matter of widespread public concern. Even with an abundant and varied food supply, malnutrition (among all socioeconomic levels) does exist in this country. These nutritional needs are greatest and most specific during fetal development. The fetus cannot, as does a parasite, extract all its nutritional needs from the maternal stores and is not necessarily completely protected in the presence of poor maternal nutritional health (**5**). A restriction of the maternal diet, therefore, can and often does affect the growth and development of the fetus and young baby.

Wartime experiences prove that nutrition can indeed have an effect on the outcome of pregnancy. Comparable studies were made on the outcome of pregnancies during the siege of Leningrad in 1941–1943 (**6**) and a period of semistarvation in Holland during the winter of 1944–1945 (**7**). In Leningrad, an 18-month period of starvation was reflected in a doubled fetal mortality rate and a decrease in the average birth weight. Prematurity increased to 41 percent of total live births, and 9 percent of the full-term and 31 percent of the premature infants died in the neonatal period. Infants conceived before and born during a seven-month time of semistarvation in Holland weighed, on the average, 10 percent less than infants born previously.

The effects on the fetus of a poor maternal diet depend on the length of time the mother was deprived before conception, the extent of the mother's deprivation during pregnancy, and the time during gestation when deprivation was most severe. In Holland the period of semistarvation followed a time of regulated but adequate food supply. Therefore, Dutch mothers were well nourished at the onset of their time of malnutrition. The duration of the reduced food supply was relatively short, compared to the episode in Leningrad, where long-term chronic malnutrition was followed by severe undernutrition. The reproductive capability of women in Leningrad was more dramatically affected by starvation, too, than was that of the women in Holland.

Studies in several human population groups support the benefits attributed to good maternal nurture during pregnancy (**1, 4**). These reports show that nutritional intervention, when necessary, during pregnancy can have a significant influence on the subsequent growth and development of the infant. Nutritional counseling and food supplements for women in poor nutritional condition usually result in an increase in birth weight and a decrease in the mortality rate among babies (**3, 4**).

Birth weight traditionally has been used as an index of the quality of fetal development and the status of the infant at birth (**8**). The slowing down of growth (and consequent lowering of birth weight) is one of the most frequent results of nutritional disturbances (**9**). Infants are classified as having low birth weight if they weigh 2500 g (5.5 lbs) or less at birth. This low birth weight is associated with increased neonatal mortality rates, birth defects, impaired learning ability, short stature, and other problems of growth and development (**10, 11**). One-third of all deaths in the first year of life are related to low birth weight. Fifty percent of these occur within the first 24 hours of life, and 80 percent occur within the first month. Recent investigations of low birth-weight infants distinguished between those who are premature, born before the thirty-seventh week of gestation and those who have suffered intrauterine growth retardation. The latter are full-term infants but small for their gestational age. These infants are referred to as "small for term." The potential hazards of the two conditions differ. Intrauterine growth-retarded infants show patterns similar to those of the full-term infant in liver, renal, pulmonary, and central nervous system functions. However, such infants are at risk from birth for increased mortality, greater postnatal complication, and a higher incidence of mental-motor retardation at a later age. Table 4.1 compares the perinatal and neonatal mortality rates of small-for-term infants with those for normal-size age peers and prematurely born size peers. The perinatal mortality rate of small-for-term infants is approximately 10−20 times that of the normal-weight, full-term infants but only two-thirds that of the preterm-weight peers. Neonatal mortality is 10 times that of full-size, full-term infants and less than one-half that of the preterm, similar-weight infants.

Some anatomic features of intrauterine growth retardation are listed in Table 4.2.

Does a reduction in size affect body composition, metabolic pathways, and ultimate functional ability in the intrauterine growth-retarded infant? Data on birth weight for gestational age alone do not give adequate information on the effect of malnutrition on fetal development during the prenatal period. Examinations of cell number, cell size, and body composition contribute to a better understanding of a newborn's degree of maturity.

As discussed in Chapter 3, each organ and tissue develops according to a specific time pattern, and different structures grow at different rates within individual organs. The effect of a nutritional insult on organ and tissue growth is

TABLE 4.1 PERINATAL AND NEONATAL
MORTALITY IN FETAL GROWTH RETARDATION

	Birth weight (kg)	Gestational age (weeks)	Mortality per 1000 births
Perinatal mortality:			
Behrman et al., 1971	2.00–2.25	34	125
	2.00–2.25	40	84.7
	3.00–3.50	40	4.5
Yerushalmy, 1970	2.00–2.25	34	98.3
	2.00–2.25	40	64.9
	3.00–3.50	40	5.6
Neonatal mortality:			
Behrman et al., 1971	2.00–2.25	34	87
	2.00–2.25	40	35.7
	3.00–3.50	40	2.8
Battaglia et al., 1966	2.00–2.50	34	59.8
	2.00–2.50	40	28.1
	3.00–3.50	40	3.9

Source: Reprinted with permission from J. C. Sinclair, S. Saigal, and C. Y. Yeung in *Nutrition and Fetal Development,* ed. M. Winick (**12**). Copyright © 1974 by John Wiley & Sons, Inc., New York.

TABLE 4.2 FETAL GROWTH RETARDATION–ANATOMIC FEATURES

Finding

Placenta

Weight low or normal for age[1]
Weight variable for fetal weight[2]
Decidual area–cord diameter low for age
Chorionic villous surface area low for age but variable for fetal weight

Baby

Body weight low for age
Body length and head circumference low but variable for age
Ponderal index variable for age
Organ weights variable; reduced for age
    Brain and heart reduced least
    Liver and thymus reduced most
Brain and liver weight ratio increased for body weight
Cell size in various organs reduced for age
Organ differentiation accelerated for weight (e.g., lung and kidney)
DNA composition of various organs low for age

Source: Reprinted with permission from J. C. Sinclair, S. Saigal, and C. Y. Yeung in *Nutrition and Fetal Development,* ed. M. Winick (**12**). Copyright © 1974 by John Wiley & Sons, Inc., New York.
[1]"For age" means as compared with normally grown infants of same gestational age.
[2]"For weight" means as compared with normally grown infants of same body weight (who would therefore be of shorter gestation).

determined by the severity, duration, and stage in the life cycle at which it occurs and by the specific nutrients missing from or lacking in the diet. The biochemical and cellular response of infants who were malnourished *in utero* has been studied (**13, 14**) and virtually all this research indicates that most, if not all, fetal organs are affected by maternal undernutrition. The thymus, spleen, liver, and adrenal glands appear more drastically affected than the kidneys, heart, skeleton, and brain. Both cell size and cell number appear to be reduced in fetal growth retardation. It is not known to what extent this reduction in cell number and size impairs cellular metabolism and function.

Up to 50 percent of the fetally malnourished infants who survive are estimated to have congenital abnormalities (**15**), an indeterminate number suffering from permanent physical, neurological, or mental defects. A major complication in the intrauterine growth-retarded infant is the development of an abnormally low blood sugar level or hypoglycemia. The full-term infant of normal birth weight has large stores of liver glycogen permitting the maintenance of normal blood sugar levels for relatively long periods following birth. Markedly depleted glycogen stores in the intrauterine growth-retarded infant at birth, however, can result in the development of extremely low blood sugar levels soon after birth. Neonatal hypoglycemia limits the availability of glucose for cerebral metabolism and may result in brain damage to some low birth-weight infants during the first few days of life. Therefore, injections of glucose at birth are becoming common procedure for newborns identified as intrauterine growth retarded.

The total serum protein and serum albumin levels are low for gestational age in infants suffering from intrauterine growth retardation. Serum immunoglobulin G levels at birth are also lower than normal in these infants, and this may be an important predisposing factor to infection.

Do low birth-weight infants ultimately reach their inherited potential height? This question cannot be answered since knowledge about the physical growth of low birth-weight infants is incomplete. The child's mature height, however, does not seem to be influenced by a moderate degree of fetal malnutrition. There is some evidence, though, that with a birth weight of 2000 g or less some degree of retardation in physical size persists into adulthood (**16**). There may, therefore, be a birth weight below which normal development postnatally is not possible because of an irreversible cellular deficit caused by malnutrition *in utero*.

The National Center for Health Statistics reported that the infant mortality rate in the United States for 1976 was 15.1 per 1000 births (**17**). This figure is lower than the 1975 rate of 16.1 per 1000 and the lowest ever recorded in the United States. It is higher, however, than that recorded in many other industrialized nations. In 1976 the United States ranked nineteenth in a list of 20 countries with the lowest infant mortality rates (**18**). Low birth-weight infants contribute significantly to this relatively high infant mortality rate.

The Apgar scoring system is a useful aid in evaluating the probability of the survival or death of an infant. This system, introduced in 1953 (**19**) and evaluated

TABLE 4.3 ACRONYM OF THE APGAR SCORE[1]

Sign	Score		
	0	1	2
Appearance	Blue, pale	Body pink; arms and legs blue	Completely pink
Pulse (heart rate)	Absent	Below 100	Above 100
Grimace (reflex irritability or response to stimulation of sole of foot by glancing slap)	No response	Grimace	Cry
Activity (muscle tone)	Limp	Some flexion of extremities	Active motion
Respiration (respiratory effort)	Absent	Slow; irregular	Good, strong cry

Source: Reprinted with permission from L. J. Butterfield and M. J. Covey, *Journal of the American Medical Association, 181:*353, 1962 (**21**). Copyright © 1962 by the American Medical Association, Chicago.

[1]Evaluated 60 seconds after complete birth. Each sign is scored and scores totaled. Sum of 10 indicates best condition; babies scoring in range of 4–6 usually require some form of resuscitator. Most babies are vigorous and score in range from 7 to 10.

in 1962 (**20**), is based on several factors that are measured immediately after the birth of the child (Table 4.3).

MALNUTRITION AND BRAIN DEVELOPMENT

The concept that malnutrition during critical periods of brain development can cause irreversible damage is relatively new, and very little research exists regarding the effect of fetal growth retardation on the mental development of the human. There is a great deal of concern, though, that retardation in overall physical growth *in utero* may be paralleled by a retardation in mental development and that these cannot be repaired postnatally (**22, 23**).

Three percent of children born in the United States do not achieve the intellect of a 12-year-old child. Many of these are low birth-weight infants, and it is estimated that in addition to physical retardation, approximately one percent is affected with defects of intellect and neuromuscular disturbances that may be related to the fetal environment (**24, 25**).

The results of both animal experiments and human studies show that a critical period of brain growth exists during which malnutrition may produce irreversible damage (**26–30**) even when present in a mild form and for a short duration. As pointed out in Chapter 3, nutritional deprivation can result in fewer cell numbers in a specific organ, smaller cell sizes, or a reduction in cell size, depending on the timing and extent of the deprivation (**31**).

In humans, the critical period for the growth and development of the brain and other components of the central nervous system appears to begin during the last months of intrauterine life and extends into the early postnatal years (**32**). At birth the brain adds weight at a rapid rate, increasing from 25 percent of its adult weight at birth to 70 percent in one year. Growth then continues more slowly until final size is achieved. Therefore, in the human the period of vulnerability of the brain extends from the prenatal period, beyond the first year of life, and into the preschool years.

Few studies exist on the effect of malnutrition on the cellular growth of the human brain, since much of our present data was derived from animal studies and uncontrolled postnatal human studies. Indirect evidence does show that cell division in the brain of the human fetus may be retarded by maternal undernutrition (**33**). Three separate patterns of cell growth have been observed in the brains of infants who died of malnutrition in the postnatal period (Figure 4.1). Infants suffering from "marasmus" (severe protein-calorie malnutrition during the first year of life) showed a reduction in the total brain cell number when compared to normal, well nourished infants who had died accidentally (**34**). The marasmic infants with normal birth weights showed a 15–20 percent reduction in the number of brain cells. Brain cell number, however, was reduced 66 percent in those marasmic infants who weighed less than 2000 g at birth. The data suggest that the low birth-weight infant is more susceptible to the effects of neonatal malnutrition than is the normal weight infant or that a significant amount of malnutrition has already occurred *in utero*. Children who died from "kwashiorkor" (severe protein malnutrition) during the second or third year of life showed a normal brain cell number but a reduction in cell size. Other studies comparing the biochemistry of brain development in low birth-weight infants with that in infants of appropriate weight for gestational age show a reduction in cell size in the

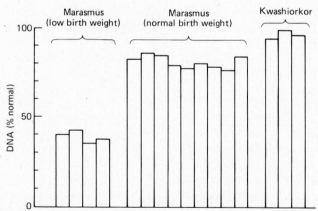

Figure 4.1 *Human-brain DNA after different types of malnutrition. The DNA content is expressed as a percentage of normal human-brain DNA in age-matched controls: each bar represents one patient. Kwashiorkor is seen to have essentially no effect on brain DNA. Infants dying of marasmus who had a normal birth weight demonstrate a 15 to 20 percent reduction in DNA content. Infants dying of marasmus who weighed less than 2000 g at birth demonstrate a 60 percent reduction in DNA content. (Source:* Reprinted with permission from M. Winick, *Federation Proceedings 29,*1510–1515, 1970.)

cerebrum and brain stem and a reduction in cerebellar cell number in low birth-weight infants (**35**).

Some studies show that low birth-weight infants develop cognitive and psychomotor skills at a slower than normal rate (**24, 25**). It is premature to conclude, though, that the observed delay in the development is due to a decrease in brain cell number as a result of intrauterine malnutrition (**24**). Malnutrition can be implicated as a cause of mental deficiency, but it is difficult to isolate malnutrition as the sole cause (**36**−**39**). Low birth-weight infants tend to belong to a lower socioeconomic group and not only suffer lack of good nutrition but also have poor housing conditions, poor educational facilities, poor health care, and many other problems, all of which may affect intellectual performance.

Recent studies in which previously malnourished children were rehabilitated indicate that both nutrition and environmental stimulation were important in the long-term development of the child. Nutritional rehabilitation of Korean children raised their heights and weights to the expected norm or above (**40**). When placed in middle-class American homes, these children were stimulated environmentally to such a degree that their intelligent quotient (IQ) was raised 40 points above children who were rehabilitated nutritionally but not environmentally. Investigators in another study reported that improvements in nutrition increased the activity of the child and in turn enhanced mother-child interaction and modified the child's behavior (**41**). Therefore, it seems convincing that rehabilitation programs for malnourished children should include medical, nutritional, and educational components (**42**).

THE ANEMIAS OF PREGNANCY

Anemia is the most commonly recognized nutrition-related complication of pregnancy in the United States (**18**). Nutritional anemia is characterized by a lower than normal hemoglobin concentration resulting from a deficiency of one or more essential nutrients, including iron, folic acid, vitamin B_{12}, and protein.

Iron

Estimates are that 95 percent of all anemias in pregnancy are caused by iron deficiency (**43**). A relatively large increase in blood volume accompanies pregnancy, along with increasing needs for iron. The total amount of available iron necessary for fetal demands and extra hemoglobin mass during a single pregnancy is at least 800 mg and must be supplied from dietary intake and/or liver, spleen, and bone marrow stores. The magnitude of iron stores determines the ability to cope with increased iron requirements during pregnancy. Normal levels of storage iron of 1000 mg would supply sufficient iron to meet all the requirements of pregnancy and maintain normal hemoglobin concentration. Research, however, shows that only 20 percent of women enter pregnancy with sufficient iron stores. Sixty percent of women have reduced stores; a further 20 percent, almost no iron stores (**44**).

The average American diet provides about 6 mg of iron per 1000 kcal, but approximately 10 percent of the iron is absorbed. If maternal storage depots and/or dietary intake are insufficient to meet fetal demands, iron is shifted from the maternal hemoglobin pool and iron-deficiency anemia can result. Iron from dietary sources is generally insufficient to meet the needs of pregnant women, so daily supplements of 30−60 mg of iron are recommended during the second and third trimester to protect maternal stores (**18**).

Normal hemoglobin concentration ranges from 12.0 to 15.4 g per 100 ml of blood, with an average value of 13.7 g (**8**). Traditionally, with the usual increase in blood volume during pregnancy, slight or moderate decreases in hemoglobin levels were expected and were considered physiologically normal rather than representative of an iron deficiency (**45**). A hemoglobin concentration of 10 g per 100 ml was considered acceptable as a result of marked "hypervolemia" (an increase in total plasma volume, accompanied by a much smaller increase in total red cell volume). More recent evidence demonstrates that changes in serum iron levels and total serum iron binding capacity are consistent with an iron deficiency when hemoglobin levels fall below 11.5 g per 100 ml in pregnant women. According to these studies bone marrow estimates of storage iron show iron stores to be depleted when hemoglobin levels are less than 11.5 g per 100 ml, and that the administration of an adequate iron supplement allows for the maintenance of normal hematological values throughout pregnancy. If iron is available, the bone marrow has little difficulty increasing the hemoglobin mass to keep pace with the physiological increase in blood volume (**43**). Therefore, the frequent occurrence of anemia during the prenatal period has led many investigators to feel that few, if any, of these cases can be considered physiological in origin. The majority are due to true iron deficiency, and nutritionists, therefore, recommend that the hematological standards considered normal for nonpregnant women should also apply during pregnancy (**43**).

Folic Acid

The prevalence of a second deficiency, that of folic acid, is receiving increasing attention, since deficiencies of iron and folic acid frequently coexist. Approximately 30 percent of pregnant women show a folic acid deficiency (**46**). This can develop because of increased requirements for the vitamin, impaired absorption, insufficient dietary intake, and increased fetal demands or a combination of any or all of these factors (**47**). Low serum folic acid levels can be associated with spontaneous abortion in early pregnancy, increased risk of hemorrhage, fetal abnormalities, increased incidence of toxemia, and premature delivery. A folic acid deficiency leads to the development of megaloblastic anemia in 2.8 percent of pregnancies in the United States, and the infants born of such mothers usually have low folate stores themselves at birth.

Megaloblastic anemia can be controlled and prevented by the administration of small amounts of folic acid during the last trimester of pregnancy. Folic acid supplements of 30 mcg per day usually give beneficial results, and the average supplementation level is approximately 300 mcg per day (**1**). Vitamin supplements do not contain folic acid in amounts greater than RDA levels because of the risk of neurological damage when folic acid is taken in the presence of a vitamin B_{12} deficiency. Also, folic acid may mask the symptoms of pernicious anemia by producing hematological improvements without affecting the progression of neurological lesions (**47**).

Vitamin B_{12}

Pernicious anemia as a result of vitamin B_{12} deficiency during pregnancy is relatively rare. It may occur, however, in pregnant women who are strict vegetarians and avoid all animal protein, including eggs and the dairy products that contain dietary vitamin B_{12}.

THE TOXEMIAS OF PREGNANCY

Toxemia is a term frequently applied to all hypertensive disorders of pregnancy (**1**). The term is used in this text in reference to the toxemias of pregnancy, preeclampsia and eclampsia. Preeclampsia is characterized by high blood pressure, edema, and the presence of protein in the urine. It may appear after the twentieth week of pregnancy. "Eclampsia" refers to the occurrence of one or more convulsions in a patient, with the symptoms indicative of preeclampsia. Toxemia is primarily a disorder of women in their first pregnancy and is more common among the very young and those over 30 years of age.

Toxemia leads to excessive perinatal mortality (**48**), with a small size for gestational age being the chief abnormality in those infants who die. The disturbance of normal growth in these infants is because of fetal malnutrition. The abnormalities seen in the infants of toxemic mothers are very similar to those seen in infants with known placental insufficiency. Studies of organ and cell development show that, in these cases, body length, brain, heart, and lung weights are near normal size. Adrenals, liver, spleen, and thymus, however, are disproportionately small. The organs are subnormal in size largely because of small cell sizes and some reduction in the total number of cells. The duration of toxemia has a direct relation to the total decrease in body weight of the infant. The longer toxemia continues the greater is the degree of intrauterine growth retardation of the infant.

Infants of toxemic mothers frequently show mental and motor abnormalities later in life, and the decrease in brain growth may well be the cause of these functional disturbances. Those infants most retarded in growth sometimes develop hypoglycemia in the neonatal period. A reduction in cell number and size in liver cytoplasm may lead to the inadequate development of enzymes essential for gluconeogenesis and thus a deficiency of liver glycogen. Hypoglycemia in the perinatal period may damage the central nervous system.

The maternal death rate from toxemia decreased from 52.2 per 100,000 live births in 1940 to 6.2 per 100,000 live births in 1965 (Figure 4.2). Severe toxemia of pregnancy is still a significant problem in some parts of the country, however, occurring most frequently among women in lower socioeconomic groups, particu-

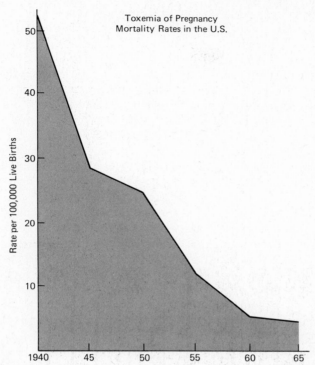

Figure 4.2 *Toxemia of pregnancy mortality rates in the U. S. (Source:* Reproduced with permission from R. M. Shank in *Nutrition Today* magazine, P. O. Box 1829, Annapolis, Maryland 21404, © Summer 1970.)

larly in the southeastern states (**1**). Poor nutrition may be a factor in the etiology of toxemia, since these women often have substandard diets.

The role of nutrition as a causative factor in the development of toxemia is not clear and has been the subject of much controversy (**1**). Calories, sodium, and protein all come under suspicion (**18**). Eclampsia cases subsided during World War I in Germany and Austria-Hungary, and it was assumed that the women's inadequate diet, which resulted in a low weight gain, protected them against toxemia. Without further study physicians then widely advocated a low calorie diet and limited weight gain during pregnancy to help prevent toxemia (**49**). Several generations of physicians followed this tradition of restricting weight gain for pregnant women. Then in 1970 the Committee on Maternal Nutrition concluded that there was not enough evidence to support the existence of a cause-effect relationship between high caloric intake, weight gain, and the incidence of toxemia (**1**). According to this study, the practice of drastic dietary measures that may be detrimental to the fetus is not justified.

Patterns of abnormal weight gain, rather than total weight gain per se during pregnancy may be related to the development of toxemia. The disorder is more severe in women who are markedly underweight at conception and who fail to gain normally during the prenatal period (**50**). It is also seen frequently in those who are obese at the time of conception and then gain weight excessively.

Edema and an abnormal retention of sodium are associated with preeclampsia, and studies show that the condition of a preeclamptic patient worsens when excess salt is consumed. For this reason the practice of routinely restricting sodium intake during pregnancy is widespread (**51**). Diuretics are commonly recommended in conjunction with dietary salt restriction. No justification, however, has been found for such routine salt limitations or for the use of diuretics to limit weight gain and avoid edema (**18**). Too, an insufficient intake of sodium may place excessive stress on the normal sodium conservation mechanism (**51**). For this reason, sodium intake should not be rigidly limited for the healthy pregnant woman (**51**).

Only in pathological conditions does the retention of sodium and water become excessive. The Committee on Maternal Nutrition questions the wisdom of stressing the physiological adaptive mechanism of the kidney by restricting sodium content in the diet. The committee suggests that the widespread practice of restricting salt intake to cut down on fluid retention may be potentially dangerous for healthy, pregnant women and should be discouraged (**1**). Many nutritionists feel that additional information is needed about the relation of sodium to blood volume expansion under varying conditions and about the metabolism of sodium during normal pregnancy and in toxemia.

"Proteinuria" is one of the major symptoms of toxemia, but little research is available to determine its cause or the possible role that dietary protein plays in its development (**1**). Originally, protein intake during pregnancy was restricted to prevent the formation of toxic amines. This practice is not followed today, and it is generally believed that improvements in dietary habits, particularly with relation to protein intake, are a causative factor in the decreased incidence of toxemia in this country. Much work remains to be done on protein metabolism during pregnancy and the role of dietary protein in the prevention and treatment of toxemia.

Some evidence exists that there may be an interrelationship between the metabolism of vitamin B_6 and the development of toxemia. A vitamin B_6 deficiency is linked with abnormalities of tryptophan metabolism as indicated by an increased urinary excretion of xanthurenic acid. The excretion of xanthurenic acid, a metabolite of vitamin B_6, is excessive in patients with preeclampsia. The administration of 10−25 mg of vitamin B_6 daily will correct the abnormal tryptophan metabolism but does not seem to change the course of toxemia (**52−54**). Other studies show a reduced vitamin B_6 content in placentas from toxemia patients (**55**).

MATERNAL WEIGHT GAIN

Much of the information available about the influence of nutrition on the outcome of human pregnancy is based on observed correlations between maternal and infant weights. These data show a positive correlation between maternal weight gain during pregnancy, maternal prepregnancy weight, and the infant's weight at birth (**56**). Maternal weight and weight gain are crude indices of nutritional status, and birth weight is a crude index of fetal development. Weight gain alone during pregnancy, however, is not a definite indicator of adequacy or inadequacy of the diet, nor does it indicate final newborn size. The nutritional quality of the diet as well as weight gain must be equally considered as important to fetal growth and development.

For many years physicians followed a routine practice of restricting weight gain during pregnancy to between 10 and 14 lb. This concept started during World War I when a low weight gain was assumed to be associated with a low incidence of toxemia. This practice has been seriously questioned since the mid-sixties, however. The Committee on Maternal Nutrition concluded in 1970, in fact, that the limitation on weight gain during pregnancy may actually contribute to the relatively high infant mortality rate in the United States (**1**).

The most desirable weight gain for normal pregnant women is estimated by using three different approaches: (1) 24 lbs are estimated as the ideal total weight gain, measured by information from normal pregnancies; (2) 24 lbs are also estimated to be the ideal weight gain, based on the relationship between normal maternal weight gain and an ideal infant birth weight; (3) a desirable weight gain can be calculated from the average weights of the identifiable components of normal pregnancy (**1**). The reproductive weight gain of both maternal and fetal components is approximately 20−22 lbs (Figure 4.3). An added margin of safety brings the preferred weight gain to 24 lbs (Figure 4.4).

Obviously, no fixed or predictable amount of weight gain can be ideal for all patients. A weight gain of 20−30 lbs is generally consistent with the most

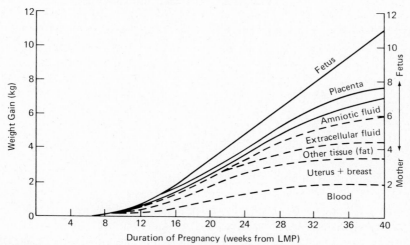

Figure 4.3 *Average pattern and components of maternal weight gain during pregnancy.* (*Source:* Reproduced with permission from R. M. Pitkin in *Nutritional Support of Medical Practice,* eds. C. Anderson, D. Coursin and H. Schneider. Copyright © 1975 by Harper & Row, Publishers, Inc., New York.)

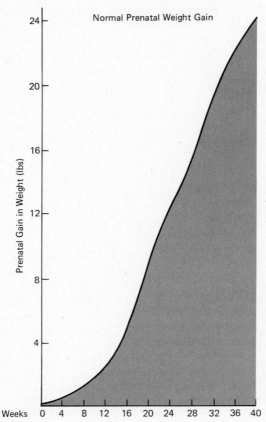

Figure 4.4 *Normal prenatal weight gain.* (*Source:* Reproduced with permission from R. E. Shank in *Nutrition Today* magazine, P. O. Box 1829, Annapolis, Maryland 21404, © Summer 1970).

favorable births, though. This results in an acceptable infant birth weight and in a postpregnancy maternal weight that is not undesirable in terms of variation from prepregnancy weight (**1**).

The pattern of weight gain during pregnancy may be of greater clinical importance than the actual total amount (**57**). Figure 4.3 indicates the normal pattern of weight gain during pregnancy. Generally, a total weight gain of 3 lbs by the end of the first trimester, 12½ lbs by the end of the second trimester, and 24 lbs at term is compatible with a favorable birth. A gain of 0.8−1 lbs per week during the second half of pregnancy concurs with the lowest overall incidence of eclampsia, low birth-weight infants, and perinatal mortality. A sudden sharp increase in weight after the twentieth week may indicate water retention and the possible onset of preeclampsia (**8**).

A normal weight prior to pregnancy is important in addition to an orderly and healthy weight increase during pregnancy to avoid certain complications. The woman who enters pregnancy 10 percent or more below the standard weight for her height and age is considered underweight. The underweight patient faces several hazards, primarily the delivery of a low birth-weight infant (**50**). The high incidence of perinatal mortality, neurological damage, and other complications associated with a low birth weight are a major concern and already have been discussed. Underweight patients often fail to gain normally during pregnancy. A gain of 1 kg or less per month during the second and third trimesters is considered inadequate and is associated with low birth-weight infants. A large percentage of patients who will gain minimal amounts of weight during pregnancy can be recognized in the first trimester, and attempts can be made to improve the gain. A moderate gain in maternal weight during the second and third trimester, following inadequate weight gain during the first trimester, can result in an increase in the mean fetal weight. The underweight woman who consumes too few calories probably has a low intake of other essential nutrients. Therefore, extensive dietary counseling is necessary for women who enter pregnancy at less than a desirable weight.

Women who weigh 10 percent or more above the standard weight for their age and height at the beginning of pregnancy are considered overweight. Many of these patients then gain an excessive amount (3 kg or more per month) during the prenatal period. This can lead to added complications during delivery, including an increased incidence of caesarian sections, prematurity, fetal mortality rate, toxemia, and hypertension (**58**). Excessive weight gain during pregnancy, if not lost after delivery, also leads to deposition of excessive fat and adds to the long-term complications of obesity and the detrimental health effects associated with it.

The overweight pregnant woman may predispose her infant to be overweight. Critical periods exist in the lifespan of an individual when fat cells increase rapidly, and one of these sensitive periods is at 31 weeks of gestation. If it is overfed during this time the fetus can develop adipose tissue characterized by a greater number of fat cells (**59**). Therefore, an infant who is overfed *in utero* may be born with more than the normal number of fat cells and start on a lifelong path toward obesity.

A restricted weight gain is usually advocated for obese women so that they can conclude their pregnancies with a net loss in weight. Some studies show that obese women can tolerate a smaller weight gain during pregnancy than normal weight women if the diet is adequate in nutrients. Other studies show, however, that even though obese patients who limited their weight gain were heavier than normal women at the end of pregnancy they frequently delivered significantly smaller children.

In addition to restricting weight gain in obese women, the physician often suggests an actual weight loss during pregnancy. Therefore, there is a need to reconsider the advisability of imposing caloric restriction programs during pregnancy. Caloric restriction is often accompanied by some restrictions in other nutrients essential for normal growth and development of the fetus. Severe caloric restriction is associated with low blood sugar, low levels of insulin, and high amino acid and ketone concentrations in the blood of the mother. If the dietary intake is restricted to such an extent that maternal reserves are depleted the catabolism of fat becomes excessive. The ketosis that may develop poses a threat to the neurological development of the fetus.

Therefore, obese women should not attempt a drastic weight reduction during pregnancy because of possible adverse effects on birth weight and neurological development of the infant (**8**). Weight loss by obese women should be undertaken either before or after pregnancy and under a physician's care. Obese women, therefore, should be cautioned to avoid gaining excess weight during pregnancy and encouraged to reduce after delivery. Although many questions about the relationship between maternal weight gain and birth weight of the infant remain unsolved, the goal of controlled weight gain is to assure a healthy outcome for both mother and infant.

TEENAGE PREGNANCY

The number of pregnant adolescent girls, specifically those under 17 years of age or less than five years postmenarchal, continues to increase in the United States. One in every 10 teenage girls will now become pregnant each year. Between 1960 and 1973 the number of births to mothers between the ages of 16 and 17 increased by 25 percent (**60**). Births to mothers under 16 years of age increased by 80 percent (**60**). Currently, the pregnancy rate in the United States for girls from 15 to 19 is higher than that in 21 other developed countries. The risks associated with teenage pregnancy are a major reason this country lags behind others of similar economic development in statistics relating to infant mortality (**60, 61**).

The nutritional needs of pregnant teenagers warrant special consideration, since the nutritional stress of pregnancy is superimposed on the normally large nutritional needs of adolescence. The average age of menarche in the United States is 13 today, with linear growth completed approximately four years later (**1**). Pregnancy before 17 is therefore occurring in a physiologically immature individual (**1**).

Few studies are available that relate to the dietary intake and nutritional status of pregnant teenagers (**62**). As a group, teenage girls have inadequate intakes of certain nutrients and, therefore, often enter pregnancy in a poor nutritional state (**63, 64**). The diets of this group are low in calories, protein, vitamin A, vitamin C, thiamin, calcium, and iron (**64–69**). The reasons for this inadequate nutrient intake frequently center around social and peer groupings (**70**). The desire to be slender leads many teenage girls to diet excessively, often to the point of becoming underweight (**63**). Others, with a compulsion to eat as the group does, consume high carbohydrate snacks and become overweight (**68, 70**). Ten to 12 percent of the adolescents who enter pregnancy are obese; a smaller proportion are underweight.

The complications of pregnancy increase for girls under 17 years of age (**60, 61**). Twenty-four percent of teenage pregnancies are complicated by excessive weight gain, and a large proportion of pregnant teenagers gain too little. Preeclampsia occurs 15 times more frequently in pregnant teenagers than in older women (**71**). The rate of stillbirths attributed to preeclampsia is 7.5 per 1000 births for mothers under 20, compared with 2.8 per 1000 for those in the 20–24 years of age bracket (**72**). Twenty-five percent of those infants born to teenage mothers also exhibit a low birth weight. Low birth infants are, therefore, two to three times more frequent among teenage mothers than among other age groups. Statistics for the percentage of newborn infants in 1973 weighing 2500 g or less and 2000 g or less show that the highest ratios, 15.7 percent at or under 2500 g and 6.6 percent at or under 2000 g, are found among infants born to mothers under the age of 15 (Figure 4.5). The corresponding ratios for mothers 15–19 are lower but not as low as for women age 20–29. Above age 29 the incidence of low birth weight increases significantly but does not reach the levels found for infants of teenage mothers (**60**). Infant mortality rates vary by maternal age in a manner similar to low birth-weight figures (Figure 4.6). Infant mortality rates among infants born to mothers under 15 are more than two times as high as for those born to women from 20 to 34 (**73, 74**).

Little research is available that can be used to base specific nutrient recommendations for the pregnant teenager (**62, 75–78**). It is known, however, that nutrient requirements in adolescence parallel the growth curve and are greater in relation to body size than those for the adult female. A failure to meet the additional nutrient demands of pregnancy during adolescence will result in an increased risk to both the mother and infant and may affect her eventual body stature. It is often difficult to improve the nutritional status of the pregnant

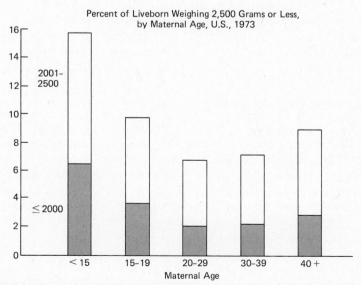

Figure 4.5 *Percent of liveborn weighing 2500 grams or less, by maternal age, U. S. A., 1973. (Source:* Reproduced with permission from *Contemporary Ob/Gyn,* June 1975, by G. Stickle and M. Paul. Copyright © 1975 by Medical Economics Company, Oradell, New Jersey.)

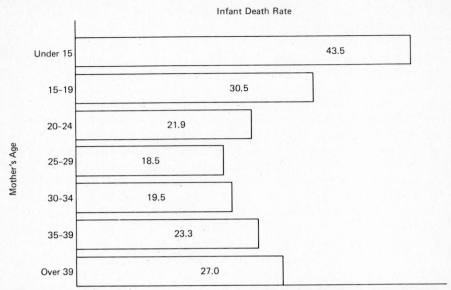

Figure 4.6 *Infant death rate by mother's age.* (*Source:* Reproduced by permission from *Perinatal Health: Challenge to Medicine and Society,* 1974, by G. Stickle. Copyright © 1974 by National Foundation—March of Dimes, White Plains, New York.)

teenager, since many do not seek medical supervision until the third trimester. Also, diets and dietary regimens commonly used in prenatal clinics are generally not suitable for adolescents. The diet of a young pregnant girl must be individualized and be developed, keeping in mind the girl's eating habits, economic status, and emotional and social needs in relation to her nutritional needs. Nutritional guidance should improve the outcome of teenage pregnancy for both mother and child.

THE USE OF DRUGS IN PREGNANCY

Until 1962 many physicians did not pay serious attention to the possibility that chemical substances passing from the mother to the fetus could be potentially dangerous. In that year thalidomide, a drug commonly prescribed for insomnia and nervous tension, was found capable of producing malformations in the fetus. Babies born to women who had taken the drug early in pregnancy were born with phocomelia or "seal limbs," foreshortened arms and legs resembling the flippers of seals. The thalidomide tragedy demonstrates strongly the hazards of taking drugs during pregnancy.

One study estimates that over 90 percent of women take at least one medication during pregnancy (**79**). The average intake is four to five medications, and four percent take 10 or more different medications. Eighty percent of these are taken without medical supervision or knowledge and include vitamin preparations, aspirin, antacids, diuretics, antibiotics, antihistamines, and barbiturates.

The fetus or infant is the potential recipient of any drug taken by the mother during pregnancy or lactation (**80**). Many drugs or chemical substances penetrate the placenta at a rate sufficient to cause significant concentrations within the fetus. Some reports have shown drugs in fetal tissues in therapeutic concentrations. Relatively little is known about the effect of specific drugs on the fetus (**81**), and equally little is known about the effects of drugs the infant may ingest through breast milk.

For years physicians have assumed that if a drug is nontoxic for the mother it will not harm the fetus. This is obviously a dangerous assumption. The kinds and amounts of toxicants to which the fetus or infant can be exposed safely are not known, nor is there a satisfactory way to determine safety. The fetus and infant do not react to chemical substances the same as the mother does. This is because the inadequate enzyme systems of the developing organism prevent it from metabolizing drugs as the mature organism can.

The mechanisms by which chemical substances interrupt the growth and development of the fetus are not thoroughly understood. Chemicals may affect the maternal tissues by decreasing the oxygen carrying capacity of the blood, altering the level of blood glucose, or decreasing the availability of essential vitamins, amino acids, trace elements, and hormones. Such effects will be felt indirectly by the fetus. Certain chemicals may specifically affect the placenta by altering the placental blood supply and interfering with the transport of oxygen, glucose, and other vital substances. In fact, any changes in placental metabolism will influence fetal development. Chemicals may also directly affect cell structure and function in the developing fetus.

The fetus is highly susceptible to chemical substances during the first three months of gestation. "Teratogenic drugs," (chemicals capable of causing malformation in the fetus) can exert their effect on the embryo within 11 days of conception. From the time of fertilization until the blastocyst becomes embedded in the placenta, teratogenic agents kill, rather than maim, the embryo. The sensitivity of the fetus is high during organogenesis (from the second or third week through the third month of gestation), and the type and extent of damage depends on timing and duration of drug administration.

The chemical substances and drugs discussed in this chapter are mentioned in the literature as being possibly teratogenic or harmful to the human fetus. The list is not inclusive, and in certain instances reports conflict and additional study is needed. Goldstein, Aronson, and Kalman (**82**) provide a more complete discussion of teratogenic drugs. In Table 4.4 material compiled by Apgar is adapted to include drugs known to be deleterious (**83**). Most of the drugs listed produce their toxic effects by placental transfer to the fetus (**84, 85**).

Antibiotics

With the possible exception of streptomycin, there is little concrete direct evidence of fetal damage by antibiotics that freely cross the placenta. Streptomycin affects the fifth cranial nerve and can damage hearing in the developing fetus. Toxic or unusual side effects produced by sulfonamides such as tetracycline in

TABLE 4.4   EFFECTS OF CERTAIN DRUGS TAKEN BY PREGNANT WOMEN

Medication	Fetal or neonatal effect
Oral progestins	Masculinization and advanced bone age
Androgens	
Estrogens	
Potassium iodide	
Propylthiouracil	Goiter and mental retardation
Methimazole (Tapazole)	
Iophenoxic acid (Teridax)	Elevation of protein-bound iodine
Sodium aminopterin	
Methotrexate (Amethopterin)	Anomalies and abortion
Chlorambucil (Leukeran)	
Bishydroxycoumarin (Dicumarol)	
Ethyl bicoumacetate (Tromexan Ethyl Acetate)	Fetal death; hemorrhage
Sodium warfarin (Coumadin Sodium, Panwarfin, Prothromadin)	
Salicylates (large amounts)	Neonatal bleeding
Sulfonamides	Kernicterus
Chloramphenicol (Chloromycetin)	"Grey" syndrome; death
Sodium novobiocin (Albamycin Sodium, Cathomycin Sodium)	Hyperbilirubinemia
Nitrofurantoin (Furadantin)	Hemolysis
Tetracyclines	Inhibition of bone growth; discoloration of teeth
Vitamin K analogues (in excess)	Hyperbilirubinemia
Ammonium chloride	Acidosis
Reserpine	Stuffy nose; respiratory obstruction
Heroin and morphine	Neonatal death
Thalidomide	Phocomelia; hearing loss; death

Source: Reprinted with permission from V. Apgar, the *Journal of the American Medical Association*, *190*, 840, 1964 (**83**). Copyright © 1964, American Medical Association, Chicago.

the pre- and neonatal period are indirect evidence of their potential danger to the fetus. Tetracycline given three weeks prior to the delivery of a premature infant has been shown to be deposited in the developing teeth of the fetus, with subsequent defects in the enamel of deciduous teeth. Sulfonamides, given near term, may result in a significant concentration of the drug in the blood of the newborn infant for several days after birth, increasing the infant's susceptibility to jaundice.

Hormones

Endocrine preparations, consisting essentially of progestational compounds, are often prescribed during pregnancy to help avert miscarriage. These preparations, however, have produced masculinization of some female fetuses, depending on the stage of pregnancy in which the drug was administered.

Anticoagulants

Anticoagulants given for the treatment of thrombophlebitis or venous thrombosis during pregnancy may result in fetal or neonatal hemorrhage and death. Aspirin, taken near term, may affect the fetal blood clotting mechanism (**86, 87**).

Tranquilizers

Mild tranquilizers can produce a variety of effects on the central and autonomic nervous system and may be teratogenic when taken during the early months of pregnancy. An increasing incidence of birth defects, too, including cleft palate, are found in infants born to mothers who took these minor tranquilizers.

Narcotics

The widespread use of drugs such as narcotics, hallucinogens, and amphetamines is a subject of increasing concern to health professionals (**88**). In New York City the number of pregnant women addicted to narcotics increased by 211 percent between 1966 and 1971, and most of these were women under 25 years of age. The bearing of low birth-weight infants occurs four times more frequently among narcotic-addicted mothers than among all others (Table 4.5).

Morphine and heroin addiction can occur *in utero* with withdrawal symptoms—including convulsions, high-pitched cry, and irritability—appearing one to three days after delivery.

This information is helpful, but more study is needed to clarify other possible effects of narcotics on the newborn.

Hallucinogens

The long-range effects on the infant of hallucinogens, including LSD, mescaline, hashish, and marijuana are not documented. Broken chromosomes, however, have been observed in persons using LSD, and the fear exists that this will affect the reproductive abilities of these persons (**90, 91**). The most active component of marijuana is fat soluble and is likely to appear in breast milk (**92**).

TABLE 4.5 PERCENTAGE OF LOW BIRTH-
WEIGHT INFANTS BORN TO ADDICTED MOTHERS

Year	All New York City births	Births to addicted mothers
1966	10.4	44.9
1967	10.1	40.8
1970	9.7	43.3
1971	9.7	42.5

Source: Reprinted with permission from S. Blumenthal, L. Bergner, and F. Nelson, *Health Services Reports 88*, 416, 1973 (**89**). Copyright © 1973 Health Services Reports, Rockville, Maryland.

Alcohol

The fetal alcohol syndrome among infants born to alcoholic mothers was described in a 1973 study (**93**). This syndrome is characterized by retarded growth, small head size, facial deformities, ear and eye problems, and abnormalities of the heart. Alcohol passes through the placenta quickly and accumulates in higher concentrations in fetal tissues than in maternal tissues. The National Council on Alcoholism and the National Institute on Alcohol Abuse and Alcoholism warn that although the risk of delivering a child with congenital defects is greatest among alcoholic women, even moderate drinkers can possibly deliver defective infants (**94**).

Cigarettes

A 1972 study showed that there is a 30 percent increase in the risk of delivering a stillborn infant among women who smoke heavily and a corresponding 26 percent increase in the risk of infant death within the first few days after birth (**95**). Some researchers estimate that 4600 stillbirths each year in the United States can be attributed to the mothers' smoking. Some evidence exists, however, to show that the risk of delivering a stillborn or low birth-weight infant is reduced if a pregnant woman stops smoking by the fourth month of gestation (**95, 96**).

The exact mechanisms that reduce fetal weight after exposure to cigarettes are not yet known (**97**). A simple possibility is that cigarette smoking affects maternal appetite, diminishes maternal weight gain, and thus affects fetal growth (**98**). *The Surgeon General's Report on Smoking and Health* suggests that impairment of mothers' protein metabolism may be partially responsible for low birth weight (**99**). In addition, health professionals suppose that the smoking mothers' higher levels of carboxyhemoglobin and nicotine may decrease oxygenation of the fetus to some extent (**99**). The cyanide content of cigarettes is also suggested as a factor affecting fetal growth, since it has an effect on the vitamin B_{12} metabolism of the mother and infant (**100**). Smoking may decrease the volume of milk secreted by lactating women. In addition, 10−20 cigarettes smoked daily will pass along 0.4−0.5 mg of nicotine in each liter of milk (**92**).

Vitamins

Even vitamin preparations can be harmful to the unborn child when taken in excessive doses by pregnant women. Yet vitamins are often prescribed in conventional therapeutic doses during pregnancy, since subclinical deficiencies of certain nutrients, including vitamin C and folic acid, may produce defects in the fetus. It is extremely important that these dosages not be exceeded. Large doses of vitamin C taken by mothers precipitate the development of scurvy in infants when birth removes them from access to the vitamin the mothers are taking. One case of severe hypercalcemia and cardiovascular lesions was reported in the fetus of a woman taking excess vitamin D. These findings resemble those in experimentally produced vitamin D intoxication. Hemorrhagic disease of the newborn can occur because of a neonatal deficiency of a complex of multiple coagulation factors. The exact role of a vitamin K deficiency in the development of this disease has not been defined clearly, and routine prenatal administration of vitamin K is open to question. In view of the different opinions regarding the role of vitamin K in preventing hemorrhagic disease of the newborn it is suggested that water-soluble vitamin K analogs be given to infants after birth (**101**).

Need for Education and Research

In 1966 the FDA guidelines for the evaluation of new drugs for use during pregnancy were stricter than earlier FDA recommendations. Health professionals see a need, though, for educational programs and further research about the effects of drugs during pregnancy. It is increasingly apparent, for instance, that test results from animal experiments do not always apply to humans. Thalidomide has not been shown to be teratogenic in rabbits used in laboratory experiments. Aspirin is not known to exhibit teratogenic effects in humans, but it does exhibit such in rabbits. Most new-drug pregnancy tests are conducted with rodents. FDA encourages but it does not require that these tests be conducted with primates. Such tests might generate results more valid for the pregnant woman. Given the lack of scientific knowledge about the safety of the vast number of drugs in current use, health professionals recommend that unnecessary medication be avoided throughout pregnancy. Those who are in need of medical treatment or are already under the care of a doctor should be guided by their physician. Since certain disease conditions may affect the unborn infant it is important to weigh the benefits of medication against any possible harm to both the mother and fetus.

THE USE OF ORAL CONTRACEPTIVES—NUTRITIONAL COMPLICATIONS

Oral contraceptives are one of the most widely used type of drug in America today (**102**). In 1970 it was estimated that approximately 10 million women in the United States were using oral contraceptive steroids (**103**). Yet more and more reports appear in the literature to indicate that oral contraceptives influence many aspects of nutrient metabolism (**104**). Over 50 different metabolic changes affecting lipid, carbohydrate, protein, mineral, and vitamin metabolism have been reported with the use of these steroids (**105**).

The effect of oral contraceptives observed most often is an altered level of nutrients in the blood. Reports of increases in serum lipids (**106–109**) and increases in plasma triglycerides (**110**) have raised concerns about the development of cardiovascular problems (**111**). However, no consistent changes in plasma cholesterol, fatty acids, and phospholipids have been found (**111**).

Many women develop an abnormal tolerance to glucose while using oral contraceptives (**112–114**). The mechanisms by which carbohydrate metabolism is altered have not been defined, although slight increases in plasma levels of glucose and insulin have been noted (**112**). Concern exists, therefore, that the long-term use of oral contraceptives will lead to the development of diabetes.

Serum protein levels change with the use of oral contraceptives (**115**). Serum albumin is decreased while the globulins and fibrinogen are increased

(112). The excretion of amino acids in the urine is increased (113). In addition, protein retention is increased and may account for some of the weight gain during the early use of oral contraceptives (114).

The levels of minerals in the body are altered with the use of oral contraceptives, including an increase in serum iron, transferrin, and the total iron binding capacity (116). In fact, an improvement in iron nutriture and a decrease in iron-related anemia are frequently reported (117), probably because of a decrease in the loss of iron through menstrual flow. Copper concentrations in blood serum are increased two- or three-fold with the initiation of oral contraceptive use (109, 116–119). Also, zinc levels are decreased in the plasma but are increased in the erythrocytes (120–123). Several tentative explanations have been suggested, but none explain clearly the cause of changing zinc levels.

Vitamins A and E are significantly higher in the serum of oral contraceptive users compared to nonusers (124–126). This increase is probably related to the total increase in serum lipids in pill users. Increased serum levels of vitamin K-dependent clotting factors are found in women taking oral contraceptives, and these women show a subnormal response to anticoagulants. This may indicate a decreased requirement for vitamin K (127–128).

Some water-soluble vitamins have altered metabolism through the use of the sex steroid hormones. Preliminary work indicates that vitamin B_{12} serum levels are decreased (129, 130), perhaps indicative of an increased metabolism rate (131, 132). Most reports on folate indicate lower serum levels (133, 134). The absorption of folate is not changed, but the metabolism is altered. Although cases of megaloblastic anemia have been reported in women who used the pill from one to five years, these cases are rare (134), so there seems to be no specific benefit to be derived from routine folate supplementation. Women at risk for developing folate deficiency with the use of oral contraceptives include those on marginal intakes of folate, those with malabsorption syndromes, those with increased folate needs, and possibly those who become pregnant shortly after discontinuing use of the agents (135).

Vitamin B_6 has received considerable attention because the use of estrogen-containing oral contraceptives may produce a B_6 deficiency in certain women (136, 137). This abnormality occurs in the metabolic pathway of tryptophan conversion to niacin. Several possible theories are available to explain the abnormal metabolism, and although none is generally accepted, all indicate an increased vitamin B_6 requirement.

Plasma leukocyte and platelet ascorbic acid levels are reduced in women using oral contraceptive agents (130, 138). The lower serum levels of ascorbic acid may be related to increased serum ceruloplasmin levels in oral contraceptive users. Ceruloplasmin catalyzes the oxidation of ascorbic acid in vitro and may, therefore, contribute to the reduction of ascorbic acid levels in the plasma and tissues. The decrease in plasma and blood cell ascorbic acid could also be due to a decreased absorption or changes in tissue distribution.

It is not known to what degree the biological changes caused by oral contraceptives are undesirable. The lack of agreement on the effect of oral contraceptives on nutrient metabolism suggests that the individual response to steroid treatment is varied. Not all women receiving the drug are similarly at risk, since changes in nutrient metabolism correlate to a large extent with the nutritional status of the individual. Some women seem to benefit from routine supplements with vitamins and minerals when on the pill. Nutrient supplements, however, may not be necessary for the majority of oral contraceptive users. The need for dietary supplements is determined by the diet and other major factors affecting nutritional status.

More information is needed on the effect oral contraceptives have on the nutritional status of high-risk groups—such as girls in early adolescence or other groups of women who consume a marginal or deficient diet. Generally, the women who take oral contraceptives and eat well-balanced diets, including a wide variety of foods, do not need dietary supplements.

The nutritional complications of oral contraceptive treatment and the importance of good nutritional status as a prerequisite to childbearing should be emphasized through educational programs (**139**).

SUMMARY

The text has continually stressed the importance of maternal nutrition before and during pregnancy as it influences the child's physical and mental development for life. Only recently has it been demonstrated that malnutrition during prenatal life can affect physical and mental development and lead perhaps to permanent stunting of physical stature and mental capacity. The majority of stillbirths, premature births, neonatal deaths, low birth weights, functional limitations, and congenital defects are found among infants born to mothers with poor to very poor prenatal diets, representative of long-term habits.

Fetal malnutrition implies a reduction in nutrient supply of sufficient magnitude and duration to retard fetal growth significantly below its full genetic potential. Fetal malnutrition is characterized by small body size for gestational age and other biochemical and pathophysiological features associated with undernutrition. Retardation in overall physical growth *in utero* may be paralled by a retardation in mental development. Recent evidence suggests that significant rehabilitation of both physical and mental retardation is possible with appropriate nutrition and environmental stimulation. Intrauterine growth-retarded infants appear to be at risk from birth, with a high death rate, greater postnatal complication, and a higher incidence of mental-motor retardation at a later age.

Anemia and toxemia are two commonly recognized nutrition-related complications of pregnancy in the United States. Both disorders can result in fetal malnutrition. Toxemia leads to excessive perinatal mortality primarily because of low birth weight, and infants of toxemic mothers have an increased incidence of mental and motor abnormalities in later life. Much of the data regarding the influence of nutrition on the outcome of human pregnancy is based on observed correlations between maternal and infant weights. Thus the nutritional quality of the diet and components of weight gain must be considered as factors modifying fetal growth and development.

The number of pregnant adolescent girls continues to increase in this country, and the risks associated with teenage pregnancy have contributed to high infant morbidity and mortality rates.

The thalidomide tragedy in 1962 caused the health profession to give serious attention to the possibility that chemical substances, including alcohol and nicotine, passing from the mother to the fetus could be potentially dangerous. Oral contraceptives, one of the most widely used drugs in America today, may adversely affect certain aspects of nutrient metabolism in the user and may have long-term effects on nutritional status.

Health professionals continue to speculate about how maternal nutritional deprivation influences fetal growth. Evidence does suggest that nutritional intervention during pregnancy can have a positive influence on the subsequent growth and development of the infant. The ideal situation is for the mother to maintain excellent nutritional status from birth throughout life.

STUDY QUESTIONS AND
TOPICS FOR INDIVIDUAL INVESTIGATION

1. Does poor nutrition of the mother affect the intellectual development of her baby? What other environmental factors play a role in the delayed intellectual performance of certain infants?

2. Anemia and toxemia are two commonly recognized nutrition-related complications of pregnancy in the United States. What is the role of nutrition as a causative factor in the development of each of these disorders? What are the current theories for nutritional management of these problems? Does any controversy exist?

3. To develop an effective nutrition education program for pregnant adolescents, the educator needs to be aware of the physiological, psychological, and social needs of the individuals involved. Develop an educational instrument (questionnaire, etc.) that would help you as a nutrition educator determine the following about the pregnant teenager: (1) present state of knowledge about food and nutrition, (2) attitudes toward food, (3) current eating practices, and (4) preference about how nutrition education might be presented.

4. Studies of the outcome of pregnancy show that complications are seen more frequently in very young girls than in adults. Although age per se is a significant factor, the possible involvement of nutrition is often overlooked. Topics that might be included in the nutrition component of a health education course for pregnant teens are listed next.

NUTRITION FOR THE MOTHER
How your body digests and uses food
What calories and food nutrients mean to you
Menu planning to eat well
How to buy the most nutritious food for your money
Food preparation
Control your weight

NUTRITION FOR THE INFANT
Feeding your baby to grow strong and smart
Feeding your young child

Choose one topic and expand it into a presentation for a teenage audience. Develop goals, objectives, subject matter content, procedures, and audiovisual aids. The topics listed can be modified. For example, you may want to expand the lesson on food nutrients into more than one lesson, covering different nutrients each time.

5. Evidence indicates that the use of drugs, including alcohol and nicotine, even in moderate amounts during pregnancy, can be harmful to the developing fetus. Until recently this has been a neglected field of human nutrition. What

practical suggestions can you give for ways in which this type of education could be included in a health program? At what age would you begin this type of education?

6. Oral contraceptives constitute one of the most widely used types of drugs in America today. Recent reports indicate that some potential nutrition-related problems are associated with the use of oral contraceptive agents and that many young women lack general nutrition knowledge. With these facts in mind, do you feel that nutrition counseling sessions for women on the pill are advisable and why? What information would you include in such sessions?

REFERENCES

1. National Research Council. *Maternal Nutrition and the Course of Pregnancy.* Committee on Maternal Nutrition, Food and Nutrition Board, National Academy of Science, Washington, D.C., 1970.
2. Pitkin, R. M., H. A. Kaminetsky, M. Newton, and J. A. Pritchard. Maternal nutrition: a selective review of clinical topics. *Obstetrics and Gynecology,* 40:773, 1972.
3. Rush, D., Z. Stein, G. Christakis, and M. Susser. The prenatal project: the first 20 months of operation. In: *Nutrition and Fetal Development,* ed. M. Winick. Wiley, New York, 1974.
4. Higgins, A. A preliminary report of a nutrition study on public maternity patients. Report of a Workshop on Nutritional Supplementation and the Outcome of Pregnancy. National Academy of Sciences-National Research Council, Washington, D.C. 1972.
5. National Dairy Council. Nutritional needs during pregnancy. *Dairy Council Digest,* 145:19, 1974.
6. Antonov, A. Children born during the siege of Leningrad in 1942. *Journal of Pediatrics,* 30:250, 1947.
7. Smith, C. A. Effects of maternal undernutrition upon the newborn infant in Holland (1944–1945). *Journal of Pediatrics,* 30:229, 1947.
8. Shank, R. E. A chink in our armor. *Nutrition Today,* 5:2, 1970.
9. Bergner, L., and M. W. Susser. Low birth weight and prenatal nutrition: an interpretative review. *Pediatrics,* 46:949, 1970.
10. Shah, F., and H. Abbey. Effects of some factors on neonatal and postnatal mortality. *Milbank Memorial Fund Quarterly,* 49:33, 1971.
11. Singer, J. E., M. Westphal, and K. Niswander. Relationship of weight gain during pregnancy to birth weight and infant growth and development in the first year of life. *Journal of Obstetrics and Gynecology,* 31:417, 1968.
12. Sinclair, J. C., S. Saigal, and C. Y. Yeung. Early postnatal consequences of fetal malnutrition. In: *Nutrition and Fetal Development,* ed. M. Winick. Wiley, New York. 1974.

13. Naeye, R. L., M. M. Diener, H. T. Harcke, and W. A. Blanc. Relation to poverty and race to birth weight and organ and cell structure in the newborn. *Pediatric Research,* 5:17, 1971.

14. Winick, M. Maternal nutrition and intrauterine growth failure. *Nutrition Growth and Development, Medical Problems in Pediatrics,* 14:48, 1975.

15. Banister, R. Congenital malformations: preliminary report of an investigation of reduction deformities of the limbs, triggered by a pilot surveillance system. *Connecticut Medical Association Journal,* 103:466, 1970.

16. Coursin, D. B. Undernutrition and brain function. *Borden's Review of Nutrition Research,* 26:1, 1965.

17. National Center for Health Statistics (Advance Report, Final Mortality Statistics, 1976). Monthly Vital Statistics Report, Vol. 26, No. 12, March 30, 1978.

18. Shank, R. E. The role of nutrition in the course of human pregnancy. *Nutrition News,* 33:11, 1970.

19. Apgar, V. A proposal for a new method of evaluation of the newborn infant. *Anesthesia and Analgesia,* 32:260, 1953.

20. Apgar, V., and L. S. James. Further observations on the newborn scoring system. *American Journal of Diseases of Children,* 104:419, 1962.

21. Butterworth, J., and M. J. Covey. Epigram of the Apgar score. *Journal of the American Medical Association,* 181:353, 1962.

22. Barnes, R. H., A. Moore, I. Reid, and W. Pond. Learning behavior following nutritional deprivations in early life. *Journal of the American Dietetics Association,* 51:34, 1967.

23. Winick, M., and P. Rosso. Effects of severe early malnutrition on cellular growth of human brain. *Pediatric Research,* 3:181, 1969.

24. Eichenwald, H. F., and P. C. Fry. Nutrition and learning. *Science,* 163:644, 1969.

25. Churchill, J. A., J. W. Neff, and D. F. Caldwell. Birth weight and intelligence. *Journal of Obstetrics and Gynecology,* 28:425, 1966.

26. Winick, M. Cellular growth in intrauterine malnutrition. *Pediatric Clinics of North America,* 17:69, 1970.

27. Chase, H., J. Dorsey, and G. McKhann. The effect of malnutrition on the synthesis of myelin lipid. *Pediatrics,* 40:551, 1967.

28. Chase, H., N. Welch, C. Dabiere, N. Vasan, and L. Butterfield. Alterations in human brain biochemistry during intrauterine growth retardation. *Pediatrics,* 50:403, 1972.

29. Nutrition Foundation. Foundation scientists uncover new data linking malnutrition, mental deficiencies, 1969–1970. Nutrition Foundation Report, New York, 1970, p. 14.

30. Stewart, R. J. Experimental studies on nutrition and brain development. *Nutrition,* 28:151, 1974.

31. Winick, M., J. Brasel, and P. Rosso. Nutrition and cell growth. In: *Nutrition and Development,* Vol. 1, ed. M. Winick. Wiley, New York, 1972.

32. Winick, M. Changes in nucleic acid and protein content of human brain during growth. *Pediatric Research,* 2:352, 1968.

33. Rosso, P., J. Hormazabal, and M. Winick. Changes in brain weight, cholesterol, phospholipid and DNA content in marasmic children. *American Journal of Clinical Nutrition,* 23:1275, 1970.

34. Winick, M. Nutrition and nerve cell growth. *Federation Proceedings,* 29:1510, 1970.

35. Winick, M., P. Rosso, and J. Waterlow. Cellular growth of cerebrum, cerebellum, and brain stem in normal and marasmic children. *Experimental Neurology,* 26:393, 1970.

36. Erickson, M. T. Intelligence: prenatal and preconception environmental influences. *Science,* 157:1210, 1967.

37. Frisch, R. E. Present status of the supposition that malnutrition causes mental retardation. *American Journal of Clinical Nutrition,* 23:189, 1970.

38. Latham, M., and F. Cobos. The effects of malnutrition on intellectual development and learning. *American Journal of Public Health,* 61:1307, 1971.

39. Liang, P., T. Hie, O. Jan, and L. Giok. Evaluation of mental development in relation to early malnutrition. *American Journal of Clinical Nutrition,* 20:1290, 1967.

40. Winick, M., K. Meyer, and R. C. Harris. Malnutrition and environmental enrichment by early adoption. *Science,* 190:1173, 1975.

41. Chavez, A., C. Martinez, and T. Yasehine. Nutrition, behavioral development, and mother-child interaction in young rural children. *Federation Proceedings,* 34:1574, 1975.

42. Read, M. S. Malnutrition, hunger and behavior. I. Malnutrition and learning. *Journal of the American Dietetics Association,* 63:379, 1973.

43. Adels, M. J., and R. R. Franklin. Treatment of iron deficiency anemia in private obstetrical patients: comparison of two oral iron treatment regimens. *Journal of the Southern Medical Association,* 60:712, 1967.

44. Briscoe, C. C. The need for routine administration of iron during pregnancy. *Postgrad Medicine,* 34:1, 1963.

45. De Leeu, W. N., L. Lowenstein, and V. Hsieh. Iron deficiency and hydremia in normal pregnancy. *Medicine,* 45:291, 1966.

46. Rothman, D. Folic acid in pregnancy. *American Journal of Obstetrics and Gynecology,* 108:149, 1970.

47. Ross Laboratories. Iron and folic acid nutrition in pregnancy. A review and abstract of current literature. Ross Laboratories, Columbus, Ohio, May 1971.

48. Hendrick, D. H., and W. E. Brenner. Toxemia of pregnancy; relationship between fetal weight, fetal survival and the maternal state. *American Journal of Obstetrics and Gynecology,* 109:225, 1971.

49. Editorial. Eclampsia rare on war diet in Germany. *Journal of the American Medical Association,* 68:732, 1917.

50. Tompkins, W., D. Wiehl, and R. Mitchell. The underweight patient, an increased obstetric risk. *American Journal of Obstetrics and Gynecology,* 69:114, 1955.

51. Pike, R. L., and D. S. Gursky. Further evidence of deleterious effects produced by sodium restriction during pregnancy. *American Journal of Clinical Nutrition,* 23:883, 1970.

52. Wachstein, M., J. Kellner, and J. Ortiz. Pyridoxal phosphate in plasma and leukocytes of normal and pregnant subjects following B_6 load tests. *Proceedings, Society for Experimental Biology and Medicine,* 103:350, 1960.

53. Wachstein, M., and L. Graffeo. Influence of vitamin B_6 on the incidence of pre-eclampsia. *Obstetrics and Gynecology,* 8:177, 1956.

54. Wachstein, M., and A. Gudaitis. Disturbance of vitamin B_6 metabolism in pregnancy. *Journal of Laboratory and Clinical Medicine,* 42:98, 1953.

55. Kleiger, J., J. Evrard, and R. Pierce. Abnormal pyridoxine metabolism in toxemia of pregnancy. *American Journal of Obstetrics and Gynecology,* 94:316, 1966.

56. Eastman, N. J., and E. Jackson. Weight relationships in pregnancy. *Obstetrics and Gynecology,* 23:1003, 1968.

57. Pitkin, R. M. In: *Nutritional Support of Medical Practice,* eds. C. Anderson, D. Coursin, and H. Schneider. Harper & Row, New York, 1975.

58. Kramer, F. Overweight women—a problem in obstetrics. *Gynecology,* 164:343, 1967.

59. Brook, C., J. Lloyd, and O. Wolf. Relationship between age of onset of obesity and size and number of adipose cells. *British Medical Journal,* 2:25, 1972.

60. Stickle, G., and P. Ma. Pregnancy in adolescents: scope of the problem. *Contemporary Obstetrics/Gynecology,* June 1975.

61. Walters, J. Birth defects and adolescent pregnancies. *Journal of Home Economics,* 67:23, 1975.

62. Blackburn, M. L., and D. H. Calloway. Energy expenditure of pregnant adolescents. *Journal of the American Dietetics Association,* 65:24, 1974.

63. Hodges, R., and W. Krehl. Nutritional status of teenagers in Iowa. *American Journal of Clinical Nutrition,* 17:200, 1965.

64. Sipple, H. Problems and progress in nutrition education. *Journal of the American Dietetics Association,* 59:18, 1971.

65. Wharton, M. Nutritive intake of adolescents. *Journal of the American Dietetics Association,* 42:301, 1963.

66. Einstein, M., and I. Horstein. Food preferences of college students and nutritional implications. *Journal of Food Science,* 35:429, 1970.

67. U.S. Department of Health, Education, and Welfare. *Ten-State Nutrition Survey 1968–1970.* Government Printing Office, Washington, D.C., 1970.

68. Hampton, M., R. Huenemann, L. Shapiro, and B. Mitchell. Caloric and nutrient intakes of teenagers. *Journal of the American Dietetics Association,* 50:385, 1967.

69. Schorr, B., D. Sanjur, and E. Erickson. Teenage food habits. *Journal of the American Dietetics Association,* 61:415, 1972.

70. Huenemann, R., L. Shapiro, M. Hampton, and B. Mitchell. Food and eating

practices of teenagers. *Journal of the American Dietetics Association,* 53:18, 1968.

71. Stevenson, R. *The Fetus and Newly Born Infant.* Mosby, St. Louis, 1973.

72. Baird, D., F. Hytten, and A. Thompson. Age and human reproduction. *Journal of Obstetrics and Gynecology of the British Empire,* 65:6, 1958.

73. Stickle, G. Perinatal health: Challenge to medicine and society. National Foundation-March of Dimes, 1974.

74. Chase, H. A study of risks, medical care, and infant mortality. *American Journal of Public Health,* 63 (Supplement), 1973.

75. King, J., S. Cohenour, D. Calloway, and H. Jacobson. Assessment of nutritional status of teenage pregnant girls. I. Nutrient intake and pregnancy. *American Journal of Clinical Nutrition,* 25:916, 1972.

76. McGanity, W. J., H. M. Little, A. Fogelman, L. Jennings, E. Calhoun, and E. Dawson. Pregnancy in the adolescent. 1. Preliminary Summary of Health Status. *American Journal of Obstetrics and Gynecology,* 103:773, 1969.

77. Van de Mark, M. S., and A. C. Wright. Hemoglobin and folate levels of pregnant teenagers. *Journal of the American Dietetics Association,* 61:511, 1972.

78. Stearns, G. Nutritional state of the mother prior to conception. *Journal of the American Medical Association,* 168:1655, 1958.

79. Peckham, C., and R. King. Study of intercurrent conditions observed during pregnancy. *American Journal of Obstetrics and Gynecology,* 87:609, 1963.

80. Shinkey, H. C. The innocent child. *Journal of the American Medical Association,* 196:418, 1966.

81. Bleyer, W. A., W. Y. Au, W. A. Lange, and L. C. Raisz. Studies on the detection of adverse drug reactions in the newborn. I. Fetal exposure to maternal medication. *Journal of American Medical Association,* 213:2046, 1970.

82. Goldstein, A., L. Aronson, and L. Kalman. *Chemical Teratogenesis. Principles of Drug Action. The Basis of Pharmacology.* Harper & Row, New York, 1968.

83. Apgar, V. Drugs in pregnancy. *Journal of the American Medical Association,* 190:840, 1964.

84. Cohlan, S. Fetal and neonatal hazards from drugs administered during pregnancy. *New York Journal of Medicine,* 64:493, 1964.

85. Lucey, J. Drugs and the intrauterine patient. Birth Defects; Orig. Article Ser, 1:46, 1965.

86. Bleyer, W. A., and R. T. Breckenridge. Studies on the detection of adverse drug reactions in the newborn. II. The effects of prenatal aspirin on newborn homeostasis. *Journal of the American Medical Association,* 213:2049, 1970.

87. Hauron, M. Alcohol in pregnancy. *Maternal/Newborn Advocate,* 4:7, 1977.

88. Zelson, C., E. Rubio, and E. Wasserman. Neonatal narcotic addiction. 10 year observation. *Pediatrics,* 48:178, 1971.

89. Blumenthal, S., L. Bergner, and F. Nelson. Low birth weight infants associated with maternal heroin use. *Health Services Reports,* 88:416, 1973.

90. Cohen, M., M. Marinello, and W. Back. Chromosomal damage in human leukocytes induced by Lysergic Acid Diethylamide. *Science,* 155:1417, 1967.

91. Irwin, S., and J. Egozcue. Chromosomal abnormalities in leukocytes from LSD-25 users. Science, 157:313, 1967.

92. Arena, J. Contamination of the ideal food. *Nutrition Today,* 5:2, 1970.

93. Jones, K., D. Smith, A. Streissguth, and N. Myrianihopoulos. Outcome in offspring of chronic alcoholic women. *Lancet,* 1:1076, 1974.

94. American Medical Association. Even moderate drinking may be hazardous to maturing fetus. Medical News Section, *Journal of the American Medical Association,* 237:2585, 1977.

95. Butler, N., H. Goldstein, and M. Ross. Cigarette smoking in pregnancy: its influence on birth weight and perinatal mortality. *British Medical Journal,* 1:127, 1972.

96. Schwartz, D. Smoking and pregnancy: results of a prospective study of 6,989 women. *European Journal of Clinics and Biological Research,* 90:867, 1972.

97. Baric, L., C. MacArthur, and M. Sherwood. A study of health educational aspects of smoking in pregnancy. *International Journal of Health Education,* 19:1, 1976.

98. Davies, D., O. Gray, P. Ellwood, and M. Abernathy. Cigarette smoking in pregnancy: Associations with maternal weight gain and fetal growth. *Lancet,* 21:385, 1976.

99. Department of Health, Education, and Welfare. Surgeon General's Report on Smoking and Health. *FDA Drug Bulletin,* February–March 1979.

100. McGarry, J., and J. Andrews. Smoking in pregnancy and vitamin B_{12} metabolism. *British Medical Journal,* 2:74, 1972.

101. Committee on Nutrition, American Academy of Pediatrics. Vitamin K supplementation for infants receiving milk substitute infant formulas and for those with fat malabsorption. *Pediatrics,* 48:483, 1971.

102. Mishell, D. R. Current status of contraceptive steroids and the intrauterine device. *Clinical Obstetrics and Gynecology,* 17:35, 1974.

103. Hodges, R. E. Nutrition and the pill. *Journal of the American Dietetics Association,* 59:212, 1971.

104. Theuer, R. C. Effect of oral contraceptive agents on vitamin and mineral needs: a review. *Journal of Reproductive Medicine,* 8:13, 1972.

105. Warren, M. P. Metabolic effects of contraceptive steroids. *American Journal of Medical Science,* 265:5, 1973.

106. Beck, P. Contraceptive steroids: modification of carbohydrate and lipid metabolism. *Metabolism,* 22:841, 1973.

107. Wynn, V., and J. Doar. Some effects of oral contraceptives on carbohydrate metabolism. *Lancet,* 2:761, 1969.

108. Stokes, T., and V. Wynn. Serum lipids in women on oral contraceptives. *Lancet,* 2:677, 1971.

109. Alfin-Slater, R. B., and L. Aftergood. Lipids and the pill. *Lipids,* 6:693, 1971.

110. Inman, W. H., M. P. Vessey, B. Westerholm, and A. Engelund. Thromboembolic disease and the steroidal content of oral contraceptives: a report to the Committee on Safety of Drugs. *British Medical Journal,* 2:203, 1970.
111. Lowenstein, E. Oral contraceptives and cardiovascular disease. *Lancet,* 2:1365, 1966.
112. Spellacy, W. N. Metabolic effects of oral contraceptives. *Clinical Obstetrics and Gynecology,* 17:53, 1974.
113. King, J. Nutrition during oral contraceptive treatment. *Contemporary Nutrition,* 2:1, 1976.
114. Yen, S., and P. Vella. Carbohydrate metabolism and long-term use of oral contraceptives. *Journal of Reproductive Medicine,* 3:25, 1969.
115. Musa, B., R. P. Does, and U. S. Seal. Serum protein alterations produced in women by synthetic estrogens. *Journal of Clinical Endocrinology,* 27:1463, 1967.
116. Burton, J. L. Effects of oral contraceptives on hemoglobin, packed-cell volume, serum iron, and total iron binding capacity in healthy women. *Lancet,* 1:979, 1967.
117. Zadel, J. A., C. D. Karabus, and J. Fielding. Hb concentrations and other values in women using an intrauterine device or taking corticosteroid contraceptive pills. *British Medical Journal,* 4:708, 1967.
118. Margen, S., and J. C. King. Effect of oral contraceptive agents on the metabolism of some trace minerals. *American Journal of Clinical Nutrition,* 28:392, 1975.
119. Briggs, M., J. Austin, and M. Staniford. Oral contraceptives and copper metabolism. *Nature,* 225:81, 1970.
120. Schenker, J., S. Hellerstein, E. Jungreis, and W. Polishuk. Serum copper and zinc levels in patients taking oral contraceptives. *Fertility and Sterility,* 22:229, 1971.
121. Schenker, J. G., E. Jungreis, and W. Z. Polishuk. Oral contraceptives and correlation between serum copper and ceruloplasmin levels. *International Journal of Fertility,* 17:28, 1972.
122. O'Leary, J. A., and W. N. Spellacy. Zinc and copper levels in pregnant women and those taking oral contraceptives. *American Journal of Obstetrics and Gynecology,* 102:131, 1969.
123. Halsted, J. A., B. M. Hackley, and J. C. Smith. Plasma zinc and copper in pregnancy and after oral contraceptives. *Lancet,* 2:249, 1968.
124. Roe, D. A. Nutrition and the contraceptive pill. In: *Nutritional Disorders of American Women,* ed. M. Winick. Wiley, New York, 1977.
125. Gal, L., C. Parkinson, and I. Kraft. Effect of oral contraceptives on human plasma vitamin A levels. *British Medical Journal,* 2:436, 1971.
126. Wilde, J., C. Schorah, and W. Smithells. Vitamin A, pregnancy and oral contraceptives. *British Medical Journal,* 1:57, 1974.
127. Mellette, S. J. Interrelationships between vitamin K and estrogenic hormones. *American Journal of Clinical Nutrition,* 9:109, 1961.

128. Scrogie, J., H. Solomon, and P. Zieve. Effect of oral contraceptives on vitamin K-dependent clotting activity. *Clinical Pharmacology and Therapeutics,* 8:670, 1967.

129. Briggs, M., and M. Briggs. Oral contraceptives and vitamin nutrition. *Lancet,* 1:1234, 1974.

130. Smith, J., G. Goldsmith, and J. Lawrence. Effects of oral contraceptive steroids on vitamin and lipid levels in serum. *American Journal of Clinical Nutrition,* 28:371, 1975.

131. Shojania, A. Effect of oral contraceptives on vitamin B_{12} metabolism. *Lancet,* 2:932, 1971.

132. Wertalik, L., E. Metz, A. Lo Buglio, and S. Balcerzak. Decreased serum B_{12} levels with oral contraceptive use. *Journal of the American Medical Association,* 21:1371, 1972.

133. Pritchard, J. A., P. J. Whalley, and D. E. Scott. The influence of maternal folate and iron deficiencies on intrauterine life. *American Journal of Obstetrics and Gynecology,* 104:388, 1969.

134. Streiff, R. Folate deficiency and oral contraceptives. *Journal of the American Medical Association,* 214:105, 1970.

135. Pietarinen, G., J. Leichter, and R. Pratt. Dietary folate intake and concentration of folate in serum and erythrocytes in women using oral contraceptives. *American Journal of Clinical Nutrition,* 30:375, 1977.

136. Rose, D. P., R. Strong, P. W. Adams, and P. E. Harding. Experimental vitamin B_6 deficiency and the effect of estrogen-containing oral contraceptives on tryptophan metabolism and vitamin B_6 requirements. *Clinical Science,* 42:465, 1972.

137. Rose, D. P. The influence of estrogens on tryptophan metabolism in man. *Clinical Science,* 31:265, 1966.

138. Rivers, J. M., and M. M. Devine. Plasma ascorbic acid concentrations and oral contraceptives. *American Journal of Clinical Nutrition,* 25:684, 1972.

139. Nordquest, M., and E. Medved. A nutrition counseling session for college women on the pill. *Journal of Nutrition Education,* 7:29, 1975.

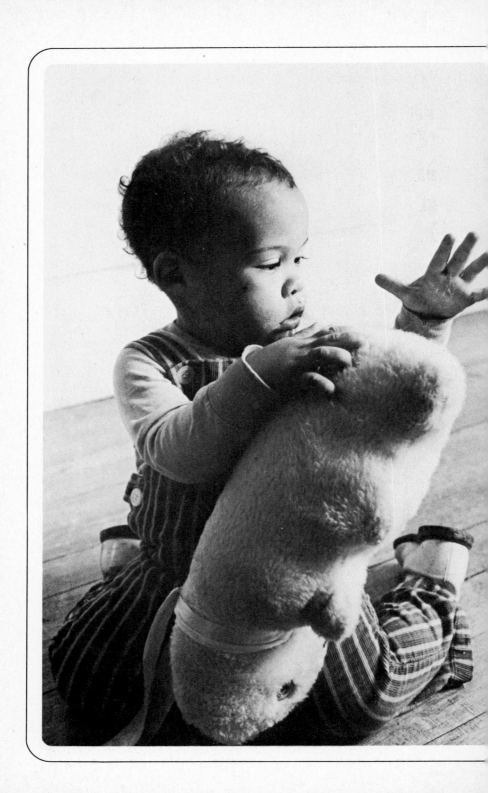

CHAPTER 5

PATTERNS OF POSTNATAL GROWTH AND DEVELOPMENT

Growth, which begins with conception and continues until maturity, is complex and dependent on genetics, time, nutrition, and other environmental factors. Chapter 3 discussed the growth and development of the fetus and the development of the biochemical and physiological processes essential for continued growth and health. This chapter presents concepts and information about the physical growth of the child during the postnatal period or from birth to maturity.

"Growth" can be regarded as the physiological gain of new tissue, reflected by increases in protein and water in the body. During growth, the body increases in size, including weight, height, and volume. An increase in weight alone, however, does not necessarily indicate growth because of the possibility of fat deposition and accompanying changes in the water content of the body. In terms of the physiological processes, those that are anabolic are dominant over the catabolic ones during growth (**1, 2**).

Growth does not proceed at a constant rate but goes through times of rapid change, or growth spurts, and periods of less pronounced changes. Immediately after birth, the growth rate declines as the infant adapts to a different environment. Following this period of adaptation, the growth rate accelerates for a time, then slows during childhood, and accelerates again during adolescence (**1, 2**). A general curve depicting human growth during postnatal life illustrates the periods of marked change as well as periods of steady growth (Figure 5.1).

PATTERNS OF GROWTH

Growth can be characterized, also, into linear and exponential phases. *Linear phases* are those periods of growth during which there is a passive accumulation

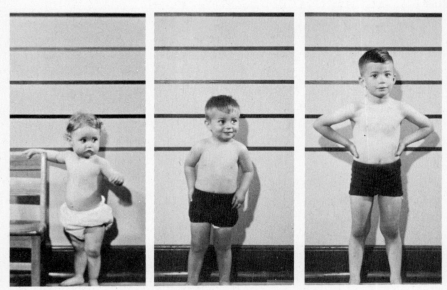

Growth of normal children at 11 months, 2½ years and 4½ years.

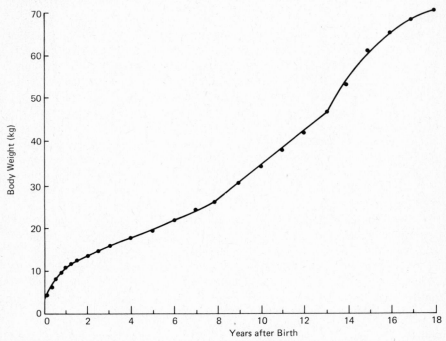

Figure 5.1 *Human growth curve during postnatal development. Growth expressed as increase in body weight (kilogram) with age. (Source:* Reproduced with permission from A. K. Laird in *Growth* 31, 345, 1967. Copyright © 1967 by Growth Publishing Company, Lakeland, Florida.)

of new products. *Exponential phases* are the times during which the products of growth reproduce themselves and lead to further growth. In the human, the periods of development from birth to approximately 6 years of age and the adolescent growth spurt are exponential in character. All other periods represent linear growth (**1**).

Human growth can be characterized further as "cephalocaudalic," the upper part of the body maturing before the lower part. The head matures before the neck, the neck before the chest, and so on. Arms mature before legs and even

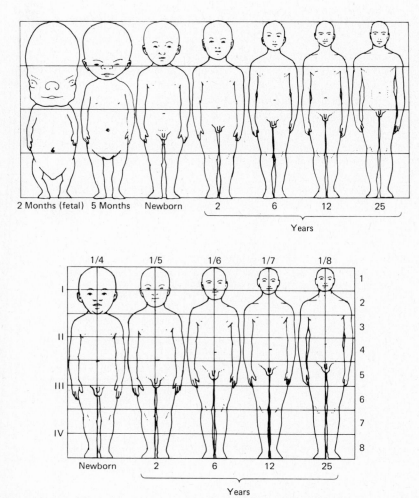

Figure 5.2 *Changes in the proportions of the human body during growth. The upper part of the figure compares prenatal and postnatal changes. The lower part of the figure expresses changes in relation to head length throughout growth.* (*Source:* Reproduced by permission from R. E. Scammon in the *American Journal of Physical Anthropology 10,* 329, 1927. Copyright © 1927 by Wistar Institute of Anatomy and Biology, Philadelphia.)

the upper arms before the lower arms. This principle follows throughout the span of human development and applies to the biochemical, as well as to the physical processes (**1**). Changes in relative sizes of the body parts are illustrated in Figure 5.2.

Major parts of the body follow definite growth patterns, but the patterns are different (**5**). Organs and tissue follow four types of growth patterns (Figure 5.3):

1. *General*   The body as a whole, organs concerned with respiration, circulation, digestion, and excretion. This growth pattern is essentially the same as the growth curve of the human (Figure 5.1).
2. *Neural*   The central nervous system: sight, hearing, and so forth. Growth is rapid during the early postnatal period, slows during infancy and childhood, and ceases by the time of puberty.
3. *Genital*   Growth typical of the sex organs. There is very little growth during infancy and childhood but very rapid growth and development just prior to puberty, and until maturity.
4. *Lymphoid*   Growth pattern of tissues such as the thymus, tonsils, adenoids, and lymph nodes and tissues. These tissues exhibit very rapid growth throughout infancy and childhood, attain maximum sizes about the time of or prior to puberty, and through involution decrease in size to adult norms.

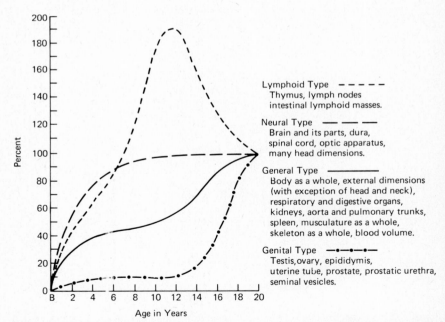

Figure 5.3 *Differential rates of growth by organs and other tissues, expressed as percent of mature size. (Source:* Reproduced by permission from the *Measurement of Man,* by J. A. Harris, C. M. Jackson, D. G. Paterson and R. E. Scammon. Copyright © 1930 by University of Minnesota Press, Minneapolis.)

DEVELOPMENT OF ORGANS AND SYSTEMS

"Development" implies an increase in complexity and function, while "growth" is indicative of an increase in size. Both growth and development are involved in the maturation of organs and tissues. Development, like growth, follows the general craniocaudal direction toward maturity. The following (Table 5.1) provides an indication of the relative increase in organs and tissues from birth to maturity (**5**).

In the following sections, the major groups of organs, tissues, and systems are discussed briefly in the context of growth and development.

Enzyme Systems

Enzymes are catalysts within cells and are necessary for the complex, but orderly, series of reactions essential for life, growth, and almost all physiological processes. They appear in cells as needed in response to the presence of the substances on which they act. Nutritional factors are important in the production or appearance of enzymes (**7**). Enzymes seem to become active in response to the presence of specific substrates, to the ability of cofactors such as certain vitamins, and to changes in postnatal dietary habits or food intake (**8**).

Muscle

During the early period of postnatal development, muscle fibers increase in both number (hyperplasia) and size (hypertrophy). From the middle of prenatal (fetal) life to early maturity, muscle growth represents the largest gain in the body. At the mid-prenatal period, it comprises 16 percent of body weight; at birth, between 20 and 25 percent; at early adolescence, 33 percent; and at early maturity, 40 percent (**2**).

TABLE 5.1 INCREASES IN WEIGHT OF
ORGANS AND TISSUES FROM BIRTH TO MATURITY

Approximate increase	Tissue or organ
30–40 times	Somatic muscle
	External genital organs
	Gonads
	Pancreas
25–30 times	Uterus
20–25 times	Body as a whole
	Skeleton
	Respiratory system
15–20 times	Heart
	Liver
	Lymphatic system
10–15 times	Thyroid gland
	Kidneys
5–10 times	Pituitary gland
Less than 5 times	Nervous system

Maximum muscle growth occurs relatively late and actually follows the maximum gain in height. A person's strength doubles between the twelfth and sixteenth years, and there is, contrary to myth, consistent and steady improvement of motor ability and coordination. This occurs during the time of rapid gain in muscle tissue (**2**).

Muscle is the major tissue, in terms of sheer mass, in the body, and changes in muscle cells reflect, or suggest, cellular changes in other tissues (**1**). The increases in muscle cells follow different patterns in the male and female (Figure 5.4). In the male, muscle cell increase is described by a quadratic equation and occurs primarily between ages 5 and 16 years. In one group of children maximum growth and increases in cell number began at about age 10.5 and continued to approximately age 16. During that period, cell number doubled, and the size of muscle cells in the male increased in a linear fashion from infancy to maturity (**9**).

The number of muscle cells increases in a linear pattern in females (**9**). This increase in cell size is more rapid in the girl after about age 3.5 and plateaus around age 10.5. At about age 14 the cell size of the male equals that of the female and surpasses the cell size of the female during the rapid growth spurt of

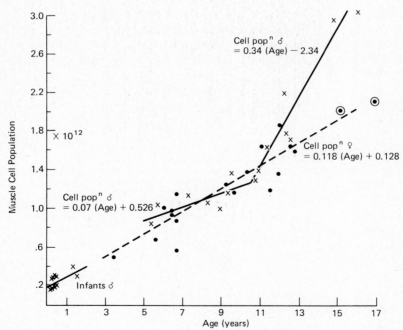

Figure 5.4 *Muscle cell number in males (×) and females (●).* (*Source:* Reproduced with permission from *Human Growth,* by D. B. Cheek. Copyright © 1968 by Lea and Febiger, Philadelphia.)

adolescence (**9**). During postnatal growth, the cell number increases by a factor of 14 in the male and by a factor of 10 in the female.

Cutaneous Structures

The skin of the newborn is thin and covered with a cheeselike material (*vermix caseosa*) that seems to protect the infant from infection. The infant also is covered with fine hair. The first hair of the head is lost and later replaced, with considerable variation, with permanent hair. All hair growth is heavy during adolescence, its appearance being influenced by sexual development (**2**).

The sweat and sebaceous glands, present in the fetus, begin to function at approximately a month of age. These glands are important in the regulation of body temperature, and subsequent development becomes significant during adolescence (**2**).

Skeleton

The human skeleton, including connective tissue, cartilage, and bone, passes through growth and development phases. The process of "chondroplasia," the growth of cartilage, progresses in a linear manner (**2**). "Osteogenesis" is the process of bone growth and epiphyseal development. Both linear growth (chondroplasia) and maturation (osteogenesis) are involved in the skeleton's increase. The duration of the cartilage, or linear, phase provides a rough indicator of the rate of growth, since the more rapidly growth occurs the less time is spent in the cartilage phase (**2**).

Bone growth provides an aid in evaluating physical development of the individual (**10**). A person's height is a general indicator of skeletal or linear growth with a major component being the development of the tubular bones. For example, the normal growth of a long bone, such as the radius, indicates linear growth (Figure 5.5). During the first year, the average increase of the radius is about 0.25 cm per month, but by the latter half of the second year the average rate of growth is approximately 0.12 cm per month (**11**).

Development of the skeleton depends on (1) growth of the areas undergoing ossification and (2) the deposition of calcium in those areas. These various centers of ossification develop at a predictable and definite schedule throughout the period from conception to maturity. All primary ossification centers for the tubular bones are present prior to birth, but the secondary centers appear after birth (Figures 5.6 and 5.7).

Considerable variation is found in the rate of bone development, but definite racial and sex differences exist. Bone development, for instance, is more rapid in the black than in the Caucasian. Also, in early childhood the bone growth of the female is faster than that of the male.

The skull is relatively soft at birth and is much larger than the face of the infant, but during early infancy the bones of the skull are molded and flattened. The cranium is composed of several bones that are joined or closed during

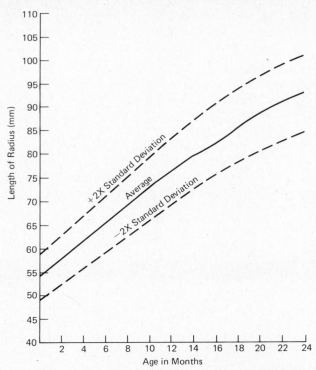

Figure 5.5 *Growth of the radius during the first two years of life. (Source:* Reproduced with permission from P. V. Woolley, Jr., and R. W. McCammon in *Journal of Pediatrics 27,* 229–235, 1945. Copyright © 1945 by C. V. Mosby Company, St. Louis, Missouri.)

normal development, although complete closure does not occur until near puberty (**2**).

Central Nervous System

Brain growth is very rapid from birth through early childhood. The brain attains about 50 percent of its total size by 1 year of age; by 3 years of age, 75 percent, and by 7 years of age, 90 percent. More gradual growth occurs during the ages 7–10, with a final small increase during adolescence. This brain growth and development occur in three stages: (1) cellular proliferation, (2) cellular hypertrophy, and (3) deposition of myelin and elaboration of the dendritic processes (**2**).

The central nervous system does not undergo a rapid growth spurt during adolescence. The fetus at 8 months has the neurons of the adult. Myelinization is initiated about the fourth fetal month but is not completed until the child is several years old. In fact, the myelin sheath continues to thicken for many years (**2**).

The spinal cord continues to develop for a long time, doubling in weight during the first 6 months of the infant's life. The cord weight has increased by a

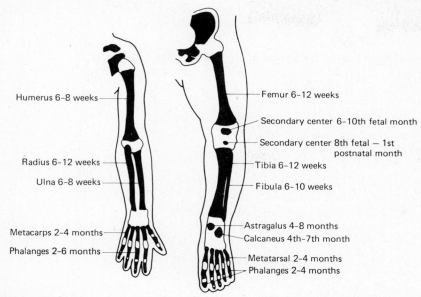

Figure 5.6 *Average time of appearance of the primary ossification centers in the arm and leg of the fetus. (Source:* Reproduced with permission from *Pediatric X-Ray Diagnosis,* 6th edition, by J. Caffey. Copyright © 1972 by Year Book Medical Publishers, Inc., Chicago.)

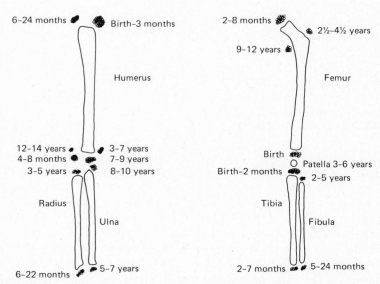

Figure 5.7 *Average time of appearance of the secondary ossification centers in the arm and leg. (Source:* Reproduced with permission from *Growth and Development of Children,* 7th edition, by G. H. Lowrey. Copyright © 1978 by Year Book Medical Publishers, Inc., Chicago. [From several sources])

147

factor of 4 at age 5, and in the adult is about eight times the original birth weight (**13**).

Development of Sensory Characteristics

The growth and development of the senses should be examined separately rather than as a general process.

The tactile sense follows the cephalocaudal progression during development. From birth to 12 to 16 months, the sensation to touch and feel becomes stronger. The reactions of the infant become more specific and precise during this time (**2, 14**).

At birth the visual function is poor, and the eyes are small and hyperopic. The adult or mature size of the eyes is attained at approximately 12–14 years. Visual acuity, however, improves from about 20/70 at 2 years to 20/30 at 5 years and to 20/20 at approximately 7 years of age (**2, 15**).

The sensation of hearing is present in the infant as soon as the amniotic fluid is cleared from the ear. The auditory sense is acute within a few days after birth, and by 6 months, the infant can focus on the origin of sound and can distinguish familiar sounds and voices (**2**).

The capacity to taste is present at birth and is well established by 2–3 months. At that point in his or her development, the infant can detect differences in the taste of foods (**2, 14**).

Circulatory System

The heart grows very slowly during the initial four months of gestation but more rapidly after that. Little change occurs in the heart during the first 6 weeks after birth, but then growth becomes steady (**2**). By the end of the first year, the heart doubles in size and increases by a factor of 4 by age 5 and by a factor of 6 by age 9. Although certain components change with age, all the normal elements of heart function are present at 5 weeks of fetal age (**16**). The heart rate declines from about 140 at birth to about 80 at age 14–18 (Table 5.2), but blood pressure increases with age (Table 5.3).

Arteries and veins grow and develop in response to the body areas they serve.

The total blood volume does not change much in relation to body weight throughout life, although there is a general decrease in volume per weight. The normal range in the infant is 80–110 ml/kg body weight. Blood volume declines to 75–90 ml/kg in the older infant and child and to 70–85 ml/kg in the adult.

Hemopoietic System

Development of the various components of the blood is important to the health and well-being of the infant and child. In the fetal period, a gradual rise is seen in the numbers of red blood cells and in the amount of hemoglobin. Both components fall to a low point at 2–3 months of age and then increase to adult levels (**2, 17**).

Hemoglobin has a different structure in the young and is known as "fetal" hemoglobin, this structural difference causing a greater affinity for oxygen.

TABLE 5.2 AVERAGE RESTING HEART RATES FOR INFANTS AND CHILDREN

Age	Average rate
Birth	140
First month	130
1–6 months	130
6–12 months	115
1–2 years	110
2–4 years	105
6–10 years	95
10–14 years	85
14–18 years	82

Source: Reproduced with permission from Growth and Development of Children, 7th edition, by G. H. Lowrey (**2**). Copyright © 1978 by Year Book Medical Publishers, Inc., Chicago.

TABLE 5.3 AVERAGE NORMAL BLOOD PRESSURE FOR INFANTS AND CHILDREN

Age (years)	Systolic	2 SD[1]	Diastolic	2 SD
1	96	30	65	25
2	99	25	65	25
4	99	20	65	20
6	100	15	60	10
8	105	15	60	10
10	110	17	60	10
12	115	19	60	10
14	118	20	60	10
16	120	16	65	10

Source: Reproduced with permission from Growth and Development of Children, 7th edition, by G. H. Lowrey (**2**). Copyright © 1978 by Year Book Medical Publishers, Inc., Chicago.
[1]Standard deviation.

"Adult" hemoglobin appears during gestation, and the relative percentages change quickly following birth. At birth the ratio of fetal : adult hemoglobin is about 80 : 20, but the proportion is 5 : 95 at 20 weeks of age (**18**). The average values for the concentration of red blood cells, hemoglobin, and for the volume of cells in the blood are summarized in Table 5.4.

The blood provides the circulatory means to transport a wide variety of essential nutrients, metabolites, enzymes, and hormones throughout the body. These are normal constituents of blood and reflect the functions of the essential systems of the body. A comparison of these normal constituents reflects, also, the growth and development of the human organism from birth to maturity (Table 5.5).

TABLE 5.4 AVERAGE NORMAL BLOOD VALUES AT DIFFERENT AGES

Age (years)	Red cells (million/cmm)[1]	Hemoglobin (g/100 ml)	Hematocrit (ml/100 ml)
1	4.5	11.2	35.0
2	4.6	11.5	35.5
3	4.5	12.5	36.0
4	4.6	12.6	37.0
5	4.6	12.6	37.0
6–10	4.8	12.9	37.5
11–15	4.8	13.4	39.0
Adults, female	4.8 ± 0.6	14.0 ± 2.0	42.0 ± 5.0
Adults, male	5.4 ± 0.8	16.0 ± 2.0	47.0 ± 5.0

Source: From Wintrobe (**17**). Reprinted with permission from Clinical Hematology, 7th edition, by M. M. Wintrobe (**17**). Copyright © 1974 by Lea & Febiger, Philadelphia.
[1]Cubic millimeter.

TABLE 5.5 NORMAL VALUES FOR CONSTITUENTS OF BLOOD[1]

Substance	Premature	Neonate	Infant	5–15 years
Aldolase, IU	(6.0–18.0)	(7.2–20.0)	(3.6–10.0)	(1.8–4.9)
Ammonia, mcg/100 ml	(100–250)	(90–100)	(45–80)	(45–80)
Urea Nitrogen, mg/100 ml	(20–47)	19 (10–30)	(6–20)	(6–15)
Nonprotein nitrogen, mg/100 ml	(24–63)	45 (25–62)	35 (25–45)	(25–35)
Uric acid, mg/100 ml	3.25	3.5 (2.7–5.1)	3.0	3.0
Amino acid nitrogen, mg/100 ml		(3.0–4.0)	(3.0–4.5)	(3.0–4.5)
Creatinine, mg/100 ml	(0.5–3.0)	(1.0–2.0)	(1.0–2.0)	(1.0–2.0)
Serum protein, gm/100 ml	5.6 (4.5–6.0)	6.1 (5.0–6.9)	5.9 (5.0–6.6)	(6.5–8.0)
Albumin	(2.5–3.5)	(3.0–4.5)	(3.8–5.0)	(4.5–6.0)
Globulin	(1.0–2.2)	(1.3–2.4)	(1.4–2.4)	(2.0–3.0)
Gamma globulin	(0.5–0.9)	(0.8–1.0)	(0.3–0.6)	(0.9–1.3)
Fibrinogen	0.4	(0.2–0.4)	(0.2–0.4)	(0.2–0.4)
Glucose (fasting), mg/100 ml	(27–90)	(47–102)	(70–120)	(70–120)
Total lipids, mg/100 ml		(100–600)	470	(500–700)
Cholesterol, mg/100 ml	(45–100)	(45–170)	(70–180)	(130–240)
Electrolytes, mEq/l				
Total base	159 (152–171)	153 (148–160)	152	152
Sodium	(138–159)	144	144	144
Potassium	(4.0–7.0)	(4.0–7.0)	(4.0–5.5)	(4.0–5.5)
Chloride	(104–120)	(102–110)	(100–107)	(100–107)
Bicarbonate	(12.7–25.3)	(18–27)	(23–28)	(23–28)
Serum calcium, mg/100 ml	(7.8–9.0)	(8.0–10.0)	(10–12)	(10–12)
Serum phosphorus, mg/100 ml	(6.0–8.5)	(6.5–8.5)	6.0	5.0
Phosphatase, Bodansky units	—	(7–10)	(9–15)	(5–13)
Serum bilirubin, mg/100 ml	(1.5–7.5)	(1.4–6.0)	(0.2–0.8)	(0.2–0.8)

Lactic acid, mg/100 ml	(15–30)	17	10	10
Protein-bound iodine, µg/100 ml[2]	(5–10)	(5–10)	(4.5–9.0)	(4.0–8.0)
17-ketosteroids, µg/100 ml	—	(60–300)	(0–50)	(0–120)[3]
17-OH (hydroxy) steroids, mcg/100 ml	—	(5–10)	(5–15)	(5–15)
Iron, serum, mcg/100 ml	—	(60–140)	(30–90)	(50–100)
Lactate dehydrogenase, IU	—	(308–1500)	(200–800)	(100–180)
Phospholipids, mcg/ml	—	(1.0–1.8)	(2.0–3.5)	(2.4–4.4)
Transaminase				
SGOT,[4] units	—	(10–120)	(5–50)	(5–45)
SGPT,[5] units	—	(10–90)	(5–50)	(5–50)

Source: Reproduced with permission from Growth and Development of Children, 7th edition, by G. H. Lowrey (2). Copyright © 1978 by Year Book Medical Publishers, Inc., Chicago.

[1]Average figures are given as a single value; the range is enclosed in parentheses. Data from various sources and the Pediatric Laboratory, University of Michigan, East Lansing.
[2]µg represents microgram.
[3]The higher levels are found during and after adolescence.
[4]SGOT = Serum glutamic oxaloacetic transaminase.
[5]SGPT = Serum glutamic pyruvate transaminase.

Lymphatic System

The lymphatic system follows a unique pattern as the number of lymph nodes and the amount of lymphoid tissue increase steadily to puberty and then are reduced to adult levels or sizes. Development of the lymphatic system occurs with the maximal incidence of acute infections, both respiratory and alimentary. The increase occurs also during the period of maximum growth in height and weight.

By the fourth month of fetal life, the spleen has the general structural characteristics of the adult spleen. At birth it is larger in relation to body size than at any other time, and as growth continues, the weight of the spleen increases by about 12 times to adult size. The spleen does not, however, like other components of the lymphatic system, atrophy during adult life. The major functions of the spleen are to produce immunoglobulins and to depress growth of invading bacteria. Both these functions are most important in the early years (**2**).

During the initial 6 months of infancy, the thymus doubles its original weight of about 12−15 g and triples its weight by seven years. The thymus atrophies after puberty.

Generally, lymphoid tissues function to protect the entire system through the formation of antibodies and through the filtering of toxic substances from the circulation. During infancy and childhood, the lymphoid tissues respond to infection by rapid swelling and hyperplasia.

Respiratory System

The larynx is about one-third of its mature size at birth and, in relation to other body parts, is larger than at maturity (**2**).

The lungs grow and develop in relation to general body size. Breathing is initiated when the maternal oxygen supply to the fetus is interrupted, and within 30 minutes after birth, the lungs have most of their total capacity and are free of fluids. During infancy, the rate and depth of breathing are variable, but respiration rates stabilize with subsequent development (Table 5.6).

Digestive System

Parts of the digestive system mature at different rates. Salivary glands attain maturity at approximately the third month of life, increasing in weight until the child is about 2 years old. At this point, the glands are similar histologically to the adult (**15**).

From birth until age 10−12 years the position of the stomach changes and attains adult shape and position. The capacity of the stomach is limited by distension capacity: at birth, 30−90 ml; at 1 month, 90−150 ml; at 1 year, 210−360 ml; at 2 years, 500 ml; and in late childhood, 750−900 ml (**2, 15**).

The small intestine is approximately 300−350 centimeters (cm) in length in the newborn, increasing by 50 percent during the first year and doubling in length by puberty (**15**). Parts of the large intestine are relative in size to the adult throughout the period of growth and development.

The liver of the infant is immature physiologically, compared to the adult. The lobulated structure is poorly developed at birth but is completely developed in early childhood (**2**).

TABLE 5.6 RESPIRATION RATE, TIDAL AIR
AND VITAL CAPACITY IN INFANTS AND CHILDREN

Age	Rate/minute	Tidal air (cc)[1]	Vital capacity (liters)[2]
Premature	40–90	12	—
Newborn	30–80	19	—
1 year	20–40	48	—
2 year	20–30	90	—
3 year	20–30	125	—
5 year	20–25	175	1.0
10 year	17–22	320	2.0
15 year	15–20	400	3.7
20 year	15–20	500	3.8

Source: Reproduced with permission from *Growth and Development of Children,* 7th edition, by G. H. Lowrey (**2**). Copyright © 1978 by Year Book Medical Publishers, Inc., Chicago.
[1]Cubic centimeters.
[2]These represent mean figures from several sources for both sexes. Vital capacity for boys averages about 6 percent greater than for girls.

Urinary System and Water Balance

Several systems aid, affect, or influence the kidney. Among these are the lungs, the pituitary, adrenal cortex, and other systems involved in the control of water and electrolyte balance (**2**).

The extracellular fluid volume of the newborn is significantly larger than that of the adult. The relative percentage, expressed as a percentage of total body water, is 43 versus 25 percent in the adult. The extracellular fluid volume, however, decreases during two periods of rapid growth: early infancy and adolescence.

TABLE 5.7 AVERAGE
DAILY SECRETIONS OF URINE
IN INFANTS AND CHILDREN

Age	Ml/24 hours
1 and 2 days	15–50
3–10 days	50–300
10 days–2 months	250–400
2 months–1 year	400–500
1–3 years	500–600
3–5 years	600–750
5–8 years	700–1000
8–14 years	700–1500

Source: Reproduced with permission from *Growth and Development of Children,* 7th edition, by G. H. Lowrey (**2**). Copyright © 1978 by Year Book Medical Publishers, Inc., Chicago.

Exchange of fluid is more rapid in the infant than in the adult, with an excretion in the range of 600–700 ml per day, representing about 20 percent of total body fluids and about 50 percent of extracellular fluids. Daily urinary excretion is approximately 2000 ml or about five percent of total body fluids in the adult. Water loss is less effectively controlled during infancy, thus severe dehydration, particularly during illnesses, is more likely than in the older child or adult (**2**). Average daily secretions of urine are summarized in Table 5.7. Most kidney functions attain mature status by 1 year of age, and the kidney continues to increase in size to the time of puberty.

The following provides information about the usual changes in weights of different organs. Changes in weight or size reflect generally increasing functions and maturity of each system or organ (Table 5.8).

TABLE 5.8   AVERAGE WEIGHTS OF
ORGANS AT DIFFERENT AGES (WEIGHTS IN GRAMS)

	Newborn	1 year	6 years	Puberty	Adult
Brain	350	910	1200	1300	1350
Heart	24	45	95	150	300
Thymus	12	20	24	30	0–15
Kidneys (both)	25	70	120	170	300
Liver	150	300	550	1500	1600
Lungs (both)	60	130	260	410	1200
Pancreas	3	9	—	40	90
Spleen	10	30	55	95	155
Stomach	8	30	—	80	135

Source: Reproduced with permission from *Growth and Development of Children,* 7th edition, by G. H. Lowrey (**2**). Copyright © 1978 by Year Book Medical Publishers, Inc., Chicago.

GROWTH STANDARDS

Several growth standards have been developed and are in use now. Most of the standards, however, are not generally representative of the population, since they are based on relatively few subjects from particular or special population groups (**19**). Thus use of a specific growth chart may lead the inexperienced person to incorrect conclusions. Continued use of any given standard, though, permits a fairly realistic assessment of growth as the user attains a feeling for the particular standard or growth curve in relation to the population being served or assessed.

The most appropriate curves for assessing growth of infants, children, and youth in the United States appear to be those recently developed by the National Center for Health Statistics (**20**). These guidelines are based on representative samples of the U.S. population and the general consensus of experts in nutrition, pediatrics, and physical growth. These growth curves provide reliable, recent guides for assessing growth and physical development and should assist in the identification of infants and children with abnormalities affecting growth and development.

Growth curves were developed for two age ranges: (1) birth to 36 months and (2) 2½−18 years, with different curves for males and females. Further, the growth patterns were divided into seven percentile groups based on observed data.

Use of Growth Charts

Effective use of the growth curves in assessing growth and development of infants and children requires an understanding of the measures and a realistic interpretation of these measures by the user.

Measurements should be made in the same manner as the base or reference data were obtained. Each measure must be carefully checked and confirmed, since, when dealing with a growing child, the information cannot be rechecked later. Also, it is essential to know the exact chronological age of the child, since most measures are related to age.

The growth charts developed by the National Center for Health Statistics are based on the following type of information: from birth to 36 months the weights represent nude weights, and the length is recumbent, not standing, and without shoes (see Figure 5.8).

This recumbent length is greater than standing height by as much as 2 cm, or 1 in., in younger children. At age 4−5 years, the difference is about 1 cm or ½ in. Recumbent length is measured using a table or special board with either wood

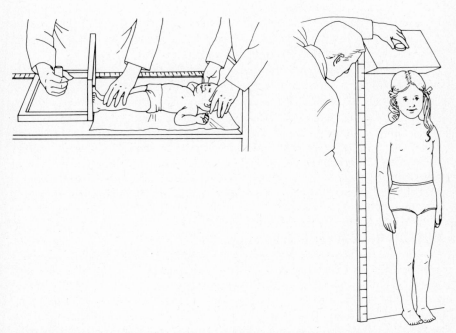

Figure 5.8 *Measurements of the recumbent length of the infant and standing height of the child. (Source:* Reproduced from the Public Health Service, Center for Disease Control, 1974, Atlanta, Georgia.)

or metal tape calibrated in millimeters and one-quarter inch increments. A movable foot piece that remains vertical to the scale or tape permits accurate measurement of the infant and younger child (**21**).

In children from 2 to 18 years height is measured in socks but not shoes. The appropriate way to measure standing height is to stand the child on a horizontal flat surface with the heels almost touching. The back is straight with heels, buttocks, and shoulders touching the wall on which a measuring stick or tape is mounted. A block is placed on the crown of the head to make the measurement of height (**19, 22**).

Weights of children are taken in light garments, without shoes, the clothing weighing from 0.05 kg at age 2 to 0.3 kg at age 18. The individual user may desire to check weights of the so-called "reference" clothing or evaluate each child under similar conditions over a period of time.

The following provides the growth and development curves for males and females and for the two age groupings used by the National Center for Health Statistics.

Interpretation of Growth Charts

The timing of specific changes and growth is unique for each child, although the pattern of growth and development follows a general trend. The growth charts (Figures 5.9−5.16) provide general guides for assessing growth in terms of height (or length), weight, weight for height, and head circumference. These charts are useful in plotting growth data for individual children in relation to general trends. Knowing that the child is tall or short is not as important as recognizing that the child is maintaining a relatively consistent distribution, weight for height, and is not shifting across percentiles of height and weight (**19, 21**).

Infants and children who are in the twenty-fifth to seventy-fifth percentile are probably normal in growth and development. Those who are between the tenth and twenty-fifth or between the seventy-fifth and ninetieth percentile may or may not be normal. Factors such as genetics, nutrition, and environment may be significantly influencing the growth of these children. Particularly significant, though, are shifts in percentile. These may be indicative of medical and/or nutrition problems and erratic growth. For example, a child usually in the sixty-fifth percentile but found to be in the fortieth percentile at an annual physical examination should be checked further for potential or real physiological problems (**23**).

Useful Physical Measurements

Several physical measures or calculations are useful in evaluating the growth and development of infants and children. Some common ones, other than height and weight, are discussed in the following sections.

Head circumference is an important measure in the infant, for it may indicate development and growth of the brain. This measure is also useful in diagnosing either micro- or macrocephaly (also hydrocephaly). Relatively small variations exist in the head circumference of most infants under normal cir-

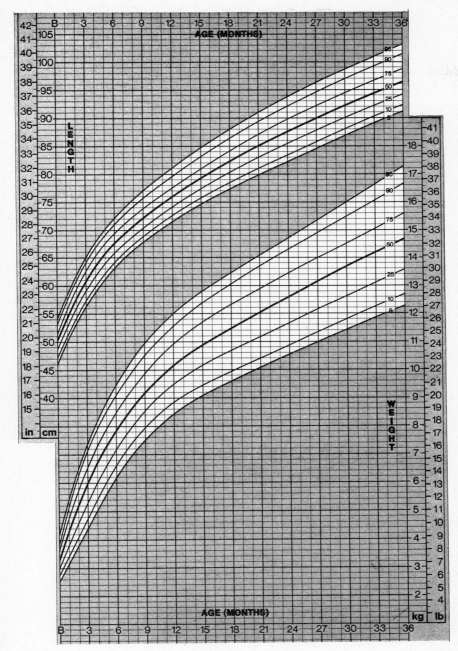

Figure 5.9 *Heights and weights of boys from birth to 36 months.* (*Source:* Reproduced from the National Center for Health Statistics [20].)

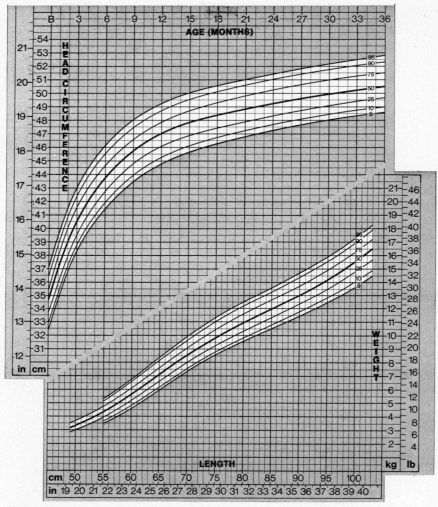

Figure 5.10 *Head circumference and weight for height of boys from birth to 36 months.* (*Source:* Reproduced from the National Center for Health Statistics [20].)

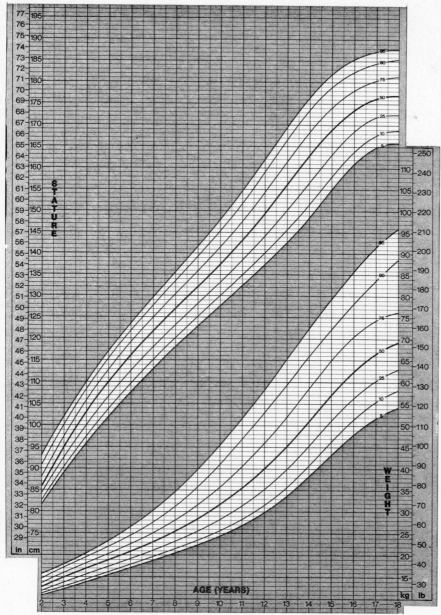

Figure 5.11 *Heights and weights of boys, 2 to 18 years. (Source:* Reproduced from the National Center for Health Statistics [**20**].)

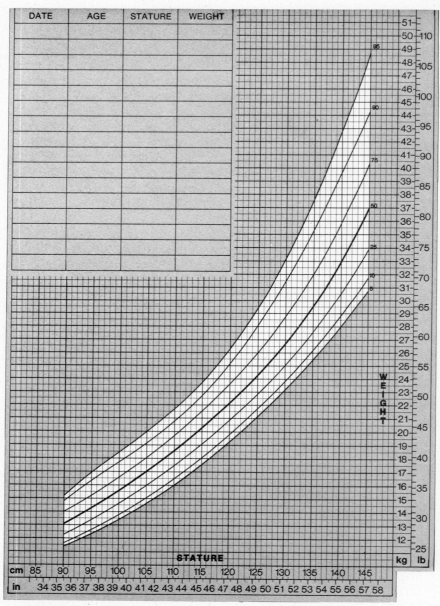

Figure 5.12 *Weight for height for boys. (Source:* Reproduced from the National Center for Health Statistics [20].)

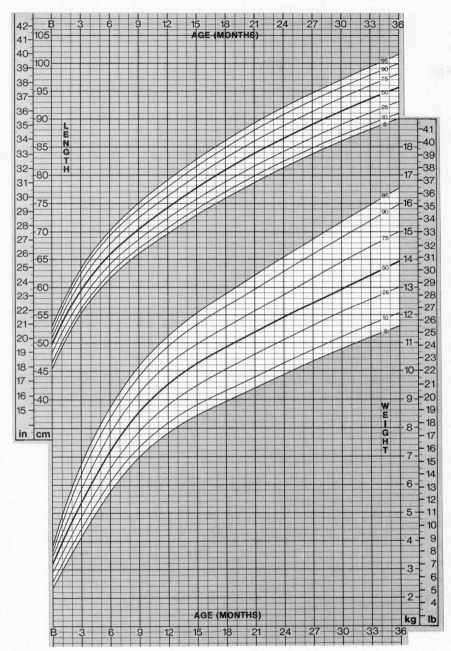

Figure 5.13 *Heights and weights of girls from birth to 36 months. (Source:* Reproduced from the National Center for Health Statistics **[20]**.)

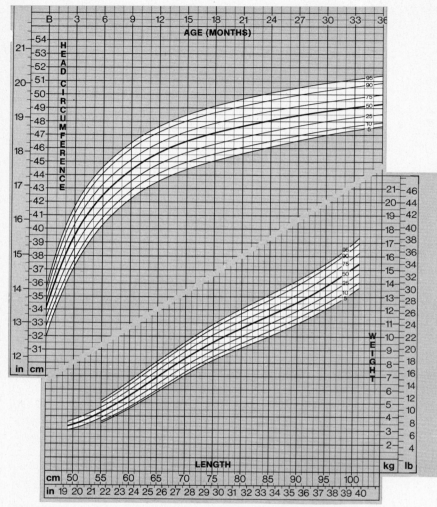

Figure 5.14 *Head circumference and weight for height of girls from birth to 36 months.* (*Source:* Reproduced from the National Center for Health Statistics [20].)

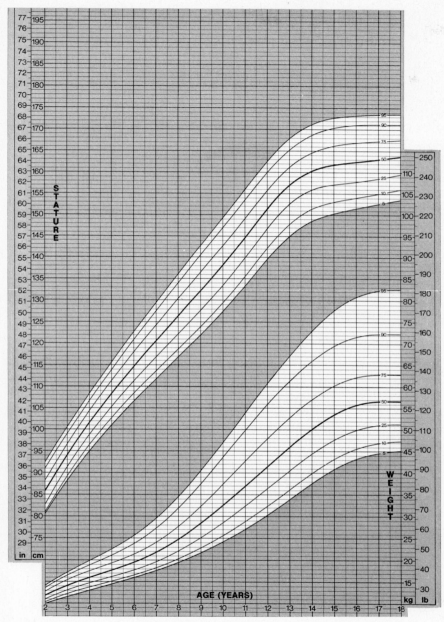

Figure 5.15 *Heights and weights of girls, 2 to 18 years.* (*Source:* Reproduced from the National Center for Health Statistics [**20**].)

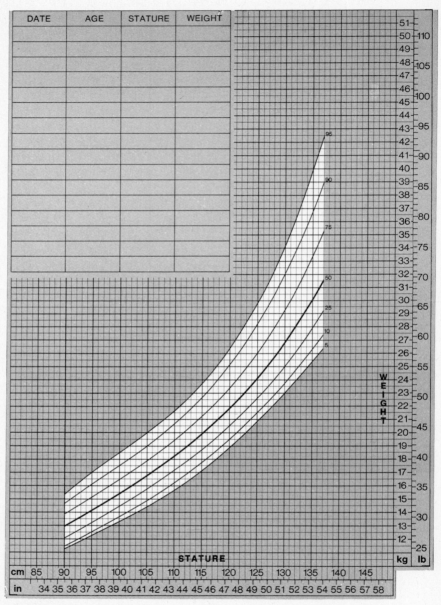

Figure 5.16 *Weight for height for girls.* (*Source:* Reproduced from the National Center for Health Statistics [20].)

cumstances, affected only slightly by race or geographic origin. The average head circumferences of American children are given in Table 5.9, and normal data may be found also in Figures 5.10 (males) and 5.14 (females). This indicates that males usually have a larger head circumstance than females. It is fairly well documented that children with head circumferences below 2 standard deviations (SD) of the mean or approximately in the lower 2 or 3 percent have some degree of mental retardation (**24**). Exceptions to this generalization would include infants with birth defects that result in poor growth.

Head circumference is measured by passing a tape over the most prominent part of the occiput and above the supraorbital ridges (**2**) (Figure 5.17). This occipitofrontal diameter provides an estimate of the degree of maturity at birth (**2**). Further changes in the shape of the head from birth to maturity are significant (Figure 5.17).

"Sitting height," the height of the upper portion of the body that is measured while sitting erect, is an indication of changes in body proportions. At birth, it represents about 70 percent of total height. This figure decreases as the lower part of the body, including the legs, catches up. In the adult, sitting height is approximately 50 percent of total height.

TABLE 5.9 AVERAGE HEAD CIRCUMFERENCES OF AMERICAN CHILDREN

Age	Mean In.	Mean Cm	Standard deviation In.	Standard deviation Cm
Birth	13.8	35	0.5	1.2
1 month	14.9	37.6	0.5	1.2
2 months	15.5	39.7	0.5	1.2
3 months	15.9	40.4	0.5	1.2
6 months	17.0	43.4	0.4	1.1
9 months	17.8	45.0	0.5	1.2
12 months	18.3	46.5	0.5	1.2
18 months	19.0	48.4	0.5	1.2
2 years	19.2	49.0	0.5	1.2
3 years	19.6	50.0	0.5	1.2
4 years	19.8	50.5	0.5	1.2
5 years	20.0	50.8	0.6	1.4
6 years	20.2	51.2	0.6	1.4
7 years	20.5	51.6	0.6	1.4
8 years	20.6	52.0	0.8	1.8
10 years	20.9	53.0	0.6	1.4
12 years	21.0	53.2	0.8	1.8
14 years	21.5	54.0	0.8	1.8
16 years	21.9	55.0	0.8	1.8
18 years	22.1	55.4	0.8	1.8
20 years	22.2	55.6	0.8	1.8

Source: Reproduced with permission from *Growth and Development of Children*, 7th edition, by G. H. Lowrey (**2**). Copyright © 1978 by Year Book Medical Publishers, Inc., Chicago.

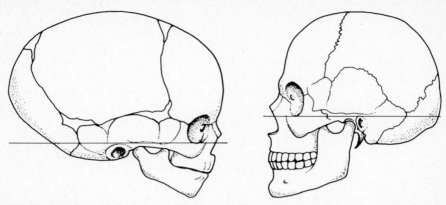

Figure 5.17 *Skull of infant (left) and an adult drawn to the same scale. Horizontal line crosses the same bony landmark. (Source:* Reproduced with permission from *Growth and Development of Children,* 7th edition, by G. H. Lowrey. Copyright © 1978 by Year Book Medical Publishers, Inc., Chicago.)

The "width-length index," the pelvic bicristal diameter divided by standing height, is a fairly reliable guide for estimating body build. The index decreases gradually from birth to puberty in boys but increases prior to puberty in girls (Table 5.10), indicating the eventual body changes at puberty (**2, 25**).

Lean Body Mass

Lean body mass represents the bulk of active metabolic tissue of the body. It excludes nonessential fatty or adipose tissue but includes the fat present with normal tissue development. It also includes the skeleton, muscle, and organs. Lean body mass increases throughout the growth period, but the change or

TABLE 5.10 WIDTH-LENGTH INDEX FOR MALES AND FEMALES FROM BIRTH TO PUBERTY

Age	Boys	Girls
Under 1 year	0.173	0.175
1 year	0.168	0.172
3 years	0.166	0.168
5 years	0.161	0.161
7 years	0.159	0.159
9 years	0.157	0.159
11 years	0.157	0.161
13 years	0.156	0.163
15 years	0.155	0.164

Source: Reprinted with permission from W. P. Lucas and H. B. Pryor, *Journal of Pediatrics 6,* 533, 1935 (**25**). Copyright © 1935 by C. V. Mosby Co., St. Louis, Missouri.

increase is much more dramatic in the male during the adolescent growth spurt (**26**). Until that time, the lean body mass is similar for the sexes (Figure 5.18).

Cessation of Growth

It is difficult to know when growth has ceased. Height is a useful, and easy to obtain, index, although others, such as lean body mass, will also provide information (Table 5.11). The usual age (fiftieth percentile) is about 21 years for males and 17 years for females, but considerable variation exists for both sexes (**27**).

Obese Children

Children who are obese are not typical of the average or normal child, since the obese child does not have the typical growth spurts. In some respects, the growth spurt of an obese child, particularly the accumulation of adipose cells, is a continuous one.

Fat depots develop differently in the obese child, and these differences are apparent by age 2. The obese child has significantly more and larger adipose cells than the nonobese child. Thus both the numbers and size of adipose cells are involved and develop differently in obese and nonobese children (**28**). Adipose cell numbers are shown in Figure 5.19 and cell size in Figure 5.20 as they relate to age.

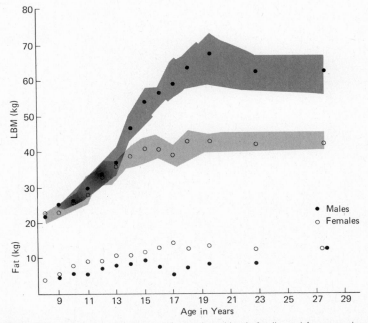

Figure 5.18 *Changes in lean body mass (upper) and body fat (lower) for normal males (●) and females (O) during the adolescent growth spurt and early adulthood. Points are at the fiftieth percentile; shaded areas indicate the twenty-fifth and seventy-fifth percentiles.* (*Source:* Reproduced with permission from G. B. Forbes in *Growth 36,* 325, 1972. Copyright © 1972 by Growth Publishing Company, Lakeland, Florida.)

TABLE 5.11   CHRONOLOGICAL AGE AT WHICH
GROWTH IN HEIGHT CEASED IN MALES AND FEMALES

	Percentiles		
	Tenth	Fiftieth	Ninetieth
Males (years)	18.4	21.2	23.5
Females (years)	15.8	17.3	21.1

Source: Reprinted with permission from A. F. Roche and
G. H. Davila, *Pediatrics 50,* 875, 1972 (**27**). Copyright ©
1972 by American Academy of Pediatrics, Boston, Massachusetts.

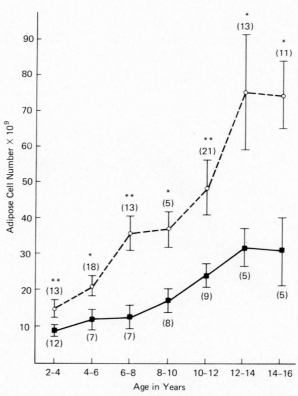

Figure 5.19 *Adipose cell number in relation to obese (○) and nonobese (■) children.
Groups are significantly different where asterisks are placed.* (*Source:* Reproduced with
permission from J. L. Knittle in *Nutrient Requirements in Adolescence,* eds. J. I. McKigney
and H. N. Munro. Copyright © 1976 by the MIT Press, Massachusetts Institute of
Technology, Cambridge, Massachusetts.)

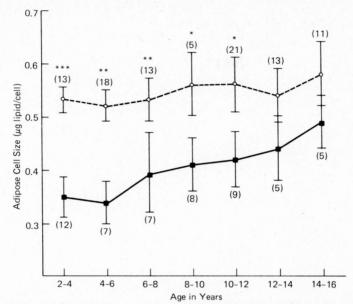

Figure 5.20 *Adipose cell size in obese (○) and nonobese (■) children. Asterisks indicate that groups are significantly different. (Source:* Reproduced with permission from J. L. Knittle in *Nutrient Requirements in Adolescence,* eds. J. I. McKigney and H. N. Munro. Copyright © 1976 by the MIT Press, Massachusetts Institute of Technology, Cambridge, Massachusetts.)

Two physical measures provide an indication of the trend toward obesity in the growing child (**21**). The fatfold is regarded by some as superior to the parameters of weight for age or weight for height in assessing obesity. It is usually measured using the left triceps and the left subscapular regions. The left triceps is used when only one measure is to be made. Because of the difficulties in measuring skinfolds or fatfolds, two measures are made at each site and an average value calculated. Accurate, dependable calipers are available for the purpose of measuring fatfolds.

Measuring the circumference of the arm, when combined with the triceps fatfold, provides a method to quantitate muscle fat and fat bulk. Arm circumference is measured at the midpoint of the upper left arm, with the arm hanging loosely by the side of the subject and using a metal, fiberglass, or laminated tape. For precision, tapes that stretch should be avoided. The following (Table 5.12) may be used as a guide to assess obesity in children.

From age 2 to ages 12–14, the obese child experiences a rapid increase in the number of adipose cells but not a significant enlargement in cell size. No significant changes occur in the nonobese child in either cell number or size from ages 2–10. Increases are seen, however, in both number and size of adipose

TABLE 5.12 APPROXIMATE LIMITS FOR MID-UPPER ARM CIRCUMFERENCE AND TRICEPS SKINFOLD

Age	Arm Circumference (Third to Fifth Percentile)[1]		Triceps Fatfold (mm) (Ninetieth to Ninety-seventh Percentile)[2]	
	In.	Cm	Boys	Girls
Birth	3.5	9	10	10
3 months	4	10	11	11
6 months	4.5	11.5	12	12
9 months	5	12	13	13
12 months	5	13	14	14
2 years	5	13	13	13
3 years	5	13	13	13
4 years	5.25	13.5	13	13
5 years	5.25	13.5	13	13
6 years	5.5	14	12	15
7 years	5.5	14	13	16
8 years	5.75	14.5	14	17
9 years	6	15	14	18
10 years	6.5	16	16	20
11 years	6.5	16.5	17	21
12–16 years	7–8	17–20	18–20	22–25

Source: Reprinted with permission from A. J. Zerfas and C. G. Neumann, *Pediatric Clinics of North America 24,* 253, 1977 (**21**). Copyright © 1977 by W. B. Saunders Co., Philadelphia.
[1]Values below these suggest undernutrition.
[2]Values above these suggest obesity.

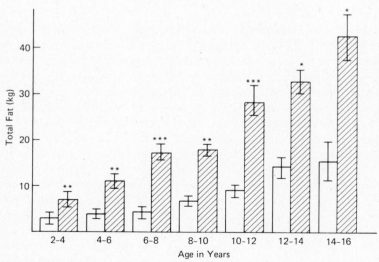

Figure 5.21 *Fat depots of obese (shaded bars) and nonobese (open bars) children. Asterisks indicate that groups are significantly different. (Source:* Reproduced with permission from J. L. Knittle in *Nutrient Requirements in Adolescence,* eds. J. I. McKigney and H. N. Munro. Copyright © 1976 by the MIT Press, Massachusetts Institute of Technology, Cambridge, Massachusetts.)

cells after age 10. The proliferation of cells appears to be the major problem in the development of obesity (**28**). The obese have a greater number of adipose cells at all ages (Figure 5.21). By 10–12 years of age, the obese child may have numbers of cells that exceed those in the nonobese adult. Even by age 6, some obese children have cell numbers that are greater than those of normal adults. The accumulation of fat depots are significantly greater in the obese child (Figure 5.21), that is, in those who exceed their "ideal" weight by 30 percent or more.

SUMMARY

The growth and development of the child during the postnatal period are as dependent on environmental influences as they are during prenatal life. Following birth the growth rate declines as the infant adapts to the new environment. It then accelerates for a time, slows during childhood, and accelerates again during adolescence. The development or increase in complexity and functional capacity of organs and systems continues to maturity.

Muscle fibers increase in both number and size during the early postnatal period, with maximum growth occurring relatively late, following the attainment of maximum height. Bone growth is a valuable indicator of physical development in the individual. Brain growth is rapid from birth through early childhood, and by age 7 the human brain has reached 90 percent of its potential development. Sensory characteristics, including touch, sight, hearing, and taste, develop at different rates following birth. The growth of the heart is continuous from about 6 weeks following birth to age 9. The lymphatic system follows a unique pattern of growth, increasing in size to puberty and then decreasing to the adult level. The lungs continue to grow and develop in relation to body size. Different parts of the digestive system grow and mature at different rates.

Each child follows his or her own unique pattern of growth and development. The patterns do follow a general trend, however; and growth charts provide general guides for assessing growth in terms of height, weight, and weight for height. Children whose measurements fall in the twenty-fifth to seventy-fifth percentile range according to these charts are probably growing and developing in a normal fashion. Children whose measurements fall outside these ranges may be, but are not necessarily, abnormal in growth.

Several growth standards are in general use to evaluate growth and development in children. The growth curves developed by the National Center for Health Statistics appear to be appropriate for assessing the growth of infants, children, and youth in the United States. The effective use of these growth charts requires an understanding of the measures used and a realistic interpretation of the statistics. Measures are also available to assess the tendency toward obesity in children.

This chapter has explored normal growth and development and commonly accepted criteria used to evaluate growth and development. Various nutritional aspects of the growing years are discussed in detail in following chapters.

STUDY QUESTIONS AND TOPICS FOR INDIVIDUAL INVESTIGATION

1. Choose one of the organs or systems in the body—for example, enzyme systems, muscle, skeletal system, central nervous system, sensory characteristics—mentioned in this chapter. Trace the organ's or system's growth and development from birth to maturity. When are the most rapid changes occurring? Why is proper nutrition vital during those times when very rapid growth is occurring?
2. Look at the following data. Using the appropriate growth chart, decide whether the child is growing normally.

NAME	AGE	SEX	WEIGHT (kg)	HEIGHT (cm)
Rose	4.2 months	F	3.81	59.5
Steve	22.4 months	M	6.32	72.0
Ann	18.0 months	F	23.10	79.5
John	10.0 years	M	35.0	141.0

Can you make a diagnosis of nutritional status using only weight and height measures? If you cannot, please explain. What additional information should you have?
3. If possible visit a local school. Choose one class. Make height and weight measures on each child. Do the children all fall into the normal range according to the growth charts presented in this chapter? Determine the variability within the class.
4. Are growth charts such as those developed by the National Center for Health Statistics a useful guideline and/or an absolute criteria for judging the nutritional status of infants and children? Explain the answer you give.

REFERENCES

1. Timiras, P. S., and T. Valcana. Body growth. In: *Developmental Physiology and Aging,* ed. P. S. Timiras. Macmillan, New York, 1972.
2. Lowrey, G. H. *Growth and Development of Children,* 7th ed. Year Book Medical Publishers, Chicago, 1978.
3. Laird, A. K. Evaluation of the human growth curve. *Growth,* 31:345, 1967.
4. Scannon, R. E. The first seriatrin study of human growth. *American Journal of Physical Anthropology,* 10:329, 1927.
5. Sinclair, D. *Human Growth After Birth.* Oxford University Press, New York, 1969.

6. Harris, J. A., C. M. Jackson, D. G. Paterson, and R. E. Scannon. *The Measurement of Man.* University of Minnesota Press, Minneapolis, 1930.
7. Miller, S. A. Protein metabolism during growth and development. In: *Mammalian Protein Metabolism,* Vol. 3, ed. H. N. Munro. Academic Pess, New York, 1969.
8. Oliver, I. T., and D. Yeung. Enzyme development and nutrition. In: *Nutrition and Development,* ed. M. Winick. Wiley, New York, 1972.
9. Cheek, D. B. *Human Growth.* Lea & Febiger, Philadelphia, 1968.
10. Dreizen, S., C. N. Spirakis, and R. E. Stone. A comparison of skeletal growth and maturation in undernourished and well-nourished girls before and after menarche. *Journal of Pediatrics,* 70:256, 1967.
11. Woolley, P.V., Jr., and R.W. McCammon. Bone growth in congenital myxedemia. *Journal of Pediatrics,* 27:229, 1945.
12. Caffey, J. *Pediatric X-Ray Diagnosis,* 6th ed. Year Book Medical Publishers, Chicago, 1972.
13. Patten, B. M. *Human Embryology,* 3rd ed. McGraw-Hill, New York, 1968.
14. McGraw, M. B. *The Neuromuscular Maturation of the Human Infant.* Columbia University Press, New York, 1943.
15. White House Conference on Child Health and Protection. Growth and Development of the Child. II. Anatomy and Physiology. Prentice-Hall, Englewood Cliffs, N.J., 1933.
16. Windle, W. F. *Physiology of the Fetus.* Saunders, Philadelphia, 1940.
17. Wintrobe, M. M. *Clinical Hematology,* 7th ed. Lea & Febiger, Philadelphia, 1974.
18. Karlberg, P., and J. Lind. Studies of the total amount of hemoglobin and the blood volume in children. *Acta Paediatrics,* 44:17, 1955.
19. Food and Nutrition Board/National Academy of Sciences. Body weights and lengths or heights of children. In: *Present Knowledge in Nutrition,* 4th ed. Nutrition Foundation, Washington, D.C., 1976.
20. Committee on Nutrition Advisory to Center for Disease Control. Comparison of Body Weights and Lengths or Heights of Groups of Children, Public Health Service, Center for Disease Control, Atlanta, Ga., 1974.
21. Zerfas, A. J., and C. G. Neumann. Office assessment of nutritional status. *Pediatric Clinics of North America,* 24:253, 1977.
22. Owen, G. M. The assessment and recording of measurements of growth of children. *Pediatrics,* 51:461, 1973.
23. Hamill, P. U. V., and W. M. Moore. Contemporary Growth Charts: Needs, Construction and Application. *Dietetic Currents 3,* 1976. Ross Laboratories, Columbus, Ohio.
24. Usher, R., F. McLean, and K. E. Scott. Judgment of fetal age. II. Clinical significance of gestational age and an objective method for its assessment. *Pediatric Clinics of North America,* 13:835, 1966.
25. Lucas, W. P., and H. B. Pryor. Range and standard deviation of certain physical measurements in healthy children. *Journal of Pediatrics,* 6:533, 1935.

26. Forbes, G. B. Growth of the lean body mass in man. *Growth,* 36:325, 1972.
27. Roche, A. F., and G. H. Davila. Late adolescent growth in stature. *Pediatrics,* 50:875, 1972.
28. Knittle, J. L. Biological implications of the adolescent growth spurt. In: *Nutrient Requirements in Adolescence,* eds. J. I. McKigney and H. N. Munro. MIT Press, Cambridge, Mass., 1976.

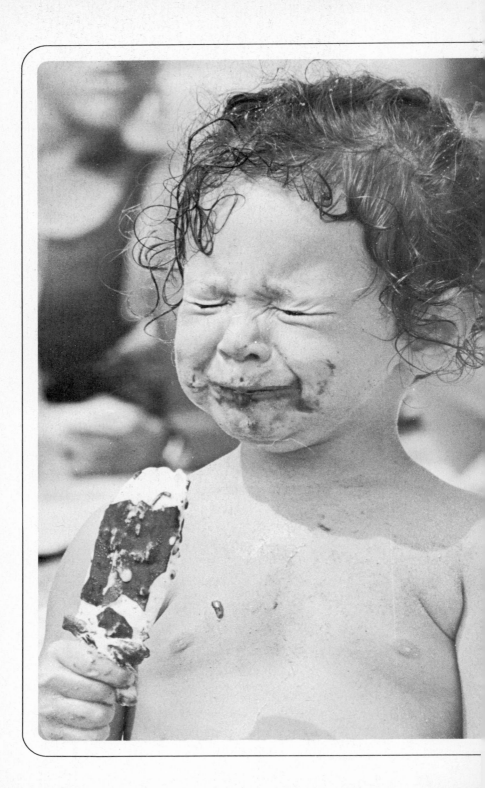

CHAPTER 6

DEVELOPMENT OF FOOD HABITS

Good nutrition is a positive factor affecting the quality of life throughout the entire life cycle and is to a large extent determined by food habits. When does good nutrition begin? Dietary practices developed during infancy and early childhood influence growth and development during the critical early years and determine lifetime eating habits. It is important for the mother to establish good food habits and wholesome attitudes toward food in the child as soon as he or she is born. Food intake patterns for a lifetime begin to take shape during these early years.

The establishment of good food habits is an area of concern to all nutritionists. Why do some children not receive or accept the best nutrition their growing bodies and minds need? Knowledge of the nutritional requirements of the growing child alone is not sufficient to answer this question. We need to know what factors influence food attitudes and practices so that we can encourage the development of habits that will allow us to implement nutrition knowledge and improve the well-being of our children. Psychological, social, and cultural factors often play a greater role in determining food consumption patterns and nutritional status than do biological factors, such as hunger or the physiological need for certain nutrients.

Food habits are the end result of all the experiences people have had with food and all the attitudes, preferences, and dislikes people have developed in relation to food. Food habits are generally classified as good when a person eats the kinds and amounts of food needed for good nutrition. Poor food habits, including eating only what a person likes, regardless of individual nutrient requirements, can result in a poor nutritional status. Food habits, good or bad, however, can be an extremely powerful force in determining what a person eats (**1**). The best way to be well nourished throughout life is to develop food habits and attitudes that are conducive to the selection of a healthy diet. Such food selection habits should begin very early in life (**2**).

THE DEVELOPMENT OF FOOD HABITS IN CHILDREN

The best time to teach good food habits is when the child is young, has a good appetite, and is naturally interested in food (**3**). Eating is one of life's first experiences and is basically instinctive. Infants, toddlers, and preschool children will generally sense that they feel hungry and need food. Infants are not born with food likes or dislikes; they learn to like or dislike certain food. For a relatively long period the infant is entirely dependent on adults for both the type and amount of food he or she eats. It is, therefore, important that the adults responsible for teaching children to develop good eating habits understand the growth and developmental patterns as well as the nutrient needs of infants. Hungry infants will react in a positive manner to food fed in a relaxed atmosphere. In the past the infant's natural rhythms of hunger have not always been relied on to determine his or her eating patterns. These patterns were more or less established under the influence of adult cultural patterns. Yet infants who are kept to an extremely rigid feeding schedule or fed food in amounts that do not satisfy them or in amounts that exceed their needs may develop negative or unhealthy attitudes toward food.

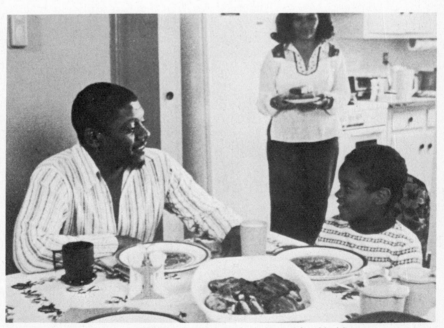

A family environment is appropriate for the teaching of good food habits.

It is best to remember that each infant is an individual and cannot be fed strictly in accordance with any one textbook description. The present trend in infant feeding is to permit the baby to set his or her own feeding schedule based more on individual hunger needs rather than on the adult clock. The daily schedule of the adult who feeds the child must also be taken into consideration, however.

The toddler and preschool child learn by example and experience what to eat and what attitudes to develop toward food. The family setting is the predominant influence on the formation of eating habits in infants, toddlers, and preschool children, although children learn from all sources to which they are exposed (**4, 5**). It is from other family members that the child first learns attitudes, feelings, and habits about food. These parental habits and attitudes toward foods, as well as food preferences and dislikes, will be reflected in the child's habits as he or she develops (**6, 7**). The home is, therefore, extremely valuable in developing and maintaining wholesome attitudes about food and good food habits. Today, however, even very young children are being exposed more and more to outside influences. Child care centers, nursery schools, mass communication, and advertising expose the child to new experiences with the sight, smell, and taste of food and bring new food ideas or patterns into the home. Advertising can be very persuasive in selling foods that may be nonnutritious if consumed in large amounts or at frequent intervals. Parents, however, still play a central role in teaching the child what foods to eat, when to eat, how much to eat, and what feelings to have toward certain foods (**8, 9**). Parental buying habits can also temper the effects of outside influences (**10**). If they are not bought and made available to the child in the home, nonnutritious foods will not be consumed regularly.

Certain characteristics of young children need to be considered if this group is to develop positive attitudes toward food. Parents need to be aware of behavioral and developmental patterns of toddlers and preschoolers if they are to provide a good environment for the development of good food habits. Several papers provide excellent discussions of eating behavior in preschool children (**11, 12**). Eating behavior changes greatly from birth to 6 years of age when appetite can vary considerably from day to day. In general the healthy infant has a good appetite. Toward the end of the first year and during the second year of life the infant may show a drop in appetite corresponding to a slowing of growth rate. The child may show growing independence by choosing not to eat. During this period it is probably best to allow the child to adjust the amounts of food he or she is able to eat at any one time. Remember that because of a smaller digestive capacity, children in this age group may not be able to eat one-third of the day's nutrient requirements at each meal. They may eat smaller meals and wish to snack as they feel hungry between meals. It is better, however, to establish a regularly scheduled snack than to allow continuous snacking. A habit of continual eating, developed in early childhood, could lead to unconscious continual eating and overweight later in life. The 3–4-year-old may dawdle over food but does show an increase in appetite over the previous year and will eat more at a sitting. Each child is an individual, of course, but will generally follow a pattern similar to that of others in his or her age group. By age 6, most children have developed a healthy, stable appetite.

The appearance of food and the way it is prepared and served will influence what the child eats and the feelings developed toward certain foods. Like adults, children prefer colorful foods. The infant and toddler, too, are sensitive to temperature and flavor extremes and are not tempted by either very hot or very cold foods. They also prefer mild-flavored foods as opposed to spicy ones. Simple, unmixed, plain foods will be eaten more readily than will casseroles, creamed foods, or stews. The gastrointestinal tract of the preschool child is often easily irritated by very sweet or rich foods, fried foods, or excessive cellulose. Young children usually prefer crunchy foods such as crackers, raw fruits, and certain vegetables. Gummy foods such as mashed potatoes, slippery foods such as custard, or stringy foods such as celery are often disliked by young children because of their textures. The ability of the child to chew will determine to some extent the texture of foods that will be eaten. Toddlers, for instance, will eat finely chopped vegetables and ground meat. By the time he or she is 4 or 5 years old, the child readily accepts diced vegetables and minced or bite size pieces of tender meats.

Feeding skills will also play a role in determining which foods young children prefer. Between 6 and 7 months of age the infant acquires the ability to grasp objects, so finger foods can be introduced at this stage. Infants grasp with a palmar grasp rather than picking an object up between the thumb and fingers as an older child will. It is, therefore, important to consider the shape of food given to the child for finger food. Plain cookies, crackers, melba toast, and teething biscuits are all good choices. Don't offer an infant sweet cookies or candy bars even if they can be easily grasped. By 1 year of age the child will have developed a more precise grasp and can hold a bottle or cup and begin to manage a spoon. During the second year children refine their eating behavior, but they will still be more skillful with their fingers than with a spoon. Don't offer elusive material such as peas or gelatin desserts during this period. Children will only become frustrated with such food items and may develop negative attitudes toward them. As they progress from the toddler stage to that of the more skilled preschooler, children begin to use a knife and fork with greater ease. They may still like to guide the food with the fingers of the other hand, however. Children at this age still enjoy finger foods. Offer them nutritious choices such as vegetable sticks, fruit sections, and sandwiches. Children will relish these with more enthusiasm than they show for the same foods in forms that require the use of a spoon or fork. Again, do not offer the child candy bars, chips, or other empty calorie foods even if they are easy to manipulate.

Poor food habits often result when food is used in ways in which it is not meant to be used. Children become confused if parents use foods in ways that have nothing to do with hunger. In some homes, for instance, food is used as an instrument of bribery to discipline or reward a child. If they are refused dessert until they eat their vegetables, children receive the message that bad-tasting vegetables are less desirable than good-tasting desserts and are conditioned to

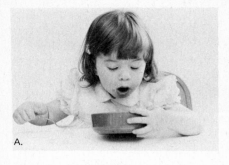
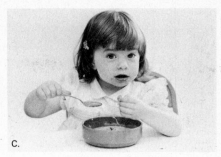
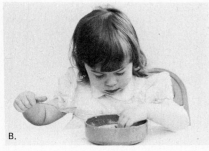
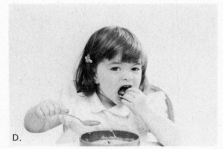

A youngster examining the texture of food.

think that sweets are special. Food should never be used by the parent to reward, bribe, or prove love to a child.

Children learn quickly that one way to gain attention is through the refusal of food, so the best way to overcome undesirable practices before they become habits may be to ignore them. Approval at the right time will teach the child what are favorable attitudes and practices. Children, especially between the ages of 2 and 4, may go on food jags and eat only one food for days at a time. Again, the child outgrows these food quirks more quickly if the parent does not pay special attention to them.

Young children may not always be eager to try new foods. New foods need to be presented in an acceptable way and in a good psychological setting. They should be introduced in small amounts, one at a time, and with foods already familiar to the child. The child may be more motivated to try a food item if other family members seem to enjoy the food. If the child does not want to try a new food the parent should not use force but could try serving the item again in a few days, perhaps prepared in a different way. New foods should preferably be served at the beginning of the meal while the child is still hungry.

Pleasurable eating experiences can help the child understand textures, tastes, colors, and shapes of different foods. Taking children grocery shopping or allowing them to help in the preparation of foods will often stimulate their curiosity about food. Desirable attitudes toward foods and good food habits will not just happen. It is the responsibility of adults to guide children in the development of good food habits. Dietary practices developed during infancy and early child-hood influence growth and development during the critical early years and largely determine lifetime eating habits. Children can be taught to enjoy good nourishing food in amounts adequate to supply essential nutrient and caloric intake to meet individual needs. Children can learn to prefer fruits and vegetables to soft drinks and high sugar snacks. Eating habits are an important part of the child's makeup for life and, therefore, deserve whatever time and effort are needed for them to develop in a desirable manner.

Outside influences play a larger role in the shaping of food habits as children grow older and begin to spend more time away from home. Young children's teachers contribute substantially to their experiences with and de-velopment of attitudes toward foods. Good school food programs can be instrumental in introducing children to a wider variety of food than they may be familiar with in the confines of their homes (**13**). The mass media and peer groups will add to each individual child's knowledge and awareness of the many roles of food in society. The child's food habits will continue to change throughout these early school years as he or she grows in both physical maturity and environmental experiences.

Dwyer, Feldman, and Mayer (**14**); Huenemann (**15**); Huenemann et al. (**16**); and Schorr, Sanjur, and Erickson (**17**) discuss nutrition and food-related con-cerns in the adolescent. It is sometimes believed that eating patterns are fairly well established by the time the child reaches adolescence. Established eating patterns, however, often change during this period of rapid growth and physiolog-ical and emotional change. Changes in food habits at this stage reflect changes in interests and attitudes, including those foods accepted by peer groups. Socializ-ing over a soft drink and snacks may be more important to the teenager than are good food habits. Adolescents may also choose different food patterns to exert their independence or to compensate for many of the conflicts associated with this period of growing up. They also sometimes develop irregular eating habits. If their likes or dislikes for certain foods are strong enough to markedly influence meal selection, adolescents' eating patterns may become so distorted that nutritional inadequacy results. The adolescent is especially vulnerable to poor nutrition habits and is sometimes difficult to reach through conventional nutrition education programs. Many of today's teenagers received a better scientific training in grade school than did previous generations of teenagers. They have been more thoroughly exposed to certain nutrition principles. However, they are also more exposed to the influence of various counter culture components, including advocates of the use of natural, organic, and health foods and countless weight control regimens that "guarantee" to solve concerns about figure control, appearance, and personality. If nutrition knowledge is limited to start with, teenagers can be extremely susceptible to the appeal of groups that promise them success in these areas. Nutrition educators need to be aware of the values teenagers hold in relation to health, nutrition, food, and eating practices. They need to develop teaching methods that will make nutrition information relevant to today's adolescents, provide them with foods they need and like to assure adequate nutrition, and at the same time meet the social needs of this age group (**18**).

FACTORS AFFECTING THE DEVELOPMENT OF FOOD HABITS

Why do people eat as they do? Eating is an activity associated with psychological, social, and cultural factors. These factors may have more influence in determining human food consumption than do biological factors such as hunger or the physiological need for certain nutrients. Food habits are an integral part of every individual's lifestyle and as such have a wide range of personal and social meanings (**19**). Food patterns reflect value systems, age, income, family size, family situation, place of residence, accessibility of food, nature of the food production system, education, religion, tradition, occupation, and social position. All these factors in some way determine food selection and food preference. The following section looks more closely at some of these factors and the ways they influence food patterns and habits.

Food is chosen on the basis of its availability and acceptability. The availability of food is determined to a large extent by the income, geographical setting, and social conditions of the consumer. Physiological, psychological, social, and cultural factors determine the acceptability of foods.

Look at some of the individual factors that affect the availability of food. Income or socioeconomic status is a major factor influencing the availability of food, often meaning the difference between steak or chopped meat for dinner. Increases or decreases in food prices with periods of inflation or recession affect people's buying power and what people serve at certain meals. Advances in technology also have affected the availability of food. Today's shopper has a much wider range of foods from which to choose than ever before. A vast array of convenience foods have entered the food picture. Geography influences growing patterns, including soil conditions, temperatures, rainfall, and length of growing season. Such factors determine what food is commonly available in certain regions of the country.

The acceptability of food varies with several factors, including sensory components. If their taste buds tell them that the flavor of a certain food is enjoyable people are likely to eat that food often. The acceptability of food is also influenced by social customs, and in most cultures people eat together to express sociability. Food is also associated with hospitality. When friends drop in most people feel the need to offer food and drink and are embarrassed if caught with nothing festive in the cupboard. Food plays a central role in national holiday celebrations and in family events such as birthdays and weddings.

Culture influences the acceptability of food and, therefore, food habits. Culture includes all the habits, beliefs, attitudes, and social forms shared by any particular group of people (**20**). It conveys certain values, attitudes, and customs that given people begin to learn from earliest childhood and that motivate their food choices. Culture also dictates acceptable eating patterns. These patterns are modified only if new practices are within the boundaries of one's culture. If they clash with cultural norms, new dietary practices are not likely to be accepted readily.

What are some of these cultural influences? Certain groups of individuals prefer foods that others reared in a different culture may not like as well or may actually reject. For example, milk is a first food and is associated with security, comfort, and good nutrition in most countries. Certain African tribes, however, refuse to drink milk. They consider milk an offensive body discharge instead of a beverage of high nutritional value. Sometimes food habits are practiced simply because it is a tradition to do so, even though the reasons certain foods are restricted or forbidden are unclear.

Food habits are also closely linked to certain religious beliefs, particularly in Judaism. Orthodox Jews base many of their eating practices on Old Testament teachings, whereas Jewish dietary laws today appear to be based on religious self-discipline. Opinions are divided about the original purpose of Jewish eating habits, although safe food practices and health were certainly valid consid-erations in a situation vastly different from today. Foods prepared according to "kosher" requirements and traditional dishes such as cheese knishes, matzo balls, and gefilte fish are eaten daily by Orthodox Jews or are used to celebrate certain religious festivals.

Definite regional differences also influence food habits (Table 6.1). The many racial groups, nationalities, and cultures in the United States make it almost impossible to describe a typical American eating pattern. Although basic nutrient requirements are the same the world over, the foods used to supply these essential nutrients vary from one region to another, depending on culturally acceptable food patterns (Table 6.2). Food customs of each culture do change but only slowly. Immigrants to America from Europe settled near others with similar backgrounds, and familiar customs, including food habits, were per-petuated. These cultural food habits, with all their ethnic implications about food and eating practices naturally were transferred from one generation to the next. An indication of the cultural food practices and preferences of many people is the popularity in the United States today of restaurants specializing in German, Italian, Mexican, and other national foods.

The twentieth century has seen the creation or expansion of another influence on the acceptability of food—the science of nutrition. It is hoped that food habits in the future will be determined to some extent by people's knowledge of the nutritional value of foods. Unfortunately, this is often the least potent factor in the establishment of food habits. Stress and tension affect people's attitudes and feelings about foods, and people often use eating as an outlet to relieve these stresses. In such situations good nutrition may not be a top priority. Again, the nutritional value of food is seldom a primary consideration in menu selection for social celebrations. In this culture, achieving and maintaining a slim figure has become a symbol of prestige for some people. For many, good health or nutrition is rarely associated with efforts to become slim. On the brighter side, an increasing proportion of the population is becoming more concerned about and

TABLE 6.1 REGIONAL FOOD PATTERNS IN THE UNITED STATES

Ethnic influence	Characteristic traditional foods	Agricultural food products
North Central		
French, Dutch, German, English, Swiss, Italian, Balkan, Scandinavian, Irish	Cherry pie, Cornish pastries (meat pies), blueberry pie and other dishes, peaches, apples	Corn, wheat, dairy products, cherries, peaches, apples, blueberries, grapes, meat, fish, beans
South		
Scotch, Irish, English (Piedmont area), French (New Orleans area), Spanish (Florida area), Blacks	Hot breads such as cornbread, biscuits, spoon bread; corn fritters, corn pone, hominy grits, black-eyed peas, leafy green vegetables (turnip tops, mustard greens, collards, cabbage) cooked with salt pork; sweet potatoes and yams; Southern fried chicken; fish such as red snapper, Maryland crab, shrimp, ham, Creole cookery (Spanish and French)	Rice, pecans, pork, chicken, corn, sweet potatoes and yams, citrus fruits
New England and Middle Atlantic		
English, Scotch, German (Pennsylvania Dutch), Irish, Dutch, French, Swedish, Spanish, others	Soups, clam chowder, fish and shellfish, dried codfish, corned beef, New England boiled dinner, Boston baked beans, simple steamed puddings, cobblers and pies, Pennsylvania Dutch dishes	Fish, haddock, red fish, flounder, sole, cod, whiting, pollock, hake, oysters, clams, root vegetables, berries
West		
Indians, Spanish, Mexican (Southwest), Chinese, Japanese, Filipinos, Hawaiians (Mid-Pacific)	Tortillas, tamales, pinto beans, chili, corn, fish and shellfish (crab, lobster), tomatoes, chili peppers, fresh vegetables, salads, avocados, artichokes, citrus fruits, ripe olives, barbecued beef and poultry, sourdough bread	Beef, wheat, rice, citrus fruits, dates, apples, pears, plums, peaches, fish, shellfish

Source: Reprinted with permission from *Changing Food Habits* by A. Dean. Extension Bulletin 613, Michigan State University, 1968 (**21**).

TABLE 6.2 FOOD SOURCES OF PROTEIN AND
VITAMIN C FOR JAPAN, CHINA, SWEDEN, AND DENMARK

	Protein	Vitamin C
Japan	Fish, beef	Citrus fruits (tangerines)
	Soybean-based products	Nasi (similar to pear and apple)
	Eggs when available	Bean sprouts
China	Pork, fish	Cabbage
	Lamb, goats	
	Shellfish	
	Fowl (duck)	
	Soybeans	
	Eggs	
	Legumes	
Sweden	Fish	Strawberries
	Meat (veal, reindeer)	Wild berries
	Dried yellow peas	Potatoes with skin
		Turnips
		Greens in season
		Cabbage
		Rose hips
Denmark	Codfish	Potatoes
	Meat (lamb)	Cabbage
	Fish pudding	Berries
	Poultry	
	Cheese	
	Eggs	
	Yellow peas	

Source: Reprinted with permission from *Changing Food Habits* by A. Dean.
Extension Bulletin 613, Michigan State University, 1968 (**21**).

more aware of the relationship between good nutrition and good health. In the future, food habits may begin to reflect more of this concern.

Food habits, then, are a way of life influenced by a multitude of factors. The next time you make what may seem to be a simple choice between hamburger or chicken or fish, consider some of the factors that may be influencing your choice.

RECENT CHANGES IN NATIONAL FOOD HABITS

Human food habits seem to be relatively inflexible. Few individuals, for example, can control obesity over a long time period, indicating how strong eating habits are. Few people will change their food habits simply because they are told that certain foods are good for them or will make them healthy. Eating patterns, however, are not static. The different forces that influence the development of food habits can bring about changes in those food habits despite any built-in conservatism an individual may have about food. Noticeable changes have indeed occurred in American eating patterns in the last few decades (**22**). When the food habits currently in vogue are compared to those of a generation ago it can be said that food habits have changed dramatically. Between 1900 and the present people learned to eat thousands of new items, changes that reflect the evolving social and physical environment in which they live.

How have our food habits as a nation changed in recent years and what factors have been major influences in effecting those changes? Since the early part of this century, several food consumption studies have been conducted under the direction of USDA (**23**). Every major USDA survey showed changes in people's food consumption patterns. Between 1935 and 1948 familiar practices in the purchasing and use of certain foods were affected greatly by major changes in the distribution and storage of food products. Cooking patterns underwent striking changes between 1955 and 1965 as many new convenience type foods became increasingly common in the marketplace (**24**). Since the last nationwide survey in 1965 many more changes in food processing, food packaging, and food products have taken place. Changes in lifestyles have created a demand for a new food technology. In addition, changes in food technology have facilitated even further changes in lifestyle that in turn have affected food consumption patterns.

As a result of these changes the realities of modern food use no longer reflect traditional household eating patterns. Family members often do not eat together. Food prepared and eaten away from home is an accepted part of people's lifestyle. Household food use alone, therefore, does not present a reliable picture of actual food consumption patterns. For this reason, a survey now being conducted is a composite of six individual surveys, each consisting of two parts: household food use and individual food intake (**25**). This current nationwide food consumption survey is expected to provide new baseline data on the composition and adequacy of diets of various segments of the population.

Changes and trends in the consumption of calories, protein, fat, and carbohydrate over the past 65 years are shown in Figure 6.1. Caloric consumption has remained fairly constant over this period, and the proportion of calories

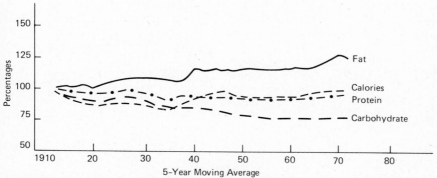

Figure 6.1 *Changes in per capita consumption of food energy, protein, fat, and carbohydrate, 1910–1973. (Source:* Reproduced with permission from W. Gortner in *Contemporary Nutrition,* November 1976. Copyright © 1976 by General Mills, Inc., Minneapolis, Minnesota.)

derived from protein is similar to the value reported for 1910. During the early part of the century, however, approximately 50 percent of the protein intake was supplied by grain and vegetable sources, with the remaining 50 percent supplied from animal products. Today, animal products supply approximately 70 percent of the protein intake. The increased consumption of meat, poultry, fish, dairy products, and eggs during this century accounts for this shift in protein consumption from vegetable to animal origin (Figure 6.2). Carbohydrate consumption has changed in the past 60 years, decreasing in amount and changing in nature (Figure 6.3). A decrease is seen in the consumption of complex carbohydrate containing foods, including fruits, vegetables, and cereal grain products. This decrease is a result of an increase in the consumption of meat and other animal protein foods at the expense of grains, fruits, and vegetables. The consumption of potatoes and cereal grains has decreased by 50 percent. The consumption of vegetables (other than potatoes) and fruits remains approximately the same, although there is an increase in the use of canned or frozen fruits and vegetables at the expense of fresh produce. Between 1940 and 1970 the annual per capita consumption of fresh fruit decreased from 139 to 78 lb. The per capita use of fresh vegetables decreased from 61 to 30 lb, and the consumption of canned and frozen vegetables increased by 15 percent during the same period.

This decrease in the overall consumption of complex carbohydrates is accompanied by a marked rise in the use of refined sugars. Since 1920 the consumption of sugar (not including that in beverages) increased about 20 percent. It is estimated that some teenagers eat 400 lb of sugar each year in carbonated beverages and snack foods. There is some evidence though, that certain of these trends in carbohydrate consumption may have modified or even reversed since 1973 because of economic factors. Inflation can bring about changes in food purchasing patterns leading to increased use of grains and grain products. However, in spite of a sharp increase in the price of sugar and sweets, the consumption of these products remains steady.

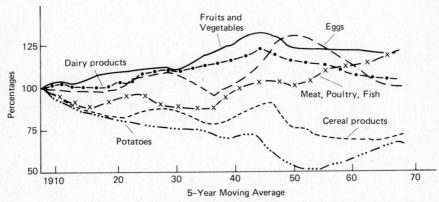

Figure 6.2 *Trends in U. S. eating habits.* (*Source:* Reproduced with permission from W. Gortner in *Contemporary Nutrition,* November, 1976. Copyright © 1976 by General Mills, Inc., Minneapolis, Minnesota.)

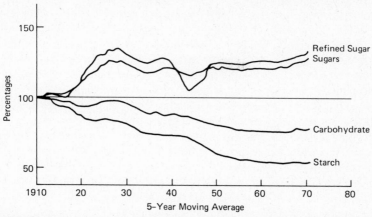

Figure 6.3 *Changes in per capita civilian consumption of sugars, starch, and carbohydrate, 1910–1973.* (*Source:* Reproduced with permission from W. Gortner in *Contemporary Nutrition,* November 1976. Copyright © 1976 by General Mills, Inc., Minneapolis, Minnesota.)

A steady increase is seen in fat consumption since the turn of the century, yet the intake of saturated fatty acids has changed only slightly. Cholesterol consumption has increased by only 10 percent. In the last 20 years polyunsaturated fatty acid intake also increased. The consumption of most vitamins and minerals remained steady over the past few decades, but the intake of calcium, vitamin C, and vitamin A actually increased. In 1941 the enrichment of flour and cereals with iron, niacin, riboflavin, and thiamin resulted in increased consumption of these nutrients.

FACTORS FACILITATING CHANGE IN FOOD HABITS

Children's food habits were the subject of several major research studies conducted in the past 20 years. The studies asked several questions: What economic, social, and cultural changes have had the greatest effect on the determination of food preferences in the young? What factors have caused food habits of the present generation to differ from those of previous generations? This research showed that food habits have become more individualistic and less related to traditional family practices. Increased urbanization, greater mobility, less formality, and other changes in lifestyles in recent years have led to a reduction in home meal preparation and family meal time, with accompanying changes in food habits.

Food Advertising

Food advertisers have successfully changed the nation's food habits by appealing to people's visual and olfactory senses and psychological and cultural makeup. The mass media, including newspapers, magazines, radio, and television, exert a tremendous influence on the changing of old food habits and the initiation of new ones. The mass media can be very effective in persuading people to buy certain food items and change their eating behaviors. Children appear especially susceptible to this type of advertising (**27, 28**). Ninety-five percent of American households have television sets, and the impact of the medium is recognized as a major factor in the development of food consumption patterns in children. What is the actual effect of television food advertising on the child, and how are responses to such advertising actually translated into food behavior?

The average youngster between the ages of 6 and 16 watches television three to four hours each day during the week and more often on weekends. During that time the child is exposed to numerous advertisements for food, drink, and vitamin products that appear to be more heavily directed to the child than to the adult. Food advertising accounts for approximately 26 percent of the commercials directed to adults, but more than 80 percent of all commercials directed primarily to the younger viewing audience are concerned with food. At the same time the average number of food items found in the supermarket increased from 900 in 1930 to more than 10,000 in the 1970s. An overwhelming amount of cookies, candies, crackers, breakfast cereals, soft drinks, and other high-sugar, high-salt snacks are now available. The common belief that Americans are the best-fed people in the world or that the American food supply is the best in the world is not always evident from the food advertised on television. The four food groups are not adequately promoted and are generally poorly represented. Forty percent of children's food commercials are for presweetened

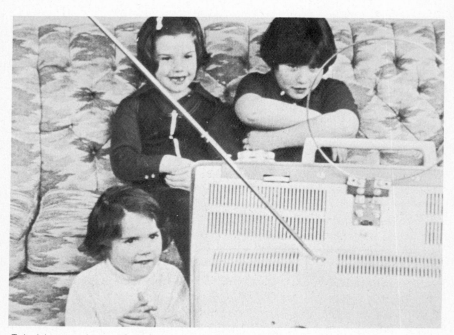

Television may be a powerful influence upon food habits.

cereals. Milk is advertised as fun, sweet, thick, and chocolatey and often made into a dessert. Somehow, the idea is being sold that milk as milk is unacceptable. The appeal of sweetness in foods is repeatedly emphasized. Vitamins are advertised as being capable of keeping children growing properly even if they aren't eating properly. The overall message associated with vitamin pills is that they compensate for poor eating habits in children. Unfortunately, few television ads even hint at proper eating habits. The fact is that children in this country, at an age when they are still young enough to be forming attitudes about food and diet, are being continually urged to eat foods that in the long term will not produce good health or healthy lifetime food habits (**29**).

Television provides a credible means through which the child learns to recognize and desire the advertised products. Younger children, especially, are most likely to believe that television ads tell the truth. They are easily influenced to either ask their parents to buy certain food items for them or even, in some instances, to purchase them with their own money. Nourishing oneself, however, is a learned skill. It must be taught. When they are given a choice of nutritious foods only, children can select a well-balanced diet. When adults preselect a variety of nutritious foods to offer children they can learn to eat and enjoy them. However, if they are offered desserts, soda, and candy bars in addition to more nutritionally desirable foods and left to their own devices, children will not generally choose a nutritious diet. The foods offered on television make it difficult for a child to chose a nutritious diet, since that diet is indeed basically unbalanced. Nutritionists do not generally oppose sweets as a minor component in an otherwise nourishing diet. They do, however, oppose the disproportionately large number of sweet foods promoted in television advertising.

The child's response to television advertising is not the only factor affecting his or her food consumption pattern. The interaction between the parent and child is critical. Very few preschool children do the family shopping. Studies show that the number of requests young children make for advertised food products increases in relation to the number of hours of television watched and decreases in relation to the number of times the parent has previously refused such requests. The response of children to food advertising is, therefore, influenced by the response of the parents themselves to such advertising. This in turn is related to parental food habits and knowledge of the nutritional value of advertised foods. Parents who are not well informed nutritionally are in a more difficult position.

Working Women
Today, 48 percent of all women in the United States work outside the home, a significant increase over past years (**30**). How has this trend affected food consumption patterns and the nutritional quality of the diet? The increase in the number of women who work outside the home to partially or fully support their families, especially working mothers, has meant a decrease in the amount of time spent in meal preparation, an increase in the use of convenience foods, an increase in the number of meals prepared and eaten outside the home, and an increase in the incidence of snacking and "eating on the run."

Fast-Food Restaurants

The growth and success of the fast-food restaurant has been phenomenal and is related to other societal changes: an increase in the number of women working outside the home, an increase in per capita disposable income, and an increase in leisure time for many people (**31**). More adolescents and families with middle and low incomes are eating fewer meals at home and more snack-type meals at fast-food restaurants than ever before (**32**). How does this change from traditional meal patterns affect the nutrient intake of fast-food patrons? What nutritional variety is actually available at fast-food restaurants?

Fast-food choices provide many essential nutrients but are high in calories, with fat supplying approximately 42 percent of the total calories. Indeed, some meals can provide over 1000 calories or up to one-half of a person's daily energy needs (**33**). The high caloric value is often found in the French fries, soft drinks, and desserts that accompany the meal. Hamburgers and French fries are generously presalted in most fast-food restaurants. The average meal may contain 80 percent of the day's requirements for sodium; yet how often do people ask for "extra salt" to accompany such a meal? There is no need to request additional packets of salt at a fast-food restaurant. Fast-food meals generally are low in vitamin A, vitamin C, calcium, and fiber (**34**). No vegetables are available, except French fried potatoes, tomatoes, and lettuce. Milk and milk shakes are on the menu, but people do not generally choose these as a beverage. The effect of fast-food eating on nutrient intake obviously depends on which foods are chosen and the extent to which an individual eats at fast-food restaurants. The nutrient composition of meals and snacks is not a cause for major concern if a person eats only one to three meals a week at a fast-food outlet (**35**). Certain nutrient deficits, however, could develop in those who eat in such an establishment more than six times a week. The persons who do eat fast-food meals frequently need to choose other meals carefully to guarantee themselves the essential nutrients without excess calories.

People who do eat at fast-food restaurants frequently should select the remainder of the day's food with special care to include dark green leafy and deep yellow fruits or vegetables as a source of vitamin A. Greens, sweet potatoes, carrots, and apricots are all good choices. Citrus fruits are excellent sources of vitamin C. Tomatoes, potatoes, greens, green peppers, strawberries, and cantaloupe also provide vitamin C in the diet. Although it is available at most fast-food restaurants, milk is not often a first-choice beverage. Milk and other dairy products should be chosen to accompany other meals.

Fiber or roughage in the diet helps move food through the digestive tract. Dietary fiber is supplied largely by whole grain cereals, fruits, and vegetables, amd more of these should be eaten throughout the day. Careful selection of food items for a fast-food meal and careful selection of food at home should allow one to enjoy good nutrition without giving up the fast-food outings. Some special hints for those with weight problems are given later in this chapter.

Nutritionists have a responsibility to encourage fast-food restaurants to improve their menus so that good sources of all essential nutrients are included in the meals. Nutrition education is also needed to make the public more aware of what are the more nutritious menu items at present and to influence consumer selection in favor of such items.

Snacking

The tendency toward snacking is another recent change in eating behavior and is, in a sense, related to the trends of eating away from home and in hurried, more casual eating patterns. Most people have a favorite snack that they enjoy eating between regular meals. This includes school children who all seem to enjoy afterschool snacks. Snacks, indeed, often replace meals and may displace other more nutritious foods in the diet. Up to one-third of the teenage population in this country skips breakfast (**36**). Small numbers may skip lunch and even dinner.

Snacks should be considered a part of the day's total food intake. Fruits, vegetables, juices, and protein foods eaten as snacks can contribute important amounts of essential nutrients and food energy to the overall diet. Many popular snack foods, however, such as chips, soft drinks, candy bars, cookies, and doughnuts, are high in sugar and salt content and supply little nutritive value to the diet. The food industry in this country encourages the demand for snack foods by introducing more and more varieties to the market. People and health professionals need to push for the development of lower calorie, more nutritious

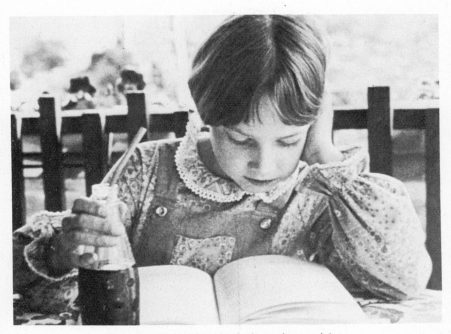

Snacking is an important part of total food intake in modern society.

snack foods to meet the needs of growing children and teenagers whose lifestyles often include eating many snacks in place of regular meals.

Vending Machines

Another major influence on the eating habits of school-age children has been the rapid proliferation of vending machines in schools over the past few years (**37**). In many instances candy, packaged cakes, cookies, and carbonated beverages are the only food choices available in these machines. Soft drink companies give special concessions to schools that sell their products, and in many schools the sale of such foods is often the major source of student activity funds. The sale of these foods is defended on the basis that they may only be harmful to those students who do not have an adequate diet and who replace more nutritious foods in the diet with vending machine items offering little nutritive value. A second defense is that students should be given the opportunity to make their own food choices. The fact remains that many students are poorly nourished. These are often the young people who are also poorly informed about good eating habits and who may not be able to make wise dietary choices when presented an option of school lunch as opposed to candy bars and soft drinks. Some school officials feel that students will simply go elsewhere to seek "nutrient deficient" foods if these are not available to them at school. This will not necessarily be true if appetizing nutritious foods are available in the school.

Until 1973, the Secretary of Agriculture had the authority to regulate the use of school vending machines and the sale of foods in competition with meals served under the National School Lunch and School Breakfast Programs. Authority was then given to state and local school districts. Some states did take steps to phase out the sale of unacceptable foods to students. The authority was returned to the Secretary of Agriculture in 1977, however, when Congress observed that few localities had taken any action in this area. A new rule on the sale of competitive foods went into effect in July 1980. This ruling identifies categories of foods of minimal nutritional value that may not be sold from the beginning of the school day to the end of the last lunch period. Foods of minimal nutritional value are defined as foods that provide less than 5 percent of the U.S. RDAs for any of eight specified nutrients per 100 calories and/or per serving. For foods that are artificially sweetened, only the per serving measure applies. The eight specified nutrients are protein, vitamin A, ascorbic acid, niacin, riboflavin, thiamin, calcium, and iron. Foods affected by this regulation include sodas, water ices, chewing gum, and certain candies. Schools are encouraged to sell more nutritious snacks, such as fresh fruit, fruit juices, vegetable juices, and whole grain products in place of the banned foods. The competitive foods regulation sets a minimum standard for use by local officials. It does not preclude local schools from setting stricter rules.

In certain localities throughout the country the sale of candy and carbonated beverages has been prohibited in some schools in response to parental concern. These less desirable snacks have been replaced with milk and fruit. Vending machines are available that will stock nutritious items such as milk and juice in cartons, fresh fruit, yogurt, and ice cream products. Other machines are designed to dispense sandwiches or hot food, such as soup, stew, and chili in individual portions. Although several companies presently market nutritious snack products for use in these vending machines, the food industry should be encouraged to develop more such appealing, nutritious snacks. Student councils should be made aware of other revenue sources besides the sale of nonnutritious food items in school.

FOOD HABITS SHAPED BY DIETARY FADS

Nutritionists, health professionals, and the public in general are becoming concerned about the increasing amount of misinformation available about foods and nutrition (**38**). Such misinformation can result in the economic and nutritional exploitation of the individual who does not have the background knowledge needed to evaluate claims made about the nutritive value of health foods, dietary supplements, or various dietary regimens (**39**). Such misinformation is often directed to that segment of the population least able to separate fact from fiction but most willing to accept what appears to be plausible—young people. The increased concern of young people about food problems, nutrition, and health has made them an easy source for exploitation by food faddists. Young people, genuinely concerned about food problems but lacking access to reliable informa-tion, sometimes adopt food fads, including organic foods, health foods, natural foods, and vegetarian diets. Without adequate knowledge, adherence to such diets can create health problems, but combating food faddism can be extremely difficult. Traditional methods of nutrition education may be inadequate if no attempt is made to understand different food fads and the underlying value systems and philosophies of groups or individuals who follow them. Health professionals should stress to young people the importance of evaluating the validity of the nutritional claims made by food faddists.

Natural, Organic, and Health Foods

Concern for health and the environment has stimulated the growth of the health food movement among many young persons. In such movements the emotional or symbolic values of food are often emphasized to a much greater extent than are scientific or nutritional values. Food choices are made on a psychological or social basis rather than on any proven health benefits. Although no federal regulations have been established regarding natural, organic, or health foods, the President's Office on Consumer Affairs suggests the following definitions: *natural foods* are foods having no added preservatives, emulsifiers, or artificial ingre-dients. *Organic foods* are natural foods grown without the use of pesticides and/or chemical fertilizers. *Health foods* are organic, natural, and other foods thought to have special properties, some of which may contain artificial chemicals (**40**).

The growing interest in natural foods can be traced to the increased interest in ecology, back-to-nature lifestyles, and concern about additives, pesticides, and drug residues in foods. The resulting demand for natural foods has more than doubled since 1970. Stores specializing in the sale of such foods increased from approximately 1200 in 1968 to over 3000 in the early 1970s (**41**). Many of the major food chains in this country, in fact, have added natural food sections in their supermarkets. In the correct sense the term "natural" refers to foods as they occur in nature. It is possible to include a large number of natural foods, defined in this sense, in the diet without becoming overly obsessed with the theories espoused by extreme food faddists. Some foods, however, can be eaten in the natural state, whereas others cannot. Raw milk, for instance, which is promoted by "naturalists" in preference to pasteurized milk, is a favored medium for bacterial growth.

The conditions required for the growth and processing of organic foods are not regulated or guaranteed. Consumers are generally led to believe that such foods are produced without pesticides and artificial fertilizers and are free of any synthetic additives. Studies show that families substituting organically grown foods for regular, nonorganic foods may pay 30–100 percent more for a similar diet (**42**). Organic fertilizers must be broken down into their inorganic constituents before nutrients can be absorbed by the plant. Therefore, plants grown with the use of chemical fertilizers or organic farming methods do not differ nutritionally in the long run.

Health foods are promoted by food faddists as having specific healing properties beyond those found in a balanced diet consisting of a variety of foods (**43**). The value of such foods is elevated to extremes. By selecting a variety of foods in adequate amounts a balance of the essential nutrients will be provided for good health. In this sense, all foods, when used in proper balance, promote physiological and psychological health and are health foods.

Zen-Macrobiotic Diet

The Zen-Macrobiotic diet represents an extreme example of the trend toward natural foods (**44**). It has become increasingly popular among young people, mainly for philosophical or religious reasons (**45**). What are the nutritional implications of following such a diet? There are ten stages of dietary restriction in the Zen-Macrobiotic diet, with a gradual elimination of animal products and fruits and vegetables at each level. The highest level is made up of a diet of 100 percent cereal products and restricted fluid intake. Scurvy and other forms of malnutrition, however, can result from adherence to this diet for only a few months. Infants and pregnant or lactating women are especially vulnerable to nutrient deficiencies on this diet. The American Medical Association's Council on Foods and Nutrition has condemned the Zen-Macrobiotic diet as unsafe (**46**).

Vegetarianism

Vegetarian diets are becoming increasingly popular, especially among young people in the United States (**47, 48**). This diet shifts away from familiar Western food patterns and toward one that excludes totally or includes only a minimal amount of animal protein. Nutritionists have some concern that this change in eating habits may adversely affect the nutritional status of young people who may not have adequate knowledge about the proper selection of a nutritious vegetarian diet (**49**). A vegetarian diet can be nutritionally adequate if foods are selected wisely and care is taken in meal planning. Humans have survived for centuries on vegetarian or near-vegetarian diets by complementing or supplementing one vegetable protein source with another vegetable protein or by combining vegetable protein with a small amount of animal protein.

A reasonably chosen plant diet supplemented with a fair amount of dairy products, with or without eggs, will meet nutrient needs. When dairy products and eggs are totally omitted from the diet, some difficulty may be encountered in obtaining certain essential nutrients. Vitamin B_{12} is one essential nutrient that is available only in foods of animal origin. Therefore, pure vegetarians will need to take a vitamin B_{12} supplement to augment their diet. If milk is eliminated from the vegetarian diet, the person will have difficulty meeting his or her dietary requirements for calcium. This is especially true for children, as well as for pregnant and lactating women whose needs are greater than those of the average person. One large serving (1 cup or 200 g) of greens such as collards, kale, turnip, and mustard provides as much calcium as one cup of milk. Cabbage, broccoli, and cauliflower will contribute smaller amounts of calcium to the diet. Vitamin D may also be low in the vegetarian diet. Fish liver oils may be advisable for infants, young children, and pregnant and nursing women. The richest sources of riboflavin are milk and milk products. Green leafy vegetables such as greens, asparagus, broccoli, brussels sprouts, and okra are good sources of riboflavin for the vegetarian but must be eaten at regular intervals to replace the riboflavin of milk. Anemia, resulting from iron deficiency, is common among growing children and women in the childbearing years who follow vegetarian lifestyles. An iron supplement is desirable in these situations.

Dietary Supplements

Certain groups of young people, athletes in particular, sometimes consume large amounts of dietary supplements in the belief that the current food supply is nutrient deficient and that certain supplements have health and curative powers (**50**). Studies show that approximately 75 percent of the public believes that supplementary vitamins and minerals furnish energy. The mass media appeal to people to use vitamin and mineral supplements based on the argument that people may develop dietary deficiencies which doctors cannot detect. These advertisements suggest that the majority of people are not capable of selecting a nutritionally adequate diet and that the only way to ensure an adequate intake of essential nutrients is to take supplements. Candy-flavored, cartoon character supplements are promoted for children, and such advertising has led to the large-scale use of vitamin-mineral supplements without medical advice.

A person can easily consume excess amounts of vitamins, especially A and D, that are stored in the body. Therefore, preparations that contain more than 3000 R.E. (10,000 IU) of vitamin A or 10 mcg (400 IU) of vitamin D in a daily dosage unit should be taken only by prescription (**51**). In addition to supplying certain nutrients out of proportion to body needs, supplements may contain nutrients that the body can synthesize itself or that are generously supplied in foods. Athletes are often encouraged to consume protein supplements. Everyone, especially athletes, needs energy to perform well when exercising. Extra protein alone, however, is not the total answer to extra energy, health, or strength. The average young person in the United States consumes sufficient protein from food sources and indeed may consume amounts in excess of that required. Excess protein will then be stored in the body as fat. Energy can be well supplied by carbohydrates and fat in the diet. Carbohydrates and fat are generally less expensive than protein foods and should be an important part of the diet of an athlete. Most protein supplements contain less protein per unit than meat and at far greater cost.

The normal healthy individual does not require vitamin, mineral, or other types of dietary supplements if an adequate diet is eaten. No one food contains all the vitamins and minerals necessary for health, but a wide variety of foods selected from the basic four food groups will provide an adequate diet, with the following exceptions. As pointed out in other sections of this text, adolescent girls and women in the childbearing years may need an iron supplement (**52**). Infants who do not receive iron-fortified formula or cereal generally need additional iron by the third month of life. Children under age 4 may show an increased need for iron beyond that supplied in the diet. Beginning in the fourth month of pregnancy, women may require supplements of 30−60 mg of iron per day and 200−400 mcg of folacin (**53**). Supplementary nutrients needed in these situations should be used only under medical supervision. No dietary supplements, however, should be used on a long-term basis in an effort to compensate for inadequate food intake or faulty food habits (**54**).

Weight Control
The amount of misinformation in the field of weight control is staggering. An ever-increasing number of fad diets promote weight reduction as an easy and painless process. American society, through fashion magazines and other media, tends to idolize the slim figure as a symbol of sex appeal and attractiveness. Many adolescent girls become dissatisfied with their body build and, even though not obese, will follow fad reduction or crash diet programs to lose weight for cosmetic rather than health reasons. Instead of increasing physical activity to accomplish her goal, the teenager generally chooses to follow a diet that may be nutritionally inadequate and dangerous to her health.

Teenagers are bombarded from all sides with revolutionary diet ideas promising miraculous permanent painless weight loss. A new diet is published almost every month in the magazines popular with teenage girls. How often have you heard a friend say, "I'm going to lose 15 lbs in two weeks by going on this great new diet"? Or "It's easy to lose weight by fasting. I just eat one meal a day. . . .That's all I need." How often have you tried those methods yourself? The average young person may find it very difficult to evaluate the nutritional adequacy of certain fad diets and dietary aids and is often unaware of the potential damage crash diets or dietary aids can do to health.

A *fad diet* is any currently popular crash diet designed for quick and easy weight loss. A rich tradition of nutrition nonsense has developed to promote the belief that certain foods or systems of dieting have value beyond that of established factors of nutritional diet therapy in the treatment of obesity. Many fad diets are promoted on the basis of unlimited consumption of certain foods. Consider these: "Eat all you want"; "Calories don't Count." The fact is that no diet will result in weight loss if the principles of the conservation of energy are ignored. Other fad diets are based on the notion that certain food combinations are less fattening than others. These emphasize certain foods that should be included in the diet and others that should be excluded. These diets are very likely to be inadequate in several essential nutrients. In recent years much popularity has been focused on "ketogenic" diets that restrict carbohydrate intake while allowing a liberal protein and fat intake. There are dangers associated with this combination of nutrients. An excessive amount of protein in the diet can cause blood protein levels to rise. In an attempt to reduce blood protein, the kidney resorbs additional water to rid the body of excess protein through excretion in the urine. The load of work performed by the kidney can increase to potentially harmful levels. A liberal fat intake can result in an elevation of blood lipid and cholesterol to undesirable levels. Such high levels can contribute to the development of blood vessel and/or heart disease. The body requires approximately 100 g of carbohydrate each day to maintain blood glucose levels, to spare the body's protein from being used as an energy source, and to insure normal body function. Carbohydrates help to retain sodium, a key regulator of fluid balance, in the body. On a low carbohydrate diet, therefore, sodium and fluid are lost rapidly. Much of the weight lost on such a diet is an illusion created by water loss and is quickly regained when carbohydrate consumption increases. Dramatic weight losses have very little meaning if the composition of such weight loss is largely water.

Other diets promote a low protein intake as the best way to lose weight. Low protein diets, however, can result in protein loss from the body, depleting muscle and organ tissues. Such a diet can result in stunted growth in the growing child.

Recently, many young people have turned to complete fasting as a means of rapid weight loss. Fasting can result in weakness, confusion, low blood sugar, low blood pressure, and high blood fat and protein, and should not be carried out for long periods without proper medical supervision. Fasting generally results in the loss of a high percentage of muscle or lean body tissue. Actual loss of fat tissues is usually less. The lean tissue (and, therefore, weight) is rapidly regained when eating is resumed. Mineral loss from the body during fasting is related to lean body mass lost. An excessive loss of water, sodium, and potassium can lead to muscle spasms.

Most recently, protein-sparing modified fasts have become extremely popular. The theory behind such diets is that they are nutritionally safe regimens which meet daily protein requirements, thus preventing or reducing lean body tissue loss. Concern exists, though, that some of the predigested protein mixtures consumed on a protein-sparing modified fast are prepared from collagen, an incomplete protein which cannot be efficiently utilized by humans. Such a diet can result in the loss of significant amounts of potassium from the body. Liquid protein diets followed without medical supervision can be hazardous to the health and normal development of the growing person (**55**).

One concern associated with fasting, especially in the case of the adolescent girl, is the possible development of anorexia or loss of the desire to eat long after a desirable amount of weight has been lost (**56**).The term "anorexia nervosa" means nervous loss of appetite. It is applied to a condition in which people actually undergo self-imposed starvation. This disorder is on the rise among weight-conscious teenagers and is much more common among girls than boys. The average anorexia nervosa patient is under 20, bright and intelligent, and from a middle or upper class family. She tends to worry about her body image and decides that losing a few pounds will improve her figure. As she loses weight and becomes thinner and thinner she finds that she cannot stop dieting and soon goes beyond desirable limits in the game of losing weight. Body weight may drop by 20–30 percent, and the girl becomes severely underweight and malnourished. The reasons for the development of anorexia nervosa differ. They are related ultimately to many of the problems of just growing up. Psychological care and medical treatment are needed to help such an adolescent return to her normal weight. The implications for the future health of a person who denies his or her body the required nutrients at a critical developmental stage have probably not been fully realized or appreciated.

Young people who are overweight need to be helped to establish realistic goals for weight reduction. They need programs geared to meet the physiological and social needs of growing children. Childhood obesity is estimated to range from 5 to 23 percent (**57, 58**), whereas 30 percent of American adolescents are overweight (**59**). Below age 6 the overfat child is encountered more frequently than the overthin child. A major environmental factor contributing to the development of obesity in the young is poor nutrition patterns (**60, 61**). Once a child does become overweight it is not necessary or desirable for him or her to lose a great deal of excess weight in a hurry. It is not recommended that a growing child be put on a diet which would interfere with normal growth in any way. The child's habits, however, must be changed from those of overconsumption and underactivity to healthy eating and exercise. In this manner, although actual weight loss does not occur, the rate of weight gain will be slowed so that growth in height eventually catches up with weight. As the child grows taller he or she will become thinner, and muscle and bone tissue will make up a larger proportion of body mass, and the percentage of body fat will decrease. Therefore, although the weight as measured on a scale has not changed, the child will look different and better. Some children, especially adolescents, are often discouraged when they do not see a drop in body weight. It must be stressed to these children that their bodies are still growing and that extreme weight reduction is not desirable. Only in the child who has already attained full normal growth or for those who are extremely overweight should actual weight reduction be considered and then only under medical supervision.

How can the situation be reversed once a child has become obese? One of the most successful methods of helping obese adults lose weight is through behavior modification (**62**). This technique recognizes that activity and eating patterns are learned behaviors. Behavior modification emphasizes the necessity to change those patterns of behavior associated with overeating and to develop more appropriate eating patterns that are conducive to weight control. Little research is available, however, on the application of behavior modification techniques with children. When dealing with young children behavioral modification procedures must be applied to both the child and parent. Older children can be taught to use the techniques themselves. A common complaint associated with most weight control diets is that they sometimes isolate the person doing the dieting. The person becomes different from the rest of the group. The dieter cannot eat what others eat or participate in social activities where eating is involved. This is a particularly difficult problem for the adolescent. Socializing with the peer group may be much more important than healthy weight control. Good times mean going for hamburgers after the movies, stopping for ice cream cones on the way home from the library, ordering pizza on Saturday night, having cookouts, and attending school dances. All these events mean eating a lot of very good and sometimes very fattening food. How do you tell teenagers that they cannot go for hamburgers or ice cream with the crowd? Obviously, you cannot. Going out for hamburgers is an integral part of the lifestyle of many teenagers. You can, however, teach the overweight adolescent behavior modification so that he or she can frequent fast-food restaurants with friends and control weight at the same time.

At one end of the spectrum are the teenagers who walk into a fast-food restaurant and feel the need to order a hamburger or superburger, French fries, a shake, and perhaps apple pie. That's a big snack, and it is loaded with calories. At the other extreme is the teenager who feels that the only way to control weight is to give up fast-food outings entirely and become a recluse. The ideal situation is for teenagers to learn to modify their behavior so that they are still able to enjoy jaunts to fast-food outlets but order a combination of foods that is relatively low in calories but provides essential nutrients.

The calories in some common fast-food sandwiches are shown in Figure 6.4. A plain hamburger with added mustard, catsup, or pickles has about 250 calories. Add a slice of cheese and the caloric content increases, but so does the protein content. Many people are tempted to order the fish sandwich because fish is low in calories. This fish, however, has added fat from deep-fat frying and added tartar sauce. Leaving the tartar sauce off the fish sandwich will decrease the caloric content by 75 calories. Superburgers all contain about 500–600 calories. Also, the caloric content of condiments served in fast-food restaurants increases the total number of calories in a meal (Figure 6.5). Catsup and sweet pickle relish have only 15–20 calories per tablespoon. Mustard has even less. However, the oil-based condiments such as salad dressing or tartar sauce have approximately 65–80 calories per tablespoon. Condiments could be omitted or used in smaller amounts, of course, to save on calories. Beverages offered at fast-food restaurants are usually high in calories but low in nutrients (Figure 6.6). Black coffee and iced tea (unsweetened) are available in most fast-food chains,

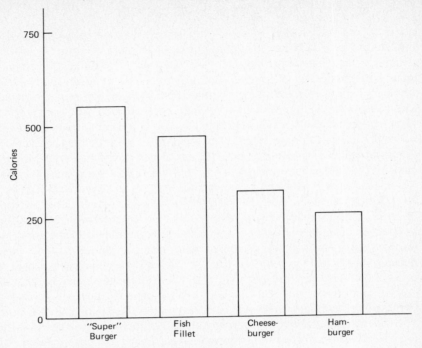

Figure 6.4 *Calories in "Fast Food" sandwiches.*

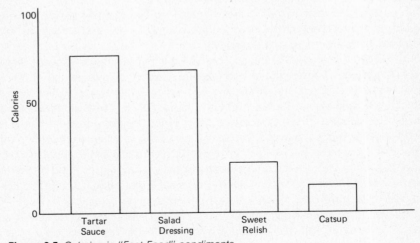

Figure 6.5 *Calories in "Fast Food" condiments.*

202

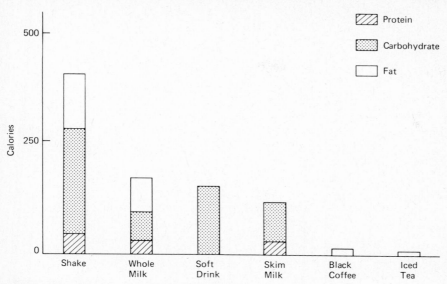

Figure 6.6 *Calories in "Fast Food" beverages.*

however, and these beverages supply no calories or nutrients. A 12 oz soft drink can add approximately 140 calories to a meal. Milk is often available and contains about 150 calories in an 8 oz serving but supplies protein and calcium as well. A shake contains approximately 330 calories, mostly in the form of sugar and thickeners. The majority of shakes available in fast-food restaurants are not milk based. (For this reason, they are called "thick shakes" or other names omitting the term "milk.") A milk shake, however, should provide additional protein and calcium. So consider both the caloric and nutrient value of foods if you are on a diet. The choice at a fast-food restaurant would be a plain hamburger or a cheeseburger and coffee, tea, or preferably milk as a beverage. This combination would supply a nutritious but not extremely high calorie meal. The caloric content of other fast-food combinations is shown in Figure 6.7.

What about afternoon stops at the ice cream store? Don't make them a daily habit, but certainly once in a while you can treat yourself to the lower calorie choices. A small vanilla cone averages 186 calories. The larger size contains 370 calories, so order the smaller one. Do not choose the fancier ice creams, since they are higher in calories. Chocolate, butterscotch, fudge, or nuts all increase the caloric count of ice cream. One scoop of any flavor sherbet contains 136 calories, whereas one scoop of flavored ice contains 129 calories. So go for ice cream with your friends, but be aware of the lower calorie choices available to you.

Some diet fads, then, are harmless; some are useless, and some are actually dangerous if followed for a relatively lengthy time. At a time when old food habits are still being replaced with new ones young people should be made

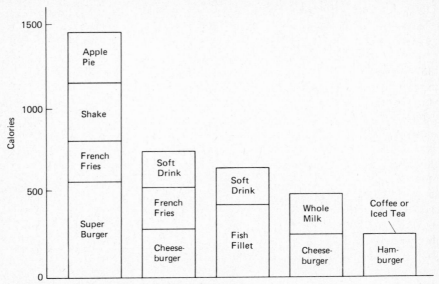

Figure 6.7 Calories in "Fast Food" combinations.

aware of the characteristics of fad dieting and the potential dangers associated with it. A weight control diet should be one which promotes good food habits that can be followed for a lifetime, supplies all essential nutrients in adequate amounts, does not socially isolate young people from their peers, and leads to successful weight control.

BETTER FOOD HABITS THROUGH NUTRITION EDUCATION

Nutritionists agree that food patterns for a majority of the American public need to change if a healthy society is to be achieved. The exact nature and extent of needed changes and how these changes should be implemented are controversial subjects, though. Nutrition education has not been in the past, and is not today, as effective as everyone would like it to be (**63**). Most changes in food habits in this country are brought about by the advertising and promotion of various food products and not by the persuasive statements of nutritionists. Dietary intake cannot be improved by teaching nutrition facts alone (**64**), since people need to understand the various factors affecting food choices, motivation, attitudes, and values. It is then the responsibility of nutrition educators to guide and promote those forces in society that will lead to dietary improvement.

No single pattern of food consumption will insure good nutritional status, since the body requires certain nutrients rather than specific food items. How then do nutrition educators influence consumers to achieve adequate nutrient intake through proper selection of a wide variety of foods? Teaching nutrition facts and concepts may be necessary and useful in some instances, but providing nutrition information alone is usually not sufficient to alter food consumption patterns. Effective nutrition education programs must deal with attitudes and habits as well as nutrition facts. Hochbaum argues against the superiority of any one nutrition education method but stresses the need to understand behavior in each situation (**65**). Increasingly, nutrition educators recognize that a greater understanding of many factors underlying people's food habits is needed if we are to improve our effectiveness as change agents (**66**). Knowledge of the behavioral patterns associated with food habits is essential if nutrition knowledge is ever to be applied widely (**65**). Understanding what factors affect food habits in certain groups is valuable in planning nutrition education programs to include those foods most likely to be accepted. The adoption of fad diets by teenagers can be the basis for meaningful dialogue and insight into developing effective nutrition education techniques (**67**). Also, nutrition educators could probably achieve significant dietary changes by approaching food advertisers and adopting some of their techniques. The successful modification of food habits ultimately depends, though, on an understanding of the basis for present food choices and the development of techniques to influence that basis. This would take into consideration the total environment, needs, and interests of each particular target group. We nutritionists also need to accept more responsibility for the proper interpretation of nutrition facts to the general public. Nutrition education in relation to new foods and new eating patterns cannot be left entirely to the food manufacturer. Stansfield and Fox suggest that there is merit in working with grocers to develop advertising, store displays, and other promotional devices focusing on the nutritional value of food (**68**).

Health professionals need to direct nutrition education efforts to food suppliers and consumers as the trend increases toward eating more foods prepared and served away from home. Further research is also needed in behavioral aspects that determine the formation of food habits and their susceptibility to change (**68–72**). To improve the nation's health through diet, nutrition educators must take advantage of every opportunity to present reliable information and effective intervention techniques through speaking engagements, written reports for the general public, the effective use of mass media, and informal contacts in our day-to-day living situations. Food patterns in the United States will not remain fixed (**73**), since a multitude of influences continually force change. Nutrition research is an ever-present influence, though, in the favor of change in food habits. As nutrition knowledge increases, food habits will change to adapt to current knowledge but will remain flexible enough to change again when necessary.

SUMMARY

Nutritional status is to a large extent determined by food habits, and children begin to develop food preferences and practices very early in life. It is, therefore, important to begin to establish good food habits and wholesome attitudes toward food as soon as an infant is born. The home is extremely valuable in developing and maintaining these good food habits. Although children will learn from all sources to which they are exposed, the family setting is the predominant influence on the formation of eating habits in infants, toddlers, and preschool childrren. Parental habits and attitudes will be reflected in the children's habits as they develop. Dietary practices developed during infancy influence growth and development during the critical early years and largely determine lifetime eating habits. As the child grows and is exposed to external influences beyond the family, the mass media and peer groups add to each individual child's knowledge and awareness of the many roles of food in society.

Food habits are an integral part of every individual's lifestyle and have a wide range of personal and social meanings. Age, income, family environment, availability of food, education, religion, tradition, and social position all determine food selection patterns. Major changes have taken place in eating patterns in the United States over the last few decades, and these changes in lifestyle have created a demand for changes in the food industry. Changes in food production and availability have in turn facilitated further changes in lifestyle, leading to more changes in food consumption patterns. Greater demand for leisure time, more women in the work force, greater per capita income, and greater mobility of the population as a whole are some of the major influences effecting these current changes in people's food habits.

An increased awareness of nutrition and its relationship to health is apparent among many young people. However, an alarming amount of misinformation on foods and nutrition is available and is often directed to this segment of the population that is least able to evaluate certain claims but most willing to accept them. This increased concern for health and the environment among young people provides an opportunity for their exploitation by food faddists and has stimulated the growth of many so-called health food movements. Health foods, organic foods, natural foods, vegetarian diets, dietary supplements, and numerous weight control regimens are among the fads readily adopted by young people. Unfortunately, young people do not fully realize the implications of denying their bodies the required nutrients at this critical developmental stage. Unwise eating habits at this age can affect the health of the present generation of children and of the one they will become parents to in the future.

We nutritionists generally agree that some change in the food intake patterns of the American population is necessary if we are to achieve a healthy society. The exact nature and extent of needed changes and how nutrition education can be improved to implement these changes, however, are controversial subjects.

STUDY QUESTIONS AND
TOPICS FOR INDIVIDUAL INVESTIGATION

1. Most people form their food habits early in life before they become conscious of good nutritional practices. Think about your own eating habits. How did those habits develop? What part would you say your home environment played in this development, your peers, television advertising, availability of food, and any other influences?

2. If you were a parent, how would you help your children to develop good eating habits? Think about external factors beyond your influence (school, peers, mass media) that might undermine, or at least differ from, your efforts. How would you deal with these?

3. Many people's eating habits develop in ignorance of good nutrition. In recent years the public has become more aware of the requisites for good nutrition. Do you think that increased knowledge will bring about substantial change in eating habits? Will people continue to eat according to old habits even though they may know better? Look more closely at some of the references on nutrition education listed at the end of this chapter. How might nutrition education programs be improved to increase the probability of enhancing change for the better?

4. Do you feel that the food industry and mass media exert considerable influence on people's eating habits? Give reasons for your answer. Can you cite anecdotal examples from your own experience to support your decision? To what extent do you feel consumers themselves are responsible for their food choices? Do you see a role for the consumer in changing the nature of the products the food industry offers or the manner in which foods are advertised? Explain your answer.

5. For your own information, watch an hour of Saturday morning children's television. Keep notes on what channels and what shows you watch. What food products are advertised? What is the style of advertising?

6. Are you aware of your own particular eating habits? Many people are not. Keep a food record for two or three days. Write down all the food you eat, amounts eaten, when eaten and where eaten. Do you eat in the company of other people? What influence do others have on the food choices you make? Do you eat less or more when eating with others? Analyze your mood when you reached for that candy bar. Were you bored, lonely, or were you hungry? What degree of hunger did you feel? Did eating change the degree of hunger in any way? Evaluate your food intake in terms of nutrient value. Have you become aware of instances when you could improve your own food habits?

7. Conduct a snack study. List your favorite snack foods. Look up the nutrient composition of the foods listed. Which of the snack foods you eat can be considered nutritious? Which of those foods have no food value other than calories? Look at the foods served in your cafeteria or dining hall. Do you

choose certain foods for their nutritional value, from habit, or because your friends choose those foods?

8. Are you confused by the multitude of books and magazines that proclaim new miracle reducing diets? Not all these diets are based on sound nutritional principles. Choose any currently popular fad diet and analyze it. Does the diet include a variety of foods based on a flexible diet plan? Does the diet include all essential nutrients? Does the diet limit caloric intake so that you expend more energy than you take in but still provide essential nutrients in adequate amounts? Does the diet recommend slow but constant weight loss at a rate of not more than 1–2 lb per week? Would the diet help you establish new eating patterns different from the patterns that led to weight gain originally? Is the diet plan readily adaptable from family meals, and is it reasonable in cost? The answer "no" to one or more of these questions indicates that the diet is probably not based on sound dietary principles.

9. Nutrition can be a topic that many teenagers enjoy discussing. An excellent aid for discussion groups with teenagers on this topic is a pamphlet developed by Concern, Incorporated, 2233 Wisconsin Avenue, NW, Washington, D.C. 20007, entitled *Nutrition: How Much Can Government Help?* The pamphlet offers a useful outline on the whole issue of diet and the need for better dietary guidelines. Questions are raised to stimulate thinking. You may wish to order a copy of this publication. Read the publication and determine how you could use it to initiate a lively interest in nutrition among teenagers.

REFERENCES

1. Mead, M. A perspective on food patterns. In: *Consumers and Food: Making Choices.* J. C. Penney Forum, Fall/Winter:2, 1977.
2. Lauda, F. Can a 3-year-old learn nutrition? *Sphere,* October:7, 1972.
3. Hill, M. Creating good food habits—start young, never quit. Yearbook of Agriculture, p. 260, 1969.
4. Fox, H., B. Fryer, G. Lamkin, V. Vivian, and E. Eppright. The North Central regional study on diets of preschool children. 1. Family environment. *Journal of Home Economics,* 62:241, 1970.
5. Mills, E. Psychological aspects of food habits. *Journal of Nutrition Education,* 9:67, 1977.
6. Douglas, R. Dinnertime dynamics. *Family Coordinator,* 17:181, 1968.
7. Dreyer, C., and A. Dreyer. Family dinner time as a unique behavior habitat. *Family Process,* 12:291, 1973.
8. Eppright, E., H. Fox, B. Fryer, G. Lamkin, and V. Vivian. Eating behavior of preschool children. *Journal of Nutrition Education,* 1:16, 1969.
9. Yperman, A., and J. Vermeersch. Factors associated with children's food habits. *Journal of Nutrition Education,* 11:72, 1979.

10. Clancy-Hepburn, K., A. Hickey, and G. Nevill. Children's behavior responses to TV food advertisements. *Journal of Nutrition Education,* 6:93, 1974.

11. Eppright, E., H. Fox, B. Fryer, G. Lamkin, and V. Vivian. The North Central regional study on diets of preschool children. 2. Nutrition knowledge and attitudes of mothers. *Journal of Home Economics,* 62:627, 1970.

12. Eppright, E., H. Fox, B. Fryer, G. Lamkin, V. Vivian, and E. Fuller. Nutrition of infants and preschool children in the North Central region of the United States of America. *World Review of Nutrition and Dietetics,* 14:269, 1972.

13. Pitt, A. Lunchtime at school. *Canadian Consumer,* October:29, 1976.

14. Dwyer, J., J. Feldman, and J. Mayer. Nutritional literacy of high school students. *Journal of Nutrition Education,* 2:59, 1970.

15. Huenemann, R. A review of teenage nutrition in the United States. *Proceedings, National Nutrition Education Conference,* USDA Miscellaneous Publication No. 1254, Washington, D.C., 1971.

16. Huenemann, R., L. Shapiro, M. Hampton, and B. Mitchell. Food and eating practices of teenagers. *Journal of the American Dietetics Association,* 53:17, 1968.

17. Schorr, B., D. Sanjur, and E. Erickson. Teenage food habits. *Journal of the American Dietetics Association,* 61:415, 1972.

18. Mapes, M. Gulp—an alternate method for reaching teens. *Journal of Nutrition Education,* 9:12, 1977.

19. Gifft, H., M. Washbon, and G. Harrison. *Nutrition, Behavior and Change.* Prentice-Hall, Englewood Cliffs, N.J., 1972.

20. Wenkam, N. Cultural determinants of nutritional behavior. *Nutrition Progress News,* July—August:1, 1969.

21. Dean, A. Changing food habits. Extension Bulletin 613. Home and Family Series. Cooperative Extension Service, Michigan State University, East Lansing, 1968.

22. Todhunter, N. Contemporary eating patterns; and some implications. National Extension Conference, Mexico City, 1972.

23. Clark, F. Recent food consumption surveys and their uses. *Federation Proceedings,* 33:2270, 1974.

24. Agriculture Research Service. Household food consumption survey 1965—66. Report Nos. 1 and 18. USDA, Washington, D.C., 1968—1974.

25. Rizek, R. USDA Food Consumption Survey. National Extension Nutrition and Food Preservation Workshop. Minneapolis, Minn., 1977.

26. Gortner, W. U. S. dietary trends and implications. *Contemporary Nutrition,* November:1, 1976.

27. Ambrosino, L. Do children believe in TV? *Children Today,* 1:18, 1972.

28. Ward, S., and O. Wackman. Television advertising and intrafamily influence: children's purchase influence attempts and parental yielding. In: *Television and Social Behavior,* U.S. Department of Health, Education, and Welfare, 1972.

29. Gussow, J. Counternutritional messages of TV ads aimed at children. *Journal of Nutrition Education,* 4:48, 1972.

30. Olson, M., and C. Bisogni. The impact of technology. In: *Consumers and Food: Making Choices.* J. C. Penney Forum, Fall/Winter:10, 1977.

31. Call, D. The changing food market—nutrition in a revolution. *Journal of the American Dietetic Association,* 60:384, 1972.

32. American Dietetic Association Position Paper on nutrition education and fast food service. *Journal of the American Dietetics Association,* 65:54, 1974.

33. Chem, L., and P. LaChance. An area of concern: the nutritive profile of fast food meal combinations. *Product Development,* October:40, 1974.

34. How nutritious are fast food meals? *Consumer Report,* 40:278, 1975.

35. Greecher, C., and B. Shannon. Impact of fast food meals on nutrient intake of two groups. *Journal of the American Dietetics Association,* 70:368, 1977.

36. Parrish, J. Implications of changing food habits for nutrition education. *Journal of Nutrition Education,* 2:140, 1971.

37. Diener, L. School vending machines. *Canadian Consumer,* October:37, 1976.

38. Bruch, H. The allure of food cults and nutrition quackery. *Journal of the American Dietetics Association,* 57:316, 1970.

39. National Dairy Council. Food faddism. *Dairy Council Digest,* 44:1, 1973.

40. Margolius, S. Health foods: Facts and Fakes. *New York Public Affairs Commission,* p. 28, 1973.

41. Wolnak, B. Health foods: natural, basic, and organic. *Food and Drug Cosmetic Law Journal,* 27:453, 1972.

42. White, H. The organic foods movement. *Food Technology,* 26:29, 1972.

43. Stare, F. Health foods: definitions and nutrient values. *Journal of Nutrition Education,* 4:94, 1972.

44. Erhard, D. Nutrition education for the "now generation." *Journal of Nutrition Education,* 2:135, 1971.

45. Rosebury, T. Zen diets. *Journal of the American Medical Association,* 218:1703, 1971.

46. Council on Foods and Nutrition. Zen-Macrobiotic diets. *Journal of the American Medical Association,* 218:397, 1971.

47. Majumber, S. Vegetarianism: fad, faith, or fact. *American Scientist,* 60:175, 1972.

48. Raper, N., and M. Hill. Vegetarian diets. *Nutrition Reviews,* 32:29, 1974.

49. Dwyer, J., L. Mayer, R. Kandel, and J. Mayer. The new vegetarians. *Journal of the American Dietetics Association,* 62:503, 1973.

50. Serfass, R. Dietary considerations for athletes. In: *Nutrition Update: Accent on Youth,* ed. B. Tanis. Proceedings of the 1978 Nutrition Education Workshop. American Home Economics Association, New Orleans, 1978.

51. McBean, L., and E. Speckmann. Food faddism, a challenge to nutritionists and dietitians. *American Journal of Clinical Nutrition,* 27:1071, 1974.

52. Food and Nutrition Board. *Recommended Dietary Allowances,* 9th rev. ed. National Academy of Sciences, Washington, D.C., 1980.

53. Committee on Maternal Nutrition, Food and Nutrition Board. *Maternal Nutrition and the Course of Pregnancy.* National Academy of Sciences, Washington, D.C., 1970.

54. Cook, C., and I. Payne, Effect of supplements on the nutrient intake of children. *Journal of the American Dietetics Association,* 74:130, 1979.

55. Mayer, J. Liquid protein: The last word on the "last-chance" diet. *Family Health/Today's Health,* January:40, 1978.

56. Bruch, H. Anorexia nervosa. *Nutrition Today,* 13(5):14, 1978.

57. Seltzer, C., and J. Mayer. An effective weight control program in the public school system. *American Journal of Public Health,* 60:679, 1970.

58. Collipp, P., B. Schmierer, J. Greensher, I. Rezvaine, and M. Halle. Childhood Obesity—to treat or not to treat. *Medical Times,* 99:155, 1971.

59. Cheek, D., R. Schultz, A. Parra, and R. Reba. Overgrowth of lean and adipose tissues in adolescent obesity. *Pediatric Research,* 4:268, 1970.

60. Hooper, P. Infantile overnutrition. *British Medical Journal,* 3:237, 1973.

61. Winick, M. *Childhood Obesity.* Wiley, New York, 1975.

62. Stuart, R., and B. Davis. *Slim Chance in a Fat World: Behavioral Control of Obesity.* Research Press, Champaign, Ill., 1972.

63. Hegsted, M. Food and nutrition policy: probability and practicality. *Journal of the American Dietetics Association,* 74:534, 1979.

64. Reaburn, J., M. Krondl, and D. Lau. Social determinants in food selection. *Journal of the American Dietetics Association,* 74:637, 1979.

65. Hochbaum, G. Human behavior and nutrition education. *Nutrition News,* 40:1, 1977.

66. Sipple, H. Problems and progress in nutrition education. *Journal of the American Dietetics Association,* 59:18, 1971.

67. Dwyer, J. Fad diets. Are they headaches or opportunities for upbeat nutrition education among teenagers? In: *Nutrition Update: Accent on Youth,* ed. B. Tanis. Proceedings of the 1978 Nutrition Education Workshop. American Home Economics Association, New Orleans, 1978.

68. Stansfield, P., and H. Fox. Grocers—nutrition knowledge and attitudes. *Journal of Nutrition Education,* 9:69, 1977.

69. Barlow, D., and J. Tillotson. Behavioral Science and Nutrition: A new perspective. *Journal of the American Dietetics Association,* 72:368, 1978.

70. Mahoney, M., and A. Gaggiula. Applying behavioral methods to nutritional counseling. *Journal of the American Dietetics Association,* 72:372, 1978.

71. Evans, R., and Y. Hall. Social-psychologic perspectives in motivating changes in eating behavior. *Journal of the American Dietetics Association,* 72:378, 1978.

72. Glanz, K. Strategies for nutritional counseling. *Journal of the American Dietetics Association,* 74:431, 1979.

73. Harrison, G. Cultures and food choices. In: Consumers and Food: Making Choices. J. C. Penney Forum, Fall/Winter:4, 1977.

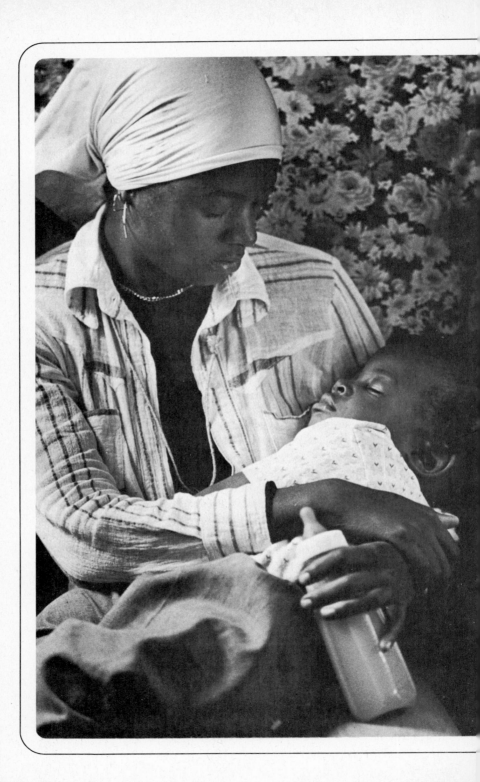

CHAPTER 7

MILK
IN
THE
INFANT
DIET

Babies are remarkable creatures. Just as remarkable is the extent of their growth and development during the first year of life. The consumption of an all-milk diet and then the transition from such a diet to one of solid foods are significant aspects of that growth and development. Feeding behaviors, like other behaviors, continually change and mature as the child grows and develops physiologically and functionally. From helpless infants, with only a sucking instinct, babies become children able to feed themselves an amazing variety of foods. This chapter and the one that follows examine nutrient intake and food habits during this critical early period of development and note what changes take place.

NUTRIENT REQUIREMENTS

The nutritional status of the young child is a major factor in determining his or her health, growth, and development (**1**). The magnitude of growth during the first year of life is secondary only to the rate of growth during the intrauterine period. As a corollary, the child's nutritional requirements per unit of body weight are greater during infancy than at any later age. Since the infant is especially vulnerable to nutritional inadequacy, it is critical that the diet supply nutrients in sufficient quantity and quality to support the rapid rate of growth and development.

A desirable and progressive increase in the infant's weight and length depends, to a large extent, on adequate nutrition. During the first 24−72 hours after birth, the infant experiences a weight loss of 5−7 oz or 140−200 g. This weight loss is partially due to fluid loss and partially to poor food intake during this time before a regular feeding pattern becomes well established (**2**). Following this initial weight loss the infant gains at a rate of approximately 6 oz or 170 g per week, and the average infant doubles its birth weight and grows 4 in (10 cm) in length by the age of 6 months (**2**). By 12 months of age the average infant weighs approximately 20 lb (9 kg) or triple its birth weight (**2**). The average length is now 28 in. (71 cm), an increase of approximately 7 in. (18 cm) or 33 percent of the average length at birth. The infant's nutrient intake during these first 12 months of life must satisfy these extremely rapid growth rate requirements and replace losses.

It is difficult to set ideal standards for infant nutrition, but the nutritional performance of infants fed human milk is generally considered the norm when assessing the performance of infants receiving other forms of food. Many unanswered questions remain in the area of infant nutrient requirements, but the nutrient intake of human infants thriving on breast milk is regarded as a reliable guide to determine infant nutritional needs, with the exception of certain minerals and vitamins.

Nutrient requirements vary with age, size, growth rate, activity level, and interaction with other nutrients in the diet. Several methods are in use to estimate nutrient requirements in infants. None of these, however, is totally satisfactory, and recommendations for nutrient intake are often based on inadequate information. As pointed out previously, nutrient requirements are usually estimated in relation to the nutrient content supplied by human milk. This method presents some problems, though. It is generally accepted that certain nutrients, in particular iron and vitamin D, are not provided by breast milk in sufficient amounts to support adequate growth (**3**). In addition the amounts of nutrients received from breast milk depend on the volume consumed and the stage of lactation. The few existing metabolic balance studies of normal full-term infants (**4, 5, 6**) are used to estimate infant requirements for protein, essential amino acids, and certain minerals. However, because of ethical considerations associated with experiments on human infants, these studies generally serve only to confirm estimates made by other approaches.

Further estimates can be made by extrapolating data derived from experiments with adult humans or with infant and adult animals. The nutrient intake of healthy infants, other than breast-fed, can also serve as a guide to nutritional requirements (**7, 8**). Information from such studies, though, often shows a wide variation in the intake of particular nutrients. The effect of intake on future growth often cannot be predicted from the little information available. This is an area needing additional and continued study.

Infant nutrient requirements also can be determined using the factorial method of adding together the requirements for growth, replacement of losses, and maintenance. This method is not useful for establishing requirements for certain nutrients (e.g., protein at various ages), but it can be used to estimate the mineral requirements of infants.

The estimated requirements, advisable intakes, and RDAs for certain nutrients during infancy are shown in Table 7.1. These RDAs are those of the

TABLE 7.1 RDAs, ESTIMATED DAILY REQUIREMENTS, AND ADVISABLE INTAKE FOR VARIOUS NUTRIENTS

Nutrient	Recommended Allowances[1]		Estimated Requirements[2]		Advisable Intakes[2]	
	0–6 months[3]	6–12 months[4]	0–4 months	4–12 months	0–4 months	4–12 months
Energy	kg × 115 (kcal)	kg × 105 (kcal)				
Protein	kg × 2.2 (g)	kg × 2.0 (g)	1.6 g/100 kcal	1.4 g/100 kcal	1.9 g/100 kcal	1.7 g/100 kcal
Sodium			2.5 mEq	2.1 mEq	8 mEq	6 mEq
Chloride			2.3 mEq	2.1 mEq	7 mEq	6 mEq
Potassium			2.4 mEq	2.0 mEq	7 mEq	6 mEq
Calcium	360 mg	540 mg	388 mg	289 mg	450 mg	350 mg
Phosphorus	240 mg	360 mg	132 mg	110 mg	160 mg	130 mg
Iodine	40 mcg	50 mcg				
Iron	10 mg	15 mg	16.5 mg	13.5 mg		
Magnesium	50 mg	70 mg			25 mg	20 mg
Zinc	3 mg	5 mg				

Nutrient	Recommended Allowances[1]		Estimated Requirements[2]	Advisable Intakes[2]
	0–6 months	6–12 months	0–12 months	0–12 months
Vitamin A	420 R.E.[5]	400 R.E.	50 R.E.	100 R.E.
Vitamin D[6]	10 mcg	10 mcg	2.5–5 mcg	10 mcg
Vitamin E	3 mg[7]	4 mg	3.3 mg	2.6 mg
Vitamin K			5 mcg	15 mcg
Ascorbic acid	35 mg	35 mg	10 mg	20 mg
Folacin	30 mcg	45 mcg	<50 mcg	50 mcg
Niacin	6 mg[8]	8 mg	4.4 mg/1000 kcal	5 mg
Riboflavin	0.4 mg	0.6 mg	<0.5 mg/1000 kcal	0.4 mg
Thiamin	0.3 mg	0.5 mg	0.2 mg/1000 kcal	0.2 mg
Vitamin B_6	0.3 mg	0.6 mg	9 mcg/g protein	0.4 mg
Vitamin B_{12}	0.5 mcg	1.5 mcg		

[1] From FNB (9).
[2] From Fomon (10).
[3] Weight, 6 kg; height 60 cm.
[4] Weight, 9 kg; height 71 cm.
[5] Retinol equivalents (R.E.). 1 R.E. = 1 mcg retinol or 6 mcg B carotene.
[6] As cholecalciferol. 10 mcg cholecalciferol = 400 IU vitamin D.
[7] Mg of α-tocopherol equivalents; 1 mg D-α-tocopherol = 1 α-T.E.
[8] (N.E.) niacin equivalent = 1 mg niacin or 60 mg dietary tryptophan.

National Academy of Sciences, FNB (**9**). In addition to these standard values, this chapter includes values for estimated requirements and advisable intakes for each nutrient discussed, as Fomon (**10**) has done in his text on infant nutrition. The estimated requirements for each specific nutrient are the least amounts of that nutrient needed to promote an optimal state of health. Because food varies widely in its nutritional value, nutritionists usually suggest intakes in excess of the estimated requirements. The three values (RDA, estimated requirement, and advisable intake) are used to give additional information about nutrient requirements for infants and toddlers. They also emphasize that the state of knowledge about nutritional requirements for infants and toddlers has not reached the point where finite recommendations are available.

Protein and Amino Acids

In developing countries, infants frequently receive an inadequate amount of protein or essential amino acids to support normal growth and health. This protein malnutrition is rarely a problem in developed countries. During the first year of life the protein content of the body increases from 11 to 14.6 percent, while body weight increases by 7 kg (**9**). The average increase in body protein is 3.5 g per day for the first four months of life and 3.1 g per day during the next eight months (**10**). The RDA for protein established by the FNB (**9**) is based on the amount of protein provided by the quantity of milk required to insure a satisfactory growth rate. This amount is estimated to be approximately 2–2.4 g of protein per kilogram per day during the first month of life, gradually decreasing to 1.5 g per kilogram by the sixth month. The RDA for protein for infants is set at 2.2 g per kilogram per day from birth to 6 months, and 2.0 g per kilogram per day from 6 to 12 months (**9**). Fomon (**11**) suggests that the protein requirement of a full-term infant fed *ad libitum* is no greater than 1.6 g per 100 kcal during the first 16 weeks of life, then decreasing to 1.4 g per 100 kcal. These estimates for protein requirement per unit of caloric intake do not differ greatly from the protein : calorie ratio of human milk which is 1.5 g per 100 kcal. Although this ratio of protein to calories may be adequate for the breast-fed infant, there is not enough information on the adequacy of this protein to calorie ratio from other protein sources used in infant feeding. Fomon (**10**), therefore, suggests that advisable protein intakes be set 20 percent higher than the estimated requirements or 1.9 g per 100 kcal for the first 4 months and 1.7 g per 100 kcal for the rest of the first year. An infant diet supplying less than 6 percent of calories in the form of protein can lead to a protein deficiency and resulting poor health (**10, 12**). On the other hand, a diet supplying greater than 16 percent of caloric intake as protein may actually be harmful to the infant and is certainly not a metabolically or economically efficient manner to supply calories (**10**).

The amino acids considered essential in the adult are also essential for the infant (**13, 14, 15**). In addition, histidine was recently established as essential for both the normal and premature infant. Cystine may also be an essential amino acid in the first few weeks of life (**16**). The amino acid requirements for infant growth and maintenance, expressed per kilogram of body weight, are two to three times greater than those of children aged 10 to 12 years and four to ten times greater than those of the adult (Table 7.2). Two grams of protein (of the quality listed in column 4, Table 7.2) per kilogram of body weight per day will meet the amino acid needs of the infant (**9**). Thirty-five percent of a dietary protein allowance of 2 g per kilogram per day should be provided as essential amino acids for the infant (**9**). The daily amino acid requirements for an infant can be provided by 1.6 g of human milk protein or 2.0 g of cow's milk protein.

Amino acid requirements for infants were first based on estimates derived from studies in which the child was fed mixtures of purified amino acids. These requirements may differ when amino acids are fed in the form of intact protein or when protein is fed at a level approaching recommended intakes (Table 7.1). The original estimates were based on a diet supplying approximately 3 g of protein per kilogram per day, a high level. Recent studies (Table 7.3) indicate that requirements do differ when amino acids are supplied as whole protein in the diet (**14, 17**). Further research is needed in the area of amino acid requirements for human infants.

Carbohydrate

Carbohydrate is generally consumed in the form of disaccharides, most commonly lactose and sucrose (**2**). On hydrolysis both these sugars yield glucose which is necessary for maintaining blood glucose levels and meeting energy requirements for infants. Dietary carbohydrate becomes important, since fetal hepatic glycogen is almost completely depleted in the first 24−48 hours of life. Only lactose yields galactose on hydrolysis. This sugar plays a unique role in the synthesis of the cerebrosides of myelin and the glycoproteins of collagen (**18**). Human milk provides about 37 percent of its calories in the form of carbohydrate,

TABLE 7.2 ESTIMATED AMINO ACID REQUIREMENTS OF MAN

Amino Acid	Requirement (mg per kg of body wt. per day)			Amino acid pattern for high-quality proteins (mg/g of protein)
	Infant (4−6 months)	Child (10−12 years)	Adult	
Histidine	33	—	—	17
Isoleucine	83	28	12	42
Leucine	135	42	16	70
Lysine	99	44	12	51
Total S-containing amino acids	49	22	10	26
Total aromatic amino acids	141	22	16	73
Threonine	68	28	8	35
Tryptophan	21	4	3	11
Valine	92	25	14	48

Source: Reprinted from Food and Nutrition Board, *Recommended Dietary Allowances,* 9th edition. National Academy of Sciences, 1980 (**9**).

TABLE 7.3 PRELIMINARY ESTIMATES OF
REQUIREMENTS FOR AMINO ACIDS BY INFANTS

Amino acid	Estimate (mg/100 kcal)[1]
Histidine	26
Isoleucine	66
Leucine	132
Lysine	101
Phenylalanine	57
Methionine	24
Cystine	23
Threonine	59
Tryptophan	16
Valine	83

Source: Reproduced with permission from *Infant Nutrition,* 2nd edition, by S. J. Fomon (**10**). Copyright © 1974 by W. B. Saunders Co., Philadelphia.
[1]Because of the manner in which these estimates were made, the true requirement for several of the amino acids is likely to be substantially less than the preliminary estimate given here.

principally lactose (**10**). Cow's milk and infant formulas, respectively, supply approximately 29 and 42 percent of calories as carbohydrate (**10**).

Fat

Fat in the infant diet represents the high energy component, the satiety factor, and the vehicle for fat-soluble vitamins and essential fatty acids. Infants are able to absorb approximately 92 percent of the fat found in human milk but only 65 percent of that present in cow's milk (**2**).

The relative importance of the type of dietary fat for young children is a subject of extensive study. It is well known that dietary fat affects the absorption of other nutrients in the diet and influences the nature of serum lipids and composition of depot fat in the body (Figure 7.1).

Approximately 55 percent of the calories in breast milk are in the form of fat. A diet with less than 30 percent of its calories as fat will be low in satiety value and may contain excessive protein and carbohydrate in relation to fat (**20**). Skim milk provides only 3 percent of calories as fat, with 40 percent as protein. Unless additional oil is given, the infant on a skim milk diet will require such a large volume of milk to meet its caloric requirements that it may establish a pattern of overeating (**21**). Therefore, infants should not be given skim milk, except on the advice of a physician (**22**). On the other hand, a diet supplying greater than 55 percent of its caloric intake as fat may lead to ketosis (**10**).

Linoleic acid is an essential nutrient for the infant. The dietary requirement for this nutrient depends on the rate of growth and the composition of the rest of the diet. Rapidly growing infants develop deficiency symptoms when linoleic acid supplies less than 1 percent of their caloric intake. These deficiency symptoms

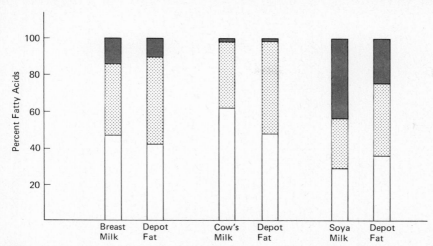

Figure 7.1 *Fatty acid composition of triglycerides of depot fat of infants aged 6 weeks compared with that of their milk feed. Polyunsaturated fatty acids,* ■■*; monounsaturated,* ▦*; saturated,* ▢*.* (*Source:* Reproduced with permission from Sweeney et al. **[19]**. Copyright © 1963 by Rockefeller University Press, New York.)

include diminished weight gain, scaly dermatitis, and an increase in total serum fatty acid content accompanied by a decrease in serum levels of linoleic and arachidonic acid (**23**). Breast milk supplies 5 percent of its calories as essential fatty acids, principally in the form of linoleic acid. This fact is taken into consideration in the establishment of recommended levels of intake. The Committee on Nutrition of the American Academy of Pediatrics recommends a minimum level of 300 mg of linoleic acid per 100 kcal in infant formula (**24**). An ideal dietary level has not been determined, though.

Calories

During infancy the child uses a large proportion of his or her energy requirements for growth. The caloric requirement per kilogram of body weight is, therefore, greater during infancy than at any other time in life. Figure 7.2 shows that the caloric percentage necessary for growth is 32.8 percent between birth and 4 months and gradually decreases to 1 percent between 2 and 3 years of age.

Table 7.4 shows the estimated chemical composition of gains between birth and 4 months of age, 4 and 12 months, 1 and 2 years, and 2 and 3 years. The synthesis of body components other than fat and protein accounts for only a very small percentage of the calories required for growth (**11**). It is assumed that the rapidly growing infant requires 7.5 and 11.6 kcal for the synthesis of 1 g of protein and 1 g of fat respectively (**1**).

The RDA for energy is set at levels that reflect the general pattern of intake for thriving infants, 115 kcal per kilogram at birth and decreasing to 105 kcal per kilogram by the first year (**9**). These amounts cover basal caloric requirements of approximately 55 kcal per kilogram, normal growth requirements of 35 kcal per

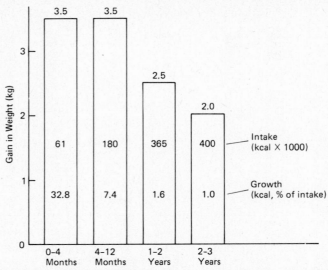

Figure 7.2 *Gain in weight of the male reference infant during various age intervals, estimated total intake of calories during each age interval and estimated percentage of calorie intake utilized for growth. (Source:* Reproduced with permission from *Infant Nutrition,* 2nd edition, by S. J. Fomon. Copyright © 1974 by W. B. Saunders Co., Philadelphia.)

TABLE 7.4 GAIN IN BODY COMPONENTS OF REFERENCE
BOY AT VARIOUS INTERVALS BETWEEN BIRTH AND 3 YEARS

Interval (Months)	Composition of Gain (gm/100 gm)			
	Water	Protein	Lipid	Other
0–4	45.3	11.4	41.6	1.7
4–12	56.6	21.0	19.1	3.3
12–24	69.4	20.3	6.8	3.5
24–36	68.5	20.9	3.4	7.2

Source: From Fomon (**10**). Reproduced with permission from *Infant Nutri-tion,* 2nd edition, by S. J. Fomon. Copyright © 1974 by W. B. Saunders Co., Philadelphia.

kilogram, and normal activity requirements of 10–25 kcal per kilogram (**20**). It is suggested that 7–16 percent of the calories in the infant diet be supplied by protein, 30–55 percent by fat, and 35–65 percent by carbohydrate (**10**). Human milk supplies approximately 7 percent of its calories as protein, 55 percent as fat, and 38 percent as carbohydrate (**10**). Most commercially prepared infant formulas in the United States supply 9–15 percent of their calories as protein, 45–50 percent as fat, and 35–46 percent as carbohydrate (**10**). Corresponding values for cow's milk are 20 percent, 60 percent, and 29 percent. Caloric requirements are probably best calculated on a weight basis initially and then modified to suit individual infant needs, body build, and degree of activity. The amount of food in a well-balanced diet that an infant will consume at fairly regular, well-spaced meals can serve as a guide to individual requirements. Healthy, well-fed infants generally adjust their caloric intake to their bodies' own natural needs.

Vitamins

The vitamins required in the infant diet are similar to those required by the older child and the adult (**2**). Because of the extremely rapid growth rate during infancy, though, these vitamins are needed in proportionally greater quantities. Although deficiency diseases related to inadequate vitamin intake have not been completely eliminated, vitamin deficiencies occurring during infancy are relatively uncommon, and the use of multiple vitamin supplements is usually unnecessary. The estimated daily requirements, advisable intakes, and the recommended daily allowances for vitamins during infancy are shown in Table 7.1.

Vitamin A.   Human milk, cow's milk, and infant formula are all relatively rich sources of vitamin A or carotene (**10**). Many strained infant foods and table food also supply vitamin A in the diet. Studies of growth and development during infancy indicate that the requirement for vitamin A is approximately 30 IU per kilogram of body weight per day (**25**). The values for estimated requirements in Table 7.1 assume an average weight of approximately 8 kg between birth and 12 months (**10**). The RDA for vitamin A is based on the average retinol content of human milk, 49 mcg per 100 ml. The healthy breast-fed infant consumes approximately 420 mcg of retinol per day (**9**). The FNB, therefore, sets the RDA for infants from birth to 6 months at 420 R.E. (1400 IU) and 400 R.E. (2000 IU) from 6 months to 1 year of age (**9**). Little is known about the requirement for the low birth-weight infant. Studies suggest, though, that the recommended intakes be similar to those of the normal full-term infant (**10**). Vitamin A deficiencies are rarely observed in the United States but do occur in cases of malabsorption syndrome or when an infant is fed a milk-free or skim milk diet not supplemented with vitamin A.

Vitamin D.   Vitamin D is one vitamin not found naturally in adequate amounts in either human or cow's milk (**10**). Studies indicate that the requirement for vitamin D during infancy is approximately 2.5 mcg (100 IU) to 5.0 mcg (200 IU) per day. The RDA is set at 10 mcg (400 IU) per day (**9**), and nutritionists generally recommend that the breast-fed infant receive a supplement of this amount each day. Evaporated milk, whole cow's milk, and most formulas are fortified with 10 mcg of vitamin D per quart. The American Academy of Pediatrics suggests a minimum formula fortification level of 1.55 mcg per 100 kcal or 10 mcg per liter and a maximum level of 2.5 mcg per 100 kcal or 16.75 mcg per liter (**24**). This latter figure technically exceeds the maximum allowance of 10 mcg per day set by the FDA to avoid the risk of hypercalcemia. The American Academy of Pediatrics feels that the higher levels are justified in the case of formulas for low birth-weight infants, where a low intake, coupled with poor fat absorption, may result in low intakes of vitamin D from formulas fortified to a level of only 10 mcg per liter (**24**).

Vitamin E.   Plasma vitamin E levels in the breast-fed infant increase steadily from 33 percent of adult levels at birth to 100 percent at 2−3 weeks of age (**9**). Thus the vitamin E content of human milk, 1.3−3.3 mg d-α-tocopherol equivalents (2−5 IU) per liter, provides an adequate intake for the healthy infant. The FNB suggests that an intake in this range should be provided in a mixed diet of solid foods and milk up to 1 year of age (**9**). RDAs are set at 3 mg α-tocopherol from birth to 6 months and 4 mg α-tocopherol from 6 to 12 months.

The vitamin E requirement is related to the polyunsaturated fatty acid (PUFA) content of cellular structures which in turn is dependent on dietary fat (**26**). A satisfactory concentration of plasma α-tocopherol of 1 mg per 100 ml (**27**) is maintained by infants fed a diet with a ratio of vitamin E to polyunsaturated fatty acids of 0.4 mg per gram (**10**). The vitamin E and polyunsaturated fatty acid content of infant formulas must be carefully monitored and adjusted to provide this ratio. Unless all the fat in an infant's formula is in the form of a highly unsaturated vegetable oil, an infant is unlikely to receive more than 7.5 g of polyunsaturated fatty acids per day. An advisable intake of 4 IU (1 mg d-α-tocopherol=1.1 IU) of vitamin E per day should, therefore, be adequate to supply the desired vitamin E : PUFA (polyunsaturated fatty acid) ratio of 0.4 mg per gram. Low birth-weight infants appear more likely to develop vitamin E deficiencies than do full-term infants, and a daily supplement of 0.5 mg per kilogram of body weight may be recommended in certain instances.

Vitamin K.   Human milk supplies approximately 15 mcg of vitamin K per liter, whereas cow's milk supplies approximately 60 mcg per liter. The infant requirement appears to be in the range of 5 mcg per day. The FNB has estimated safe and adequate intakes of 12 mcg per day from birth to 6 months and 10−20 mcg per day from 6 to 12 months (**9**). Vitamin K deficiencies have been reported in newborn infants prior to the establishment of intestinal flora and synthesis of vitamin K in the gut. Breast-fed infants appear to develop mild vitamin K deficiency within 2−3 days after birth more frequently than do those receiving formulas (**28**). Clinical symptoms of bleeding actually develop in approximately 1 of 400 of these infants (**29**). The American Academy of Pediatrics recommends that all newborn infants receive a single parenteral dose of 0.5−1.0 mg of vitamin K immediately after birth (**30**). Certain water-soluble analogues of vitamin K can produce jaundice, especially in low birth-weight infants, because of an increased breakdown of red blood cells. So such preparations are no longer recommended during the newborn period.

Thiamin.   The information on thiamin requirements during infancy is limited. Human milk provides 0.16 mg of thiamin per liter or 0.22 mg per 100 kcal. Therefore, the normal breast-fed infant receives approximately 0.12 mg of thiamin per day by the first month of life and 0.16 mg per day by the sixth month of life (**10**). Studies of the thiamin requirement in infancy in relation to the thiamin content of human milk suggest that the minimum daily requirement is approximately 0.03 mg per kilogram of body weight or 0.27 mg per 1000 kcal. The RDA is set at 0.3 mg from birth to 6 months and 0.5 mg from 6 months to 1 year (**9**).

Niacin. Human milk supplies 4.4 mg of niacin per liter. The estimated intake of the breast-fed infant is 3.3 mg per day by the first month of life and 4.1 mg per day by the sixth month (**10**). The advisable intake of niacin from birth to 3 years is set at 5.0 mg per day (**10**). The RDA from birth to 6 months is set at 6 mg per day, with approximately two-thirds being supplied by tryptophan (**9**). For infants over 6 months of age the RDA is set at 8.0 mg per day (**9**).

Riboflavin. Studies indicate that breast-fed infants receive 0.27 mg of riboflavin per day at 1 month and 0.34 mg per day at 6 months of age (**10**). Advisable intakes are set at 0.4 mg per day for the first year of life (**10**). The RDA is 0.4 mg per day for the first 6 months and 0.6 mg for the second six (**9**).

Folacin. Human milk contains approximately 2−3 mcg of folacin per 100 ml. Infant requirements are generally estimated to be less than 50 mcg per day. The RDA for folacin is set at 5 mcg per kilogram per day (**9**).

Pyridoxine. Levels of vitamin B_6 in cord blood are generally greater than those in maternal blood (**31**). The infant is, therefore, born with some vitamin B_6 stores. Human milk contains 0.01−0.02 mg of vitamin B_6 per liter during the first few days of lactation, and this value gradually increases to 0.1 mg per liter. Cow's milk contains 0.23−0.60 mg of the vitamin per liter. Clinical symptoms of deficiency are reported in some breast-fed infants receiving maternal milk with concentrations of 0.06−0.08 mg of vitamin B_6 per liter.

The vitamin B_6 requirement is related to the protein content of the diet, and requirements appear to be met when the diet supplies 0.04 mg per 100 kcal of formula or 15 mcg per gram of protein. Human milk contains 9 mcg of vitamin B_6 per gram of protein. This concentration appears to be adequate to handle the protein load received in breast-feeding and is used as a guide in developing requirements. Cow's milk contains approximately 19 mcg of vitamin B_6 per gram of protein.

Vitamin B_{12}. Little evidence is available concerning the requirement of the infant for vitamin B_{12}, but the average daily output of vitamin B_{12} in human milk is 0.3 mcg (**32**). Overt vitamin B_{12} deficiency symptoms have not been observed in infants breast-fed by mothers with adequate serum vitamin B_{12} levels. The recommended dietary allowance for this vitamin, therefore, is 0.5 mcg per day from birth to 6 months and 1.5 mcg from 6 to 12 months (**9**).

Ascorbic Acid. The supply of vitamin C is inadequate in both cow's milk and human milk, unless the mother is consuming sufficient amounts of the vitamin. The exact requirement for this vitamin is not known. If a mother is receiving adequate amounts, her baby's needs appear to be satisfied by the ascorbic acid in the breast milk, 40−55 mg per liter. The average healthy infant consumes approximately 35 mg of vitamin C from breast milk each day, and the RDA is, therefore, set at 35 mg.

Minerals

Sodium, Potassium, Chloride.   The estimated requirements, advisable intakes, and RDAs for minerals during infancy are shown in Table 7.1. Human milk provides approximately 7 mEq of sodium per liter, whereas cow's milk provides approximately 21 mEq per liter. Average intakes of sodium during the first year of life range from about 300 mg (13 mEq) per day at 2 months of age to about 1400 mg (60 mEq) per day at 12 months (**9**). Safe and adequate daily intakes are estimated to be 115–350 mg for infants from birth to 6 months of age and 250–750 mg from 6 to 12 months of age (**9**). Human milk contains 500 mg (13 mEq) of potassium per liter. Fluid cow's milk provides about 1365 mg (35 mEq) per liter. The FNB has set safe and adequate intake levels at 350–925 mg per day during the first 6 months of life and 425–1275 mg per day during the second 6 months (**9**). Chloride is found in human milk at a concentration of 11 mEq per liter. Estimated safe and adequate daily intakes for chloride are 275–700 mg for the infant up to 6 months of age and 400–1200 mg from 6 to 12 months of age (**9**).

Calcium.   At birth, mean calcium levels in cord blood are approximately 10 mg per 100 ml (**2**). In the normal newborn this level falls to 8.3 mg per 100 ml during the first 24–48 hours following birth. Seventy-five percent of breast-fed infants then show an increase in blood calcium following this initial decrease (**2**). The remaining 25 percent show no further change. Approximately one-third of those infants fed evaporated cow's milk, however, show a significant decrease in plasma calcium (**33**). Cow's milk contains approximately four to six times as much calcium as human milk in the early weeks of lactation, and the phosphorus content of cow's milk is six to eight times greater than that of human milk.

Two possibilities may explain the hypocalcemia associated with the drinking of cow's milk (**2**). First, the high phosphate content of cow's milk may interfere with calcium absorption, or an increased absorption of phosphorus may result in high plasma phosphorus levels producing a fall in plasma calcium. Second, approximately 25 percent of the fat content of cow's milk is not absorbed (**34**). Unabsorbed fatty acids may combine with calcium, forming calcium salts, and thereby decreasing calcium absorption. Breast-fed infants receiving 60 mg of calcium per kilogram (300 mg per liter of milk) retain approximately two-thirds of that amount. In contrast, infants on cow's milk formulas receive approximately 170 mg per kilogram but may retain only 25–30 percent of that amount. The breast-fed infant apparently has less calcium available to him or her, but this infant's calcium needs are usually met. The RDAs of 360 mg from birth to 6 months and 540 mg from 6 months to 1 year apply only to infants fed on formulas.

Phosphorus.   In considering a phosphorus allowance for the infant, one needs to keep in mind calcium : phosphorus ratios. The recommended amount of calcium in infant formulas is 50 mg per 100 kcal, with a calcium to phosphorus ratio between 1.1 and 2.0 (**24**). Calcium to phosphorus ratios in human and cow's milk are 2.0 and 1.2, respectively. The phosphorus intake in cow's milk may contribute to the development of hypocalcemia during the first 2–3 weeks of life.

So current evidence supports the recommendation that the calcium to phosphorus ratio in the diet during early infancy be at least 1.5 : 1 (**9**). The RDAs for phosphorus are 240 mg and 360 mg during the first and second 6 months of life, respectively.

Magnesium.   Human milk contains approximately 4 mg of magnesium per 100 ml. Cow's milk contains 12 mg of the mineral per 100 ml. The RDAs for infants are based on this information and are set at 50 mg per day from birth to 6 months and 70 mg per day from 6 to 12 months (**9**).

Iron.   The precise requirements for and the best means of providing a desirable iron intake during infancy are uncertain. The amount of iron required has been estimated using two different methods. The average body iron content at birth and at 1 year of age has been calculated, and the amount of iron that must be absorbed during the first year of life is estimated to be 0.8 mg per day, based on this method (**35**). A second method to determine requirements is to feed infants various amounts of dietary iron and observe hemoglobin concentrations. The highest hemoglobin concentrations are observed with daily iron intakes of 1.0 mg per kilogram of body weight (**36**). One milligram of iron per kilogram per day, up to a maximum of 15 mg, should be given to the normal infant, beginning at an appropriate time (generally around the third month), with respect to initial iron stores to maintain normal hemoglobin levels (**37**). Infants with low iron stores at birth or those who have suffered blood loss should have 2.0 mg per kilogram per day, beginning at 2 months of age or as soon after birth as necessary. The RDAs of 10 mg per day from birth to 6 months and 15 mg per day from 6 to 12 months are based on the average need of infants (1.5 mg per kilogram per day) during the first year of life (**9**). The iron content of an unfortified milk diet is inadequate to meet these infant iron requirements. Even on a mixed diet, iron intake will not generally be greater than 6.0 mg per 1000 kcal, unless artificially iron-enriched foods are included. To meet the foregoing requirements, iron-enriched foods are necessary during infancy. Infants should receive 1 mg of iron per kilogram per day from cereal or formula, supplemented with at least 1 mg of iron per 100 kcal. Most commercially prepared infant cereals provide 8.6–22 mg of iron per dry ounce of cereal. Many formulas are supplemented with iron at a level of 12 mg per liter, and this level is probably greater than necessary to prevent iron deficiency. Iron is less available in higher protein formulas. Iron deficiency is more common in infants fed a formula containing 2.4 percent protein than in those fed one containing 1.5 percent protein (**38**). Fortification of both types of formula to a level of 8 mg of iron per liter is associated with an absence of iron deficiency (**38**). The Committee on Nutrition of the American Academy of Pediatrics recommends that all infant formulas contain at least the level of iron found in human milk, 0.15 mg per 100 kcal or 1 mg per liter (**24**). Despite the prevalence of iron deficiency during infancy, unfortified formulas are still available in this country. The Committee on Nutrition further emphasizes the inclusion of iron-supplemented foods in the diet for at least the first 18 months of life to insure a desirable amount of iron in the diet (**37**). Further study is needed to determine how iron metabolism is affected by different levels of dietary intake, the different forms of iron in the diet, and the weight and maturity of the infant at birth.

Copper. The values of copper concentration in human and cow's milk vary considerably. The level is relatively low for both types of milk and is lower in human than in cow's milk (**39**). Full-term infants evidently need more copper than can be provided by a normal consumption of either human or cow's milk. Cow's milk is low in copper, with concentrations of 0.015–0.18 mg per liter, whereas the concentration in human milk ranges from 1.05 mg per liter at the beginning of lactation to 0.15 mg per liter at the end. Whether copper supplements in the diet are necessary becomes questionable in view of large liver stores of this mineral. Research also suggests that copper absorption from human milk is more efficient than that from cow's milk because of a zinc-copper interaction. The ratio of zinc to copper in human milk is approximately 4.0. A higher ratio in cow's milk may depress copper absorption (**40**). The FNB estimates that safe and adequate intakes of copper are in the range of 0.5–0.7 mg per day during the first 6 months of life and 0.7–1.0 mg per day during the second 6 months (**9**).

Fluorine. Fluorine is important in the infant diet because of the role it plays in tooth development. Nutritionists generally feel that infants should receive 0.1–0.5 mg of fluorine per day during the first 6 months of life and 0.2–1.0 mg per day from 6 to 12 months (**9, 41**). Nutritionists used to assume that formula-fed infants living in communities with nonfluoridated drinking water and all breast-fed infants would receive only a small amount of fluorine and would benefit from a fluorine supplement. It subsequently became evident, though, that the concentrations of fluorine in infant formulas and in certain commercially prepared infant foods are greater than had been recognized (**42, 43**). Mild enamel fluorosis is, in fact, reported in the permanent incisors of children who received fluorine supplements during infancy (**44**). Nutritionists, therefore, recommend that no fluoride supplement be given to formula-fed infants during the first 6 months of life (**45**). A supplement of 0.25 mg per day, beginning soon after birth, is still recommended for fully breast-fed infants (**43**). Recently, manufacturers have recommended the reduction of the fluorine content of commercially prepared infant formulas and cereals. Fomon et al. (**43**) suggest that if such reductions do occur, a fluorine supplement of 0.25 mg per day should also be given to infants living in areas where the fluorine content of the water is 0.3 ppm or less.

Iodine. Milk from adequately nourished mothers contains approximately 10–20 mcg of iodine per 100 kcal. The breast-fed infant receives approximately 60–120 mcg per day, sufficient for normal growth and development. The recommended dietary intake from birth to 6 months of age is 40 mcg and from 6 to 12 months of age is 50 mcg (**9**).

Zinc. Little information is available on which to base zinc requirements during infancy, and the zinc concentrations of human milk as reported in the literature vary widely. The concentration of zinc in both human and cow's milk falls from over 20 mg per liter in the colostrum to 3−4 mg per liter as lactation progresses. Both milks, however, appear to provide adequate zinc intake to full-term infants if approximately 15 percent of the amount is absorbed and retained (**39**). If the concentration of zinc in breast milk is accepted to be 3−5 mg per kilogram (**46**) the healthy breast-fed infant receives an intake of close to 3 mg of zinc or more per day for the first 6 months of life. The RDA is, on this basis, set at 3 mg per day for the first 6 months of life and 5 mg per day from 6 months to 1 year (**9**).

Water.   Fluid balance can be disturbed more easily in infants than in adults. The human infant requires more water to replace that lost through the skin, lungs, feces, and urine and to provide the small amount of water needed for active growth. These requirements range from 75 to 90 ml per kilogram of body weight per day to handle normal solute loads (**47**). Human milk, cow's milk, and almost all commercially prepared formulas contain 67 kcal per 100 ml (**20**). An infant receiving these feedings will, therefore, have a more than adequate water intake of 150−200 ml per kilogram per day (**20, 47**).

BREAST-FEEDING

Until 1900 human milk was regarded as the sole source of nutrients for the infant at birth, and it remained the primary source during the first year of life. The growth pattern and nutritional status of the healthy breast-fed infant became the reference standard for the establishment of nutritional requirements during infancy. The inability of some mothers to nurse successfully and the failure of some infants to thrive on a diet of breast milk alone eventually led to the use of modified cow's milk and the development of present-day infant formulas as substitutes for breast milk. Accompanying the use of such substitutes has been a progressive decline in the numbers of women breast-feeding their infants (**48−53**). Eighty percent of the infants in this country were being fed a commercial formula at the time of their discharge from the hospital following birth by 1970. Twenty-seven percent were partially breast-fed. Of those, only 15 percent were still receiving breast milk at 2 months of age and less than 10 percent at the age of 4 months. Recently, such organizations as La Leche League International have started a trend back toward breast-feeding, but the number of women who breast-feed their babies is still not large (Figure 7.3).

Nutrient Content of Breast Milk

As has already been pointed out, relatively little information is available on the actual nutrient intake of healthy infants. Studies that report detailed nutrient consumption and growth over a lengthy period are time consuming and the number of subjects available for such research is limited. Some information is available, derived from balance studies conducted for limited time periods on small numbers of infants. These studies, however, present conflicting results regarding the differences in weight changes, height changes, and other physical findings between infants fed breast milk, cow's milk, or infant formulas.

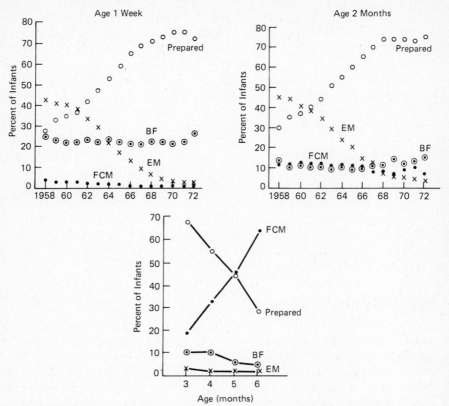

Figure 7.3 *Percent of infants in the United States between 1958 and 1972 who were breast-fed (BF), fed evaporated milk formulas (EM), commercially prepared formulas (prepared), or fresh cow milk (FCM) from one week to six months of age. (Source:* Reproduced with permission from G. A. Martinez and J. P. Nalezienski in *Pediatrics 64,* (5):686−692, 1979. Copyright © by the American Academy of Pediatrics, Evanston, Illinois.)

    Obvious differences exist in the nutrient composition of colostrum, mature human milk, and cow's milk (Table 7.5). *Colostrum* is the material secreted by the human breast for the first few days after birth before mature milk begins to be produced. It is a clear or yellowish fluid and is lower in energy value than mature milk largely because of its lower lactose and fat content. The concentrations of protein, immunoglobulins, sodium, potassium, and chloride, however, are greater in colostrum than in mature milk. Colostrum also contains slightly more vitamin A than is found in the milk secreted later in the lactation period. Colostrum is suited to the nutritional needs of the newborn infant during the first days of life and is especially important in providing the infant with some immunological defenses.

    Mature milk begins to develop from day 2 to day 10 of lactation, depending on the mother's parity and the frequency of sucking during the first few days. A major difference between mature human milk and cow's milk is the concentration

TABLE 7.5 COMPOSITION OF
COLOSTRUM, HUMAN MILK, AND COW'S MILK

	Colostrum[1]	Milk[2]	
Nutrient	(1−5 days) (100 g)	Human (100 g)	Cow's (100 g)
Kilocalorie	58	77	65
Protein (g)	2.7	1.1	3.5
Fat (g)	2.9	4.0	3.5
Carbohydrate (g)	5.3	9.5	4.9
Calcium (mg)	31	33	118
Phosphorus (mg)	14	14	93
Iron (mg)	0.09	0.1	Trace
Vitamin A (IU)	296	240	140
Thiamin (mg)	0.015	0.01	0.03
Riboflavin (mg)	0.029	0.04	0.17
Niacin (mg)	0.075	0.2	0.1
Ascorbic acid (mg)	4.4	5	1

[1]Data from FNB, National Academy of Science (**55**).
[2]Data from U.S. Department of Agriculture (**56**).

of protein found in the two types. Human milk contains approximately 1.1 g of protein per 100 ml, consisting of approximately 60 percent whey proteins (lactalbumin and lactoglobulins) and 40 percent casein (Figure 7.4). Cow's milk has a relatively higher protein concentration of 3.5 g per 100 ml, with approximately 18 percent being in the form of whey proteins and 82 percent as casein (Figure 7.4). Studies suggest that lactalbumin has a higher biological value and may be a more complete protein in terms of human requirements than casein. Metabolic balance studies, however, show that cow's milk is as effective as human milk in promoting nitrogen balance in the human infant when the protein intake is adequate. The higher ratio of whey proteins to casein in human milk does not, therefore, appear to be nutritionally advantageous to the human infant (**10**).

The digestive and metabolic capabilities of the infant are limited during the first 2−3 months of life. In the normal infant gastric secretions, pH levels, and

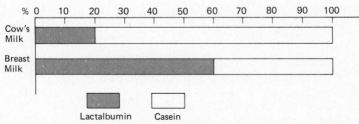

Figure 7.4 *The protein content of different types of milk.* (*Source:* Reproduced with permission from *Feeding Your Child* by L. Lambert-Lagace. Copyright © 1976 by Collier-Macmillan Canada Ltd., Cambridge, Ontario.)

enzyme activity levels remain low throughout this period. They are adequate to assure digestion of the normal quantities of protein found in breast milk. The high casein content of whole cow's milk, however, is responsible for the formation of large, poorly digested curds in an infant's stomach if the milk is not properly treated to reduce curd tension (**58**). Homogenization, acidification, and heating all help to reduce this curd tension and improve the digestibility of cow's milk. Immature renal function during the early weeks of life may impose a further limitation on the efficient use of the high concentrations of protein found in cow's milk as compared to human milk.

All eight essential amino acids are present in both types of milk in appropriate proportions and at adequate levels to promote healthy growth in the human infant (Table 7.6). In addition, cystine has recently been shown to be a possible essential amino acid in the first few weeks of life (**16**). Conversion of methionine to cystine may be limited because of low levels of the enzyme needed for conversion, especially in the premature infant and frequently in the normal infant (**58, 62**). Cystine availability may, therefore, become a rate-limiting factor for protein synthesis and growth. The cystine content of human milk is approximately twice that of cow's milk, but no concrete data are available to show that this is an advantage. In certain instances, however, the higher cystine content of human

TABLE 7.6 COMPARISON OF THE AMINO ACID REQUIREMENTS OF INFANTS AND CHILDREN WITH THE AMINO ACID CONTENT OF HUMAN AND COW'S MILK (g/16 g NITROGEN)

	Human milk	Cow's milk	Infant amino acid requirements	
			NRC/NAS[1]	Other[2]
Arginine[3]	4.1	3.7	—	—
Histidine	2.2	2.7	2.4	—
Lysine	6.6	7.9	7.7	7.5
Leucine	9.1	10.0	10.9	10.9
Isoleucine	5.5	6.5	6.6	9.2
Methionine	2.3	2.5	4.8	3.3
Cystine[3]	2.0	0.9	—	—
Total sulfur amino acids	4.3	3.4	6.2[4]	—
Phenylalanine	4.4	4.9	6.6	6.5
Tyrosine[3]	5.5	5.1	—	—
Total aromatic amino acids	9.9	10.0	—	—
Threonine	4.5	4.7	4.4	6.3
Tryptophan	1.6	1.4	1.6	1.6
Valine	6.3	7.0	6.7	7.6

Source: From National Research Council, National Academy of Sciences (**59**).
[1]Recalculated from National Research Council of National Academy of Sciences (**60**).
[2]Recalculated from L. E. Holt et al (**61**).
[3]Nonessential amino acids.
[4]Methionine requirement in absence of cystine.

milk may be responsible for the more efficient utilization of human milk protein rather than cow's milk protein by infants (**63**). Breast milk is also low in the aromatic amino acids, tyrosine and phenylalanine. Infants, especially premature infants, though, have a limited metabolic capacity to handle these compounds (**58, 62**).

A second major difference in composition between human and cow's milk is in the amount of carbohydrate present. Human milk contains approximately twice as much carbohydrate (9.5 percent) as does cow's milk (4.9 percent). The carbohydrate in both types of milk is in the form of lactose, a disaccharide that on digestion yields two monosaccharides: glucose and galactose. Galactose is a component of galactolipids essential for the development of the central nervous system. The lower lactose content of cow's milk is responsible to some extent for its lower caloric content.

Human milk is slightly higher in total fat content than is cow's milk, with milk containing 4.5 percent fat and cow's milk, 3.7 percent fat. The two milks also contain different types of fat (Figure 7.5). Breast milk has a high content of unsaturated fatty acids, particularly linoleic acid, which are essential to the cellular growth of brain tissue. Cow's milk has a high content of saturated fatty acids of moderately long chain length, 16—18 carbons. Only 2.1 percent of the fatty acids in cow's milk are in the form of linoleic acid as compared to 10.6 percent in human milk. Fats containing fatty acids 16—18 carbons in length are less readily digested than are shorter chained fatty acids, and metabolic balance studies of human infants show a higher fat absorption from breast milk than from cow's milk in the first few weeks of life.

Human milk is considerably higher in cholesterol than other milks, although it contains a wide range of concentration (**64**). A possible functional role may exist for cholesterol in breast milk and in the infant diet (**64**). The newborn infant's metabolism may require a high cholesterol diet if the necessary metabolic pathways designed to handle cholesterol are to evolve properly (**64**). Research

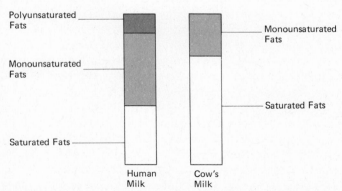

Figure 7.5 *The fatty content of different types of milk.* (*Source:* Reproduced with permission from *Feeding Your Child* by L. Lambert-Lagace. Copyright © 1976 by Collier-Macmillan Canada Ltd., Cambridge, Ontario.)

shows that at 8 years of age, children who were breast-fed as infants had lower serum cholesterol levels than a group of children who had been formula fed (**65**). Additional research is needed to confirm these findings, however.

If the mother is well nourished and the infant consumes sufficient quantities of breast milk, the requirements for vitamin A, thiamin, riboflavin, niacin, vitamin B_6, vitamin B_{12}, folacin, vitamin C, and vitamin E should be satisfied. Vitamin C is inadequate in cow's milk and should be supplemented in the diet within 2 weeks after birth. The amount of vitamin C present in breast milk of a poorly nourished mother may also be inadequate to meet her infant's requirements and need to be supplemented. Vitamin D is not present in sufficient amounts in either human or cow's milk, according to most research, and the infant's diet should be supplemented with 400 IU (10 mcg of vitamin D_3) of the vitamin per day. Chemical assays to determine vitamin D content were previously conducted only on the lipid fraction of milk. Evidence now suggests that breast milk may contain significant amounts of vitamin D in the aqueous phase (**64**). Concentrations range from 1.78 mg per 100 ml in colostrum to 0.9 mg per 100 ml in mature milk. The concentration of vitamin D in infant formulas is equivalent to this latter figure (**66**).

Cow's milk contains approximately three times as much calcium as human milk. The fat composition of human milk, however, allows for better fat and calcium absorption in the newborn. With the exception of iron and fluorine, other minerals appear to be present in both types of milk in sufficient quantities to meet requirements.

Immunological Properties of Breast Milk

Traditionally, health professionals have believed that the main value of feeding human milk to infants was because it supplied protein, calories, salts, vitamins, and fluid in proportions best suited to children's nutrient needs. An equally important advantage of breast-feeding, though, is its immunological properties (**67**). The physiological mechanism regulating resistance to infection is not fully developed in the infant at birth. The infant develops its immunological defenses slowly in the months after birth and during this time is dependent on passive immunity acquired transplacentally and provided in colostrum and breast milk. By the age of 6 weeks the infant begins to acquire active immunity, especially against the whooping cough virus. Until 9−12 months of age, however, it is relatively dependent on passively acquired immunity. Although the fetus receives immunological protection by placental transfer of immunoglobulin G *in utero*, the breast-fed infant receives additional protection (**68**). Colostrum, which is secreted in the days immediately following birth, has a high content of immunoglobulins A and E (IgA and IgE). The main function of colostrally acquired IgA is the protection of the mucous membranes of the intestinal tract. Although the definitive composition of human milk, due to its changeability, is not established until approximately three months, the major changes in the transition from colostrum to mature milk are complete by the tenth day. Breast milk secreted following that time remains rich in secretory IgA (Figure 7.6), whereas cow's milk is almost completely lacking in this component. It also provides a continuous supply of bacterial and viral

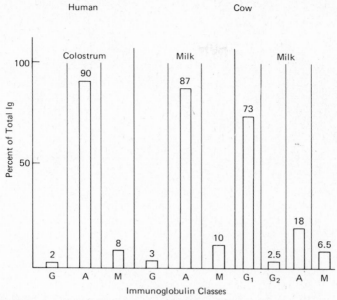

Figure 7.6 *Relative percentage of immunoglobulins in mammary secretion of the human and the cow.* (*Source:* Reproduced with permission from Ballabriga [67]. Copyright © 1976 by Nestlé Products Technical Assistance Co., Ltd., Lausanne, Switzerland.)

antibodies which increase resistance to infection from organisms entering the body through the gastrointestinal tract. These antibodies inhibit the growth of poliomyelitis, mumps, measles, and influenza viruses and provide immunity against Escherichia coli and other enteric organisms responsible for diarrhea and its subsequent dehydration in infants (**70**). Up to 6 months of age breast milk alone appears to assure maximum immunological protection and a minimum of exposure to foreign food antigens during the period in which passively acquired transplacental protection is being replaced by the infant's own immunological defenses. Studies show that until 8 months of age breast-fed infants have fewer of the respiratory and gastrointestinal tract infections often leading to poor health and sometimes severe malnutrition in artificially-fed infants (**10, 71–74**).

Further Advantages of Breast-Feeding

Several other advantages are associated with breast-feeding, including a lessening of the possibility of overfeeding and the subsequent development of obesity in the infant (**75–77**). Adequate information on the amount of milk an infant consumes when breast-feeding is not available, but breast-fed infants seem to take in fewer calories than do bottle-fed ones (**78**). The relationship of weight gain to caloric intake is shown in Figure 7.7, and the greater weight gains of infants on bottle feedings are shown in Figure 7.8. Bottle-fed babies double their birth weight more rapidly than do breast-fed babies. Breast-feeding may, therefore, be an

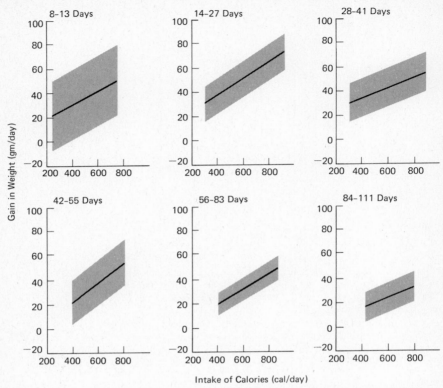

Figure 7.7 *Relation of weight gain to caloric intake of formula-fed male infants (various milk-based formulas). The center line represents the calculated regression. The shaded areas indicate the 90 percent confidence ranges.* (*Source:* Reproduced with permission from Fomon et al. [**78**])

important means of promoting sound eating habits. Overeating during infancy may lead to the establishment of undesirable eating habits that persist into later life. The breast-fed infant is less likely to establish habits of overeating. This is an area of research, however, in which information is continually changing. Genetic factors and the use of solid foods in the infant diet need to be considered also. Breast-feeding alone will not necessarily insure that an infant will not become obese later in life (**64**).

The belief that human milk protects against the development of allergies is strong, and although this belief has not been proved, favorable evidence exists to support it (**52**). Breast milk does not appear to induce allergic reactions in infants (**79**), and the absence of cow's milk in the diet at this early age eliminates the possibility of the child's developing an allergy to it. Breast-feeding in the first months of life will prevent allergic reactions in certain instances, but it will not necessarily prevent all food allergies later in life (**64**).

The advantages of breast-feeding can be demonstrated readily in areas of

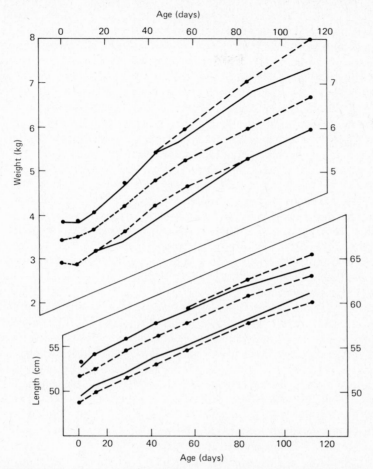

Figure 7.8 *Weights and lengths of formula-fed and breast-fed male infants between birth and 112 days of age. The heavy lines indicate the tenth, fiftieth, and ninetieth percentile values for formula-fed infants, and the broken lines include the tenth to the ninetieth percentile values for breast-fed infants.* (*Source:* Reproduced with permission from Fomon et al. [**78**])

the world where hygienic conditions are less than desirable. The use of cow's milk and artificial formulas also should be discouraged where contamination is likely because of unclean water supplies.

Possible Disadvantages of Breast-Feeding

While it is essential to emphasize the importance of breast-feeding it is also necessary to recognize possible limitations. Relatively little is known about the effects of drugs transmitted to the infant through breast milk. Any medicine or drug taken during lactation and transferred to the child in breast milk can theoretically affect the infant's development. Thus until more research is done in this field of human nutrition, the nursing mother should not use any drug in excessive amounts, including diuretics, oral contraceptives, steroids, radioactive preparations, morphine and its derivatives, hallucinogens, anticoagulants, and antithyroid drugs (**80**). Breast-feeding should not be attempted by any woman with an illness requiring large doses of any drug.

Recently, public concern has been aroused because some samples of breast-milk contain toxic environmental chemicals. Organo-chlorine pesticides such as DDT have been found in relatively large concentrations in human milk. A joint Food and Agriculture Organization/World Health Organization (FAO/WHO) meeting in 1971 set a practical residue limit for DDT content in cow's milk of 50 mcg per liter. The maximum admissible daily intake for human subjects is 0.005 mg of DDT per kilogram of body weight [**81**].) Concentrations of DDT in human milk are generally found to be well above the 50 mcg per liter limit set for cow's milk, with some reports of up to 100–220 mcg per liter (**82**). These pesticides enter the food chain when used on crops intended for human or animal consumption and become more concentrated as they progress up the food chain. It is, therefore, not surprising that human milk contains a higher concentration of DDT than does cow's milk.

Most recently, concern has been expressed over the presence of industrial chemical contaminants such as chlorinated hydrocarbons (PCBs and PBBs) in human milk (**82–84**). These chemical contaminants enter the food chain accidentally by discharge with industrial wastes into waterways or by leaching into soil and ground water from refuse dumps. Research shows that these contaminants have adverse effects in test animals and in adult humans (**83**), but no research has been conducted to investigate the effects of such contaminants on breast-fed infants. The research with test animals indicates that there may be cause for concern, but it is difficult to evaluate the health significance of such substances when consumed by the human infant.

Nursing mothers should be aware of the possibility that they may be exposed to potentially hazardous chemicals in their diet and in the environment. Any woman who has reason to believe that she has been exposed to unusually high levels of a contaminant should ask her physician for a laboratory analysis of her milk.

Employment policies and working conditions are other factors that may place certain limitations on working mothers who wish to breast-feed their infants.

The decision to breast-feed or bottle feed must be made by each individual after the advantages and disadvantages of both have been considered in relation to family lifestyle and needs. In the United States where mothers are well-fed and fetal nutrient stores are adequate, healthy infant growth during the first 4–6 months of life can usually be achieved by breast-feeding alone. It is also possible to rear an infant successfully on a milk substitute if adequate home hygiene and education are available. One method of feeding is not definitely superior to the other in the United States since good nutrition can be achieved with either method. Recently, however, several nutritionists and health professionals stated a need to promote breast-feeding to a greater extent in this country (**43, 85, 86**). In view of the unique properties of breast milk with regard to anti-infective and anti-allergenic properties, there is a need to make public health authorities, nutritionists, and nutrition program planners more aware of the advantages of human milk and to emphasize the need to reconsider the place of breast-feeding in modern infant nutrition.

INFANT FORMULAS

When breast-feeding is unsuccessful, inappropriate, or must be stopped early, infant formulas provide the best alternative to meet the child's nutritional needs. Adequate nutrition can certainly be achieved through artificial feeding with infant formulas. Only in the past 50 years have advances in technology, food processing, environmental hygiene, and pediatric nutrition made artificial feeding of infants practical for the majority of families in the United States. Human milk is now used as a standard in formula development so that infant formulas based on cow's milk or other protein sources are designed to achieve the same nutritional criteria as human milk with the addition of vitamin D and iron.

Formulas based on evaporated milk or fresh fluid whole milk with added carbohydrate were first used in the 1920s. Four-fifths of the calories in these formulas were supplied by cow's milk, with the remaining one-fifth of the calories coming from the added carbohydrate. Carbohydrate was added in the form of

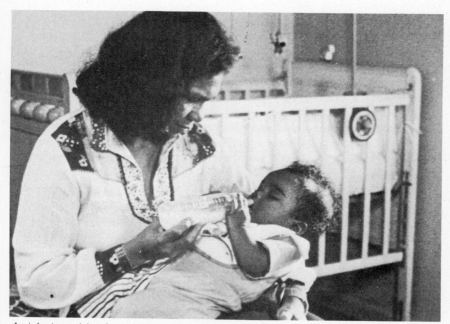

An infant receiving formula based on cow's milk.

sucrose, corn syrup solids, starch, glucose, fructose, or a combination of these. Such formulas provided 14−16 percent of their calories as protein, 36−38 percent as fat, and 46−50 percent as carbohydrate. These formulas were in common use in this country until the 1950s. They are not generally used in the United States any longer, although they are used in other countries.

These early formulas provided fat predominantly in the form of butterfat which is not readily digested by the infant. Today, the most common commercially available formulas in the United States are manufactured from nonfat cow's milk, vegetable oils, and added carbohydrate. Except for formulas developed to meet special nutritional needs most provide 7−16 percent of their calories as protein, 30−55 percent as fat, and the remaining in the form of carbohydrate. Linoleic acid is provided at a level of at least 1 percent of the caloric intake. Levels of minerals and vitamins recommended by the Committee on Nutrition of the American Academy of Pediatrics (**24**) and accepted by the FDA are added to the formulas. A vitamin-mineral supplement should be given if a formula does not supply vitamins and/or minerals in these quantities.

The Committee on Nutrition of the American Academy of Pediatrics has published proposed standards for nutrient content in infant formulas (Table 7.7). The present standards apply to formulas prepared for healthy infants but should also serve as guidelines in the preparation of formulas for infants with particular nutritional problems.

The Committee on Nutrition recommends that commercially prepared infant formulas provide a minimum of 1.8 g of protein per 100 kcal (**24**). Any proteins used in these formulas must have a protein efficiency ratio (PER) value of at least 100 percent that of casein. If a protein with a PER value of between 75 and 99 percent that of casein is used, the level of protein in the formula must be increased to compensate. No protein with a PER value of less than 70 percent that of casein can be used in infant formulas. Proteins used may be derived from a single source or a mixture of sources and may be supplemented with L-amino acids or acceptable protein hydrolysates. Any new protein proposed for use in infant formulas must undergo appropriate laboratory tests and animal and clinical trials before being placed on the market (**24**).

The level of protein supplied by breast milk is 1.6 g per 100 kcal. Most commercially prepared formulas in the United States supply 2.3 g of protein per 100 kcal. The minimum quantity and quality of protein proposed by the Committee on Nutrition promotes growth and development equal to that supported by human milk (**17, 24**). The Committee on Nutrition proposes a maximum protein content of 4.5 g of protein per 100 kcal of formula, since high protein formulas may be disadvantageous to the infant (**24**). There is no evidence that protein supplied in amounts greater than 1.8 g per 100 kcal confers any advantage for the normal infant. If higher amounts of protein are required for medical reasons, high protein formulas may be used under medical supervision and must be so labeled.

Fat in infant formulas may be in the form of natural cow's milk fat or vegetable fats such as soy, coconut, safflower, or corn oil, all of which are

TABLE 7.7 NUTRIENT LEVELS OF INFANT FORMULAS (PER 100 KCAL)

Nutrient	FDA 1971 regulations Minimum	Committee on Nutrition, 1976 recommendations Minimum	Maximum
Protein (gm)	1.8	1.8	4.5
Fat			
(Gram)	1.7	3.3	6.0
(Percentage of calories)	15.0	30.0	54.0
Essential fatty acids			
(Linoleate)			
(Percentage of calories)	2.0	2.7	—
(Milligram)	222.0	300.0	—
Vitamins			
A (IU)	250.0	250.0 (75 mcg[1])	750.0 (225 mcg[1])
D (IU)	40.0	40.0	100.0
K (mcg)	—	4.0	—
E (IU)	0.3	0.3 (with 0.7 IU/gm linoleic acid)	—
C (ascorbic acid) (mg)	7.8	8.0	—
B$_1$ (thiamin) (mcg)	25.0	40.0	—
B$_2$ (riboflavin) (mcg)	60.0	60.0	—
B$_6$ (pyridoxine) (mcg)	35.0	35.0 (with 15 mcg/gm of protein in formula)	—
B$_{12}$ (mcg)	0.15	0.15	—
Niacin			
(Microgram)	—	250.0	—
(Microgram equivalent)	800.0	—	—
Folic acid (mcg)	4.0	4.0	—
Pantothenic acid (mcg)	300.0	300.0	—
Biotin (mcg)	—	1.5	—
Choline (mg)	—	7.0	—
Inositol (mg)	—	4.0	—
Minerals			
Calcium (mg)	50.0[2]	50.0[2]	—
Phosphorus (mg)	25.0[2]	25.0[2]	—
Magnesium (mg)	6.0	6.0	—
Iron (mg)	1.0	0.15	—
Iodine (mcg)	5.0	5.0	—
Zinc (mg)	—	0.5	—
Copper (mcg)	60.0	60.0	—
Manganese (mcg)	—	5.0	—
Sodium (mg)	—	20.0 (6 mEq)[3]	60.0 (17 mEq)[3]
Potassium (mg)	—	80.0 (14 mEq)[3]	200.0 (34 mEq)[3]
Chloride (mg)	—	55.0 (11 mEq)[3]	150.0 (29 mEq)[3]

Source: From Committee on Nutrition, American Academy of Pediatrics (**24**).
[1]Retinol equivalents.
[2]Calcium to phosphorus ratio must be no less than 1.1 or more than 2.0.
[3]Milliequivalent for 670 kcal per liter of formula.

239

digested more easily. Human milk provides approximately 50 percent of its calories as fat including 5 percent as essential fatty acids. FDA regulations state that commercially prepared infant formulas must provide a minimum of 15 percent of their calories from fat (1.6 g per 100 kcal), with 2 percent of the total calories as essential fatty acids (**24**). The Committee on Nutrition recommends that the minimum level of fat be increased to 3.3 g of fat per 100 kcal (30 percent of calories) and 300 mg of linoleic acid per 100 kcal (2.7 percent of total calories) to supply an appropriate fat : carbohydrate ratio. Excess linoleic acid can lead to excessive peroxidation and increase the infant's vitamin E requirements. The present available evidence, however, is not sufficient to set an upper limit on the linoleic acid content in infant formulas. The Committee on Nutrition recommends a maximum level of 6.0 g of fat per 100 kcal (54 percent) of calories (**24**). Such an amount allows for sufficient carbohydrate and protein in the diet to prevent ketosis caused by excess fat.

Most infant formulas supply 40−50 percent of their calories as carbohydrate (**24**). Generally, one-half of the carbohydrate in infant formulas is in the form of lactose as a component of fat-free milk solids. Additional carbohydrate may be in the form of lactose, dextrose, maltose, sucrose, glycose, or corn syrup solids. Since 1970, corn syrup solids have been used more frequently than other forms of carbohydrate, since they are more economical and do not appear to alter the nutritional content when compared to lactose. When carbohydrates other than lactose are used they must be identified on the label.

Since the growth of healthy, breast-fed infants is not generally surpassed by that of healthy infants fed on artificial formulas, the average values of nutrients in human milk are considered as a rational basis for estimating minimal needs (**87**). The recommended levels for many of the vitamins and minerals present in infant formulas are therefore set at concentrations similar to those found in breast milk. Experience, however, shows that certain nutrients, in particular vitamin D and iron and, in some instances, ascorbic acid, are present in inadequate amounts in human milk to support normal growth and development (**87**).

The vitamin A content of human milk averages 250 IU per 100 kcal or 49 mcg per 100 ml, and this is the minimal level for infant formulas as recommended by the Committee on Nutrition. A maximum level of 750 IU per 100 kcal has been proposed.

The minimal level of vitamin D per 100 kcal of infant formula is set at 40 IU (1.0 mcg), and most formulas today provide approximately 62 IU per 100 kcal (400 IU per liter). In 1976 the Committee on Nutrition proposed a maximum level of 100 IU per 100 kcal or 670 IU per liter (**24**) which would exceed the maximum level of 400 IU per day allowed without prescription under present FDA regulations. The Committee on Nutrition feels that this higher level of 100 IU of vitamin D per 100 kcals should be allowed in formulas for low birth-weight infants when a reduced intake and poor fat absorption would lead to inadequate intake of the vitamin from a formula fortified with only 62 IU per 100 kcal or 400 IU per liter.

Human milk contains approximately 1.3-3.3 mg D-α-tocopherol (2−5 IU) per liter (0.3 IU per 100 kcal) (**88**). Since an increased intake of polyunsaturated fatty acids results in an increased vitamin E requirement, formulas providing a high PUFA level in the diet may deplete infant vitamin E stores (**87**). Such formulas should be supplemented with vitamin E to a minimum value of 0.3 IU of vitamin E per 100 kcal (**87**).

The ascorbic acid content of human milk varies from 2–10 mg per 100 ml (3–15 mg per 100 kcal) (**87**). Therefore, a minimum level of 7.8 mg per 100 kcal is recommended in infant formulas with conventional protein contents. The requirement for ascorbic acid during early infancy is related to the protein content of the diet, increasing as protein intake increases.

Thiamin and riboflavin are present in human milk at average levels of 25 and 60 mg per 100 kcal, respectively. Corresponding minimum levels of 25 (thiamin) and 60 (riboflavin) mg per 100 kcal have been proposed for infant formulas. A minimum level of 35 mcg of pyridoxine per 100 kcal of formula also has been suggested.

The minimum levels established for sodium, potassium, and chlorine in infant formulas are based on the average levels found in human milk and are apparently sufficient for normal growth (**24**). Maximum levels are set at levels similar to those found in cow's milk. These levels provide a higher solute load but one that can be handled by the normal infant. The ratio of sodium to potassium in formula should not exceed 1.0 (**24**), whereas the ratio of sodium, plus potassium, to chlorine should be at least 1.5. The ideal ratios are those found in human milk, 0.5 and 2.0, respectively. Experimental studies show that the ratio of sodium to potassium in the diet influences blood pressure in both animals and humans. Therefore, use of the sodium to potassium ratio of human milk reduces the risk of an excess sodium intake and possible increase in blood pressure in those infants who may be at risk for hypertensive disorders.

Minimum levels for calcium and phosphorus in infant formulas are set at 50 and 25 mg per 100 kcal respectively. The Committee recommends that the ratio of calcium to phosphorus be between 1.1 and 2.0 (**24**).

Infant formulas should contain at least 0.15 mg of iron per 100 kcal (1 mg per liter) (**24**). But, despite recommendations by the Committee on Nutrition to the contrary, formulas may still be sold unfortified with iron.

Marginal to deficient zinc intakes have been reported in some infants and children in this country (**89, 90**), so the Committee on Nutrition recommends a minimum level of 0.5 mg of zinc per 100 kcal of formula (3.2 mg per liter). As formulas are processed to reduce protein content their zinc content also may be reduced. In addition, the absorption of zinc from soy-based formulas may be less efficient than from milk-based formulas because of the high phytate content of soy protein (**90**). The present evidence, however, is not sufficient to make specific recommendations for higher zinc levels in soy-based formulas. Walravens and Hambidge report that supplementing commercial formulas with 4 mg of zinc resulted in increased daily weight gains and increased height and weight at 6 months of age in male infants when compared to controls (**91**). Female infants did not respond in a similar manner. Further studies are needed to verify the present data and confirm or deny the sex differences.

Current proposed regulations by the Committee on Nutrition allow for the addition of other nutrients to infant formulas if they are of nutritional value, safe to use, and are included at levels reasonably related to those in human milk. The present recommendations insure that all nutrients now known to be essential are present in adequate amounts. The minimum levels established by the Committee are those that promote healthy growth and development. No significant advantage is conferred by higher levels, and maximum levels have been set when excessive quantities of certain nutrients might be toxic. Levels near the minimum, in fact, are considered to be more desirable, since they reflect the composition of human milk. As knowledge of nutrition increases, information on other essential nutrients in infancy likely will become evident and revisions in these standards may be made to meet changing needs.

Formulas are available on the market in powdered, concentrated fluid, and ready-to-feed fluid forms. The powdered forms are rarely used in the United States, although they are widely used in other countries. The powdered formulas take slightly more time to prepare, but the storage life of an opened container of powdered formula is greater than that of an opened container of liquid formula. Concentrated fluid formulas contain 133 kcal per 100 ml and are designed to be mixed with equal volumes of sterile water to dilute the formula to the correct concentration. Ready-to-feed fluid formulas provide 67 kcal per 100 ml. They are more convenient than other formula types and may be slightly more expensive. Infant formulas, then, diluted to proper concentrations, provide 67 kcal per 100 ml of formula. The renal solute load in such a formula does not present a problem, provided the infant consumes at least 100 ml of formula per kilogram of body weight per day.

Several formulas have been developed for feeding infants with metabolic disorders that involve the use of specific amino acids for those with absorption problems and for those who demonstrate allergic responses to milk protein or decreased utilization of the carbohydrate lactose (**92, 94**). The majority of these formulas are prepared from protein hydrolysates, sucrose, corn oil, minerals, and vitamins. Amino acids are generally present in the free form.

Approximately 10 percent of the infants in this country today receive soy-based formulas (**10**). Originally, many soy-based formulas were prepared using soy flour, but water-soluble soy protein isolates are now in more common use and, since 1970, have essentially replaced soy flour. Studies show that the degree of processing may affect soy protein quality, resulting in lower protein efficiency ratios (PER) in these formulas (**10**). Soy protein isolate formulas supplemented with L-methionine and fed in amounts providing 1.6 g of protein per 100 kcal appear to be equivalent to cow's milk and human milk protein and contain the same percentage of calories (**17**). Therefore, the lower protein efficiency ratio may not be indicative of poorer protein quality, especially when fed at adequate levels in the diet. When it is fed at limiting levels, however, soy protein's quality may be a more critical factor.

It is possible to develop modified cow's milk formulas that are very similar in nutrient content to human milk, but some nutritionists feel that human milk cannot be satisfactorily reproduced in the laboratory. They are continuing research, though, trying to manufacture milk formulas better suited to infant needs. Studies have been designed to attempt to establish the correct osmotic coefficients, satisfactory pH levels, levels of calcium for ideal absorption, desirable fat content, and optimal protein availability. Recently, a trend has developed toward the production of "humanized" milks (**63**). In these formulas whole milk is combined with electrodialyzed whey, vegetable oils, lactose, and certain minerals. Additional vitamins and iron are added to meet RDAs. In humanized milk formulas whey is added to nonfat cow's milk to give a ratio of whey proteins to casein similar to that of human milk in the final product. Ion exchange techniques are used to remove the relatively large quantities of minerals present in whey. Minerals can then be returned in the desired amounts so that concentrations of individual minerals are similar to concentrations found in human milk. Humanized milks generally contain carbohydrate as lactose. Starch, sucrose, and corn syrup solids, however, are also used. Humanized milks are extremely close in content to breast milk, although several minor elements present in breast milk are deficient or lacking in these formulas. Extensive clinical tests show that infants handle humanized milks in a similar manner to breast milk.

MILK FEEDING FOLLOWING WEANING

Most parents discontinue formula feeding when the infant is 5 months old and begin to feed whole, skim, or "two percent" cow's milk. The question is often raised about the ideal time at which to switch an infant from formula to regular cow's milk. Digestibility is the main concern when introducing whole cow's milk into the diet. During the first 6 months of life the infant is able to absorb human milk fat and most vegetable oils adequately. Butterfat, found in cow's milk, is not readily digested during this period, though. If the infant is fed entirely on cow's milk, 50 percent of the caloric intake would be derived from butterfat. Such fat would be poorly digested and excreted in the fecal material, with a corresponding loss of calories. Average excretion of fat on such a diet is 23−36 percent of the fat intake or 12−18 percent of the caloric intake. Infants tolerate whole milk better if only five-sixths of the caloric intake comes from this source, with one-sixth coming from foods other than milk. A change in diet from infant formula to whole cow's milk is, therefore, probably best delayed until the infant is eating approximately two jars of commercially prepared strained baby foods or the equivalent in mashed table foods daily. The substitution of milk for formula may also cause a reduction in total dietary iron intake. In addition, if skim or "two percent" cow's milk is used, the infant's diet may become unbalanced with respect to the percentage of calories supplied by protein, fat, and carbohydrate. The calories supplied by skim milk may be inadequate, unless supplemented by other food sources. Nutritionists suggest that formulas should be specifically designed for the older infant to assure adequate nutrition during the second 6 months of life (**10**). Such formulas should complement other foods in the diet. Further research is needed on the nutritional needs of the older infant as formula is replaced by other foods in the diet.

SHOULD MILK DRINKING BY CHILDREN BE DISCOURAGED?

Milk serves as the major source of essential nutrients in the diet until the infant is at least 3−4 months old and often older. In the early 1970s articles appeared in the lay press suggesting that cow's milk can lead to adverse effects in some older infants and children. These articles raised questions about the desirability of feeding milk to children following the nursing period and caused some concern among parents (**21**). The American Academy of Pediatrics has, therefore, recently published a report reviewing the advantages and disadvantages of consuming cow's milk at different ages (**21**). Particular emphasis was placed on the possible occurrence of lactase deficiency in the infant and older child, the possible presence of an allergic response to milk protein, and the possible adverse effects associated with the saturated fat and cholesterol content of whole cow's milk.

Lactase, the enzyme necessary for the hydrolysis of lactose into its two component monosaccharides, glucose and galactose, is the last of the disaccharidases to develop during the period of fetal growth. Activity levels of this enzyme may be low at birth, but they generally increase rapidly and then appear to decrease after the third or fourth year of life. If enzyme activity levels do not increase sufficiently at birth, the lactose ingested in milk passes undigested to the colon. Here, the lactose's osmotic effect causes an increase in gut fluid volume. In addition the lactose undergoes fermentation by colonic bacteria, resulting in the production of lactic acid. Both these events lead to abdominal distention, cramping, and diarrhea. These symptoms are seen in children who do not tolerate lactose. The condition is more common among non-Caucasians. The American Academy of Pediatrics suggests that the problem of lactase deficiency may be significant in mass feeding programs for low-income groups in the United States and developing countries but that drinking moderate amounts of milk has no apparent adverse effect on the majority of children and is nutritionally beneficial. The Protein Advisory Group of the United Nations and the FNB of the National Research Council have concluded that, based on presently available evidence, it is not appropriate to discourage milk feeding from fear of a possible milk intolerance (**94**).

Similarly, the problem of allergy to milk protein is a controversial issue. The incidence of milk protein allergy in the general population and in infants is currently estimated to be 2 percent. Symptoms, including diarrhea, vomiting, abdominal pain, asthma, pulmonary distress, iron-deficiency anemia, and growth retardation, have all been attributed to milk protein allergy. Children who are sensitive to milk protein demonstrate allergic responses to B-lactoglobulin, α-lactalbumin, bovine serum albumin, and/or the composite casein fraction of milk. When a positive clinical reaction is observed, it is necessary to restrict or eliminate milk from the child's diet. Several milk-substituted formulas are available for those who must avoid milk entirely. These include formulas based on soy, meat, or hydrolyzed proteins that are adequately supplemented with vitamins and minerals.

In certain instances, gastrointestinal blood loss is associated with drinking fresh cow's milk (**95**). The nature of this association, magnitude, frequency, or significance of enteric blood loss has not been clearly established, though.

The possible adverse effects of the consumption of saturated fat and cholesterol from cow's milk on the development of cardiovascular disease is discussed in the next chapter.

SUMMARY

Often the idea is expressed that babies will grow up on nearly anything. Despite a widespread belief that healthy infants will thrive no matter what they are fed, there are important guidelines in infant nutrition that should not be ignored.

The infant's first food is milk. In America that traditionally has meant and still means a diet of either human or cow's milk. Breast-feeding promotes excellent development of the infant in the first few months of life if the nursing mother is well nourished. The decline in breast-feeding in this country over the past 20 years is a matter of concern among some health professionals and lay persons. An effort is being made to increase the incidence of breast-feeding at least during the early weeks of life, and in certain segments of the population breast-feeding is again becoming popular. Only now are health professionals beginning to emphasize the importance of certain nutritional and immunological benefits that breast-feeding may offer the infant.

Differences do exist between human milk and cow's milk. Advances in food technology, processing techniques, environmental hygiene, and pediatric nutrition have made possible the development of modified cow's milk formulas similar in nutritional quality to breast milk. Continuing attempts are being made to achieve further progress in manufacturing milk formulas better suited to infant needs.

Good nutrition can be achieved by either breast-feeding or formula feeding in the United States today. The decision to breast-feed or to bottle feed must be made by each family after the advantages and disadvantages of both are considered in the light of family lifestyle and needs.

STUDY QUESTIONS AND
TOPICS FOR INDIVIDUAL INVESTIGATION

1. One of the major changes in infant feeding practices that has occurred during this century is the decline in breast-feeding and the corresponding increase in artificial feeding. Conduct a survey of pregnant women in your community (childbirth classes, public health clinics, WIC clinics, etc.). How many of the women plan to breast-feed their infants? What are the women's reasons for deciding as they have? Try to determine the role that personal preferences, cultural influences, financial obligations, and so on, have played in the women's decisions. If you cannot easily conduct such a survey, you might discuss the same issues with your fellow students. What are your classmates' views on the breast- versus bottle-feeding issue?

2. Human milk was meant for babies is an old rule. Is the rule a good one? You have been asked to speak to a group of pregnant women attending a public health clinic. The topic is "Breast-Feeding as an Alternative to Formula Feeding." Consider the nutritional, immunological, and possible psychological aspects of breast-feeding in your talk.

3. The advantages of breast-feeding to the mother and infant may be lost without the understanding and encouragement of health professionals. As a nutritionist do you see a role for yourself in persuading members of the medical profession to at least make pregnant women aware of alternatives to formula feeding? Discuss what you believe to be the appropriate role of nutritionists in this type of situation.

4. Suppose you are the parent of a young infant. You are trying to decide which formula is best to use. What factors will you consider in making your decision?

5. Visit a local store or arrange to have someone bring samples of various commercially prepared infant formulas to class. Read the labels and compare formulas. What types of fats, carbohydrates, and protein sources are used in each formula? Do the formulas all contain the same vitamin and mineral supplements? Which formula do you feel is the best nutritional buy? If you were a young mother with very little background in nutrition do you feel that the information on the label would be helpful to you in making a choice between formulas? Discuss your answer with other class members.

6. Several special formulas are available for infants with digestive disturbances or special nutritional needs. Which of these formulas are available in the community in which you live? How does labeling information on the formulas differ from that on regular formulas?

7. Products known as "postformula beverages" are presently available on the market. If you can obtain one of these products compare its nutritional value with that of whole cow's milk. Is there a difference? Do you think such products are necessary from a nutritional standpoint?

REFERENCES

1. Kallen, D. Effects of nutrition on maternal-infant interaction; a symposium. *Federation Proceedings,* 34:1571, 1975.
2. Stimmler, L. Infant feeding. *Practitioner,* 204:169, 1970.
3. Brown, R. E. Breast feeding in modern times. *American Journal of Clinical Nutrition,* 26:556, 1973.
4. Straub, C. Nutritional intake of infants. II. Effect of milk or milk formula. *Journal of the American Dietetic Association,* 54:387, 1969.
5. Fomon, S. J., and C. D. May. Metabolic studies of normal full-term infants fed pasteurized human milk. *Pediatrics,* 22:101, 1958.
6. Fomon, S. J., and C. D. May. Metabolic studies of normal full-term infants fed a prepared formula providing intermediate amounts of protein. *Pediatrics,* 22:1134, 1958.
7. Maslansky, E., C. Cowell, R. Carol, S. Berman, and M. Gnossi. Survey of infant feeding practices. *American Journal of Public Health,* 64:780, 1974.
8. Cowell, C., E. Maslansky, M. Gnossi, R. Dash, S. Kayman, and M. Archer. Survey of infant feeding practices. *American Journal of Public Health,* 63:138, 1973.
9. Food and Nutrition Board, *Recommended Dietary Allowances,* 9th rev. ed. National Academy of Sciences, National Research Council, Washington, D.C., 1980.
10. Fomon, S. J. *Infant Nutrition,* 2nd ed. Saunders, Philadelphia, 1974.
11. Fomon, S. J. Nutritional requirements in relation to growth. *Mschr. Kinderheilk,* 122:236, 1974.
12. Goldman, H., O. Liebman, R. Freudenthal, and R. Reuben. Effects of early dietary protein intake on low-birth-weight infants. Evaluation at 3 years of age. *Journal of Pediatrics,* 78:126, 1971.
13. Holt, L. E., and S. E. Snyderman. Protein and amino acid requirements of infants and children. *Nutrition Abstract and Reviews,* 35:1, 1965.
14. Fomon, S. J., and L. J. Filer. Amino acid requirements for normal growth. In: *Amino Acid Metabolism and Genetic Variation,* ed. W. L. Nyham. McGraw-Hill, New York, 1967.
15. Swaminathan, M. Amino acid and protein requirements of infants, children, and adults. *Journal of Nutritional Dietetics,* 6:356, 1969.
16. Sturman, J., G. Gaull, and N. Raiha. Absence of cystathionase in human fetal liver: Is cystine essential? *Science,* 169:74, 1970.
17. Fomon, S. J., L. Thomas, L. Filer, T. Anderson, and K. Bergmann. Requirements for protein and essential amino acids in early infancy: studies with soy-isolate formula. *Acta Pediatrics Scandinavica,* 62:33, 1973.
18. Baum, J. D. Nutritional value of human milk. *Obstetrics and Gynaecology,* 37:126, 1971.
19. Sweeney, M. J., J. N. Etteldorf, L. J. Throop, D. L. Timma, and E. L. Wrenn. Diet and fatty acid distribution in subcutaneous fat and in the cholesterol-

triglyceride fraction of serum in young infants. *Journal of Clinical Investigation,* 42:1, 1963.

20. National Dairy Council. Current concepts in infant nutrition. *Dairy Council Digest,* 47(2):7, 1976.
21. Committee on Nutrition, American Academy of Pediatrics. Should milk drinking by children be discouraged? *Pediatrics,* 53:576, 1974.
22. Fomon, S. J., and E. E. Ziegler. Skim milk in infant feeding. U. S. Department of Health, Education and Welfare Publication No. (Health Services Administration) 77−5102, August 1977.
23. Pikaar, N., and J. Fernandes. Influence of different types of dietary fat on the fatty acid composition of some serum lipid fractions in infants and children. *American Journal of Clinical Nutrition,* 19:194, 1966.
24. Committee on Nutrition, American Academy of Pediatrics. Commentary on breast feeding and infant formulas, including proposed standards for formulas. *Nutrition Reviews,* 34:248, 1976.
25. Rodriquez, M. S., and M. J. Irwin. A conspectus of research on vitamin A requirements of man. *Journal of Nutrition,* 102:909, 1972.
26. Witting, L. A. The role of polyunsaturated fatty acids in determining vitamin E requirements. *Annals of the New York Academy of Sciences,* 203:192, 1972.
27. Lewis, J. S. An E/PUFA ratio of 0.4 maintains normal plasma tocopherol levels in growing children. *Federation Proceedings,* 28:758, 1969.
28. Keenan, W. J., T. Jewett, and H. Glueck. Role of feeding and vitamin K in hypoprothrombinemia of the newborn. *American Journal of Diseases of Children,* 121:271, 1971.
29. Smith, C. H. *Blood diseases of Infancy and Childhood,* 3rd edition. Mosby, St. Louis, 1972.
30. Committee on Nutrition, American Academy of Pediatrics. Vitamin K supplementation for infants receiving milk substitute formulas and for those with fat malabsorption. *Pediatrics,* 48:483, 1971.
31. Brin, M. Abnormal tryptophan metabolism in pregnancy and with the contraceptive pill. II. Relative levels of vitamin B_6—vitamers in cord and in mother's blood. *American Journal of Clinical Nutrition,* 24:704, 1971.
32. FAO/WHO (Food and Agriculture Organization/World Health Organization) Requirements of ascorbic acid, vitamin D, vitamin B_{12}, folate, and iron. Report of a joint FAO/WHO Expert Committee. WHO Technical Report. Series No. 452. WHO, Geneva, Switzerland, 1970.
33. Speirs, A. Nutritional imbalances in infancy. *Journal of the Institute for Health Education,* 9:73, 1972.
34. Southgate, D., E. Widdowson, B. Smits, W. Cooke, C. Walker, and N. Mather. Absorption and excretion of calcium and fat by young infants. *Lancet,* 1:487, 1969.
35. Schulman, I. Iron requirements in infancy. *Journal of the American Medical Association,* 175:118, 1961.
36. Sturgeon, P. Iron metabolism: A review with special consideration of iron requirements during normal infancy. *Pediatrics,* 18:267, 1956.

37. Committee on Nutrition, American Academy of Pediatrics. Iron balance and requirements in infancy. *Pediatrics,* 43:134, 1969.

38. Dallman, P. Iron, vitamin E, and folate in the preterm infant. *Journal of Pediatrics,* 85:742, 1974.

39. Widdowson, E., J. Dauncey, and J. Shaw. Trace elements in fetal and early postnatal development. *Proceedings, Nutrition Society,* 33:275, 1974.

40. Al-Rashid, R., and J. Spangler. Neonatal copper deficiency. *New England Journal of Medicine,* 285:841, 1971.

41. Guthrie, H. A. *Introductory Nutrition.* Mosby, St. Louis, 1979.

42. Wiatrowski, E., L. Kramer, and D. Osis. Dietary fluoride intake of infants. *Pediatrics,* 55:517, 1975.

43. Fomon, S. J., L. J. Filer, T. A. Anderson, and E. E. Ziegler. Recommendations for feeding normal infants. *Pediatrics,* 63:52, 1979.

44. Forsman, B. Early supply of fluoride and enamel fluorosis. *Scandinavian Journal of Dental Research,* 85:22, 1977.

45. Fomon, S. J., and S. H. Y. Wier. Prevention of dental caries. In: *Nutritional Disorders of Children. Prevention, Screening, and Follow-Up,* ed. S. J. Fomon. U. S. Department of Health, Education, and Welfare, Public Health Service, Washington, D. C., 1977.

46. Underwood, E. Trace Elements in Human and Amimal Nutrition, 3rd ed. Academic Press, New York, 1971.

47. Davidson, M. Formula feeding of normal term and low birth weight infants. *Pediatric Clinics of North America,* 17:913, 1970.

48. Meyer, H. F. Breast feeding in the United States. *Clinical Pediatrics,* 7:708, 1968.

49. Hirschman, C., and J. Sweet. Social background and breast feeding among American mothers. *Social Biology,* 21:39, 1970.

50. Berg, A. *The Nutrition Factor.* Brookings Institute, Washington, D.C., 1973, Chap. 7.

51. Jelliffe, D., and E. P. Jelliffe. Duration of breast feeding. *Lancet,* 1:752, 1975.

52. Oseid, B. Breast feeding and infant health. *Clinical Obstetrics and Gynecology,* 18:149, 1975.

53. Rivera, J. The frequency of use of various kinds of milk during infancy in middle and lower-income families. *American Journal of Public Health,* 61:277, 1971.

54. Martinez, G. Market Research Data. Ross Laboratories, Columbus, Ohio, 1973.

55. Food and Nutrition Board, *The Composition of Milks.* National Academy of Sciences, National Research Council, Publication No. 254. National Research Council, Washington, D.C., 1953.

56. U.S. Department of Agriculture, *Composition of Foods,* Agriculture Handbook No. 8. Agricultural Research Service, Washington, D.C., 1963.

57. Lambert-Lagace, L. *Feeding Your Child.* Collier-Macmillan, Canada, Cambridge, Ontario, 1976.

58. Jelliffe, E. Infant feeding practices. Associated catrogenic and commer-

ciogenic diseases. *Pediatric Clinics of North America,* 24:49, 1977.
59. National Research Council, National Academy of Sciences. *Evaluation of Protein Quality,* Publication No. 1100. Washington, D.C., 1963.
60. National Research Council, National Academy of Sciences. *Evaluation of Protein Nutrition.* Publication No. 711. Washington, D.C., 1959.
61. Holt, L., P. Gyorgi, E., Pratt, S. Snyderman, and W. Wallace. *Protein and Amino Acid Requirements in Early Life.* New York University Press, New York, 1960.
62. Hambraeus, L. Proprietary milk vs. human milk in infant feeding. *Pediatric Clinics of North America,* 24:17, 1977.
63. Muller, H. Infant nutrition today: new rationale in infant feeding? In: Nestle Research News 1974–1975. Nestlé Products Technical Assistance Co., Ltd., Lausanne, Switzerland, 1976.
64. Psiaki, D., and C. Olson. *Current Knowledge on Breast Feeding.* Extension Publication, Division of Nutritional Sciences. Cornell University, Ithaca, New York, 1977.
65. Fomon, S. J. Infant metabolic studies at Iowa State University Medical School. Seminar presented in the Division of Nutritional Sciences, Cornell University, Ithaca, New York, 1976.
66. Lakdawala, D., and E. Widdowson. Vitamin D in human milk. *Lancet,* 1:167, 1977.
67. Ballabriga, A. Immunity of the infantile gastrointestinal tract and implications of modern infant feeding. In: Nestle Research News 1974–1975. Nestle Products Technical assistance Co., Ltd., Lausanne, Switzerland, 1976.
68. Iyengar, L., and R. Selvaraj. Intestinal absorption of immunoglobulins of newborn infants. *Archives of Diseases of Childhood,* 47:411, 1972.
69. Butler, J. Immunoglobulins of the mammary secretions. In: *Lactation,* Vol. 3, eds. B. Larson and V. Smith. Academic Press, New York, 1974.
70. Ammann, A., and E. Stiehm. Immunoglobulin levels in colostrum and breast milk, and serum from formula and breast fed newborns, *Proceedings, Society for Experimental Biology and Medicine,* 122:1098, 1966.
71. Mata, L., and R. Wyatt. Host resistance to infection. Symposium on the uniqueness of human milk. *American Journal of Clinical Nutrition,* 24:976, 1970.
72. Hanson, L., and J. Winberg. Breast milk and defense against infection in the newborn. *Archives of Diseases of Children,* 47:845, 1972.
73. Grindat, J., et al. Antibodies in human milk against E coli of the sero-groups most commonly found in neonatal infections. *Acta Pediatrics Scandinavica,* 61:587, 1972.
74. Cunningham, A. Morbidity in breast-fed and artificially fed infants. *Journal of Pediatrics,* 90:726, 1977.
75. Jelliffe, D., and E. P. Jelliffe. The uniqueness of human milk. A symposium. *American Journal of Clinical Nutrition,* 24:968, 1971.
76. Taitz, L. Infantile overnutrition among artifically fed infants in the Sheffield region. *British Medical Journal,* 1:315, 1971.

77. Shukla, A., H. Forsyth, C. Anderson, and S. Marwah. Infantile overnutrition in the first year of life: a field study in Dudley, Worcestershire. *British Medical Journal,* 4:507, 1972.

78. Fomon, S. J., L. N. Thomas, L. J. Filer, Jr., E. E. Ziegler, and M. T. Leonard. Food Consumption and growth of normal infants fed milk based formulas. *Acta Pediatrica Scandinavica,* Supplement 223, 1971.

79. Eiger, M., and S. Olds. *The Complete Book of Breastfeeding.* Bantam Books, New York, 1972.

80. Arena, J. Contamination of the ideal food. *Nutrition Today,* 5:2, 1970.

81. FAO/WHO. Food and Agriculture Organization/World Health Organization. Joint FAO/WHO Meeting: Pesticide residues in food. *World Health Organization, Technical Report Series,* No. 474, Geneva, Switzerland, 1971.

82. Wilson, D., D. Locker, C. Ritzen, J. Watson, and W. Schaffner. DDT concentrations in human milk. *American Journal of Diseases of Children,* 125:814, 1973.

83. Health Advisory Council, New York State Health Planning Commission. Report of the Ad Hoc Committee on the health implications of PCBs in mothers' milk, 1977.

84. Harris, S., and J. Highland. *Birthright Denied.* Environmental Defense Fund, Washington, D.C., 1977.

85. Committee on Nutrition, American Academy of Pediatrics. Breast Feeding: *A Commentary in Celebration of the International Year of the Child.* American Academy of Pediatrics, Evanston, Ill., 1979.

86. Lackey, C. International symposium on infant and child feeding. *Nutrition Today,* 13(6):11, 1978.

87. Committee on Nutrition, American Academy of Pediatrics. Proposed changes in food and drug administration regulations concerning formula products and vitamin-mineral dietary supplements for infants. *Pediatrics,* 40:916, 1967.

88. Herting, D., and E. Drury. The vitamin E content of milk and simulated milk. *Federation Proceedings,* 24:720, 1965.

89. Anonymous. Growth and zinc deficiency. *Nutrition Reviews,* 31:145, 1973.

90. Prasad, A., and D. Oberleas. Zinc deficiency in man. *Lancet,* 1:463, 1974.

91. Walravens, P., and K. M. Hambidge. Growth of infants fed a zinc supplemental formula. *American Journal of Clinical Nutrition,* 29:1114, 1976.

92. Owen, G. Modification of cow's milk for infant formulas: current practices. *American Journal of Clinical Nutrition,* 22:1150, 1969.

93. Dean, M. A study of normal infants fed a soya protein isolate formula. *Medical Journal of Australia,* 1:1289, 1973.

94. Protein Advisory Group, United Nations. Low lactose activity and milk intake. *Protein Advisory Group,* Bulletin 2:2, 1972.

95. Anonymous. Fresh cow's milk and iron deficiency in infants. *Nutrition Reviews,* 31:318, 1973.

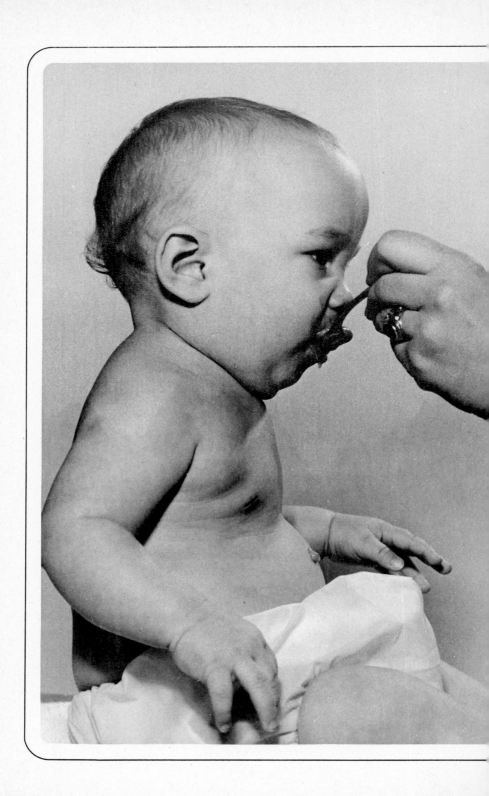

CHAPTER 8

SOLID FOODS IN THE INFANT DIET

Every parent with a newborn infant faces many questions about feeding the baby. As discussed in the previous chapter, the infant's first food is milk. Whether the baby is breast-fed or given a formula or both, the question soon raised is "Which solid foods should be introduced and when?" As the newborn thrives and grows, foods other than milk will naturally be added to the diet. Two major factors need to be considered when the matter of additional infant foods comes up. First, does the infant have nutritional requirements that can no longer be met by milk alone? Second, is the infant physiologically capable of handling foods other than milk?

Prior to a discussion of solid foods in the infant diet, the reader should note that several physiological changes take place as the infant develops in these early weeks and that those changes affect eating patterns and food intake. At birth, the baby's digestive system is not yet fully mature. All the enzymes necessary for the digestion of a wide variety of foods are not yet completely active. Milk, however, is assimilated easily during this period. Several individuals have made extensive studies of feeding behavior in infants, giving descriptions of sucking, suckling, and swallowing (**1–4**). The development of feeding behavior or the child's ability to consume food and the manner in which he or she suckles, swallows, chews, and so on is related to the maturation of the central nervous system. The acquisition of feeding skills follows a predictable sequence.

EARLY FEEDINGS

The baby is born prepared to suck and swallow and does so reflexively. Newborn infants will suck as soon as their lips contact a nipple. The sucking instinct is imperfect at first, and the first feedings require patience on the part of the parent. More mature sucking develops in the first weeks of life. One of the most important aspects of feeding at this early age is a pleasant, relaxed atmosphere. Young infants cannot always see their surroundings, but they can feel the way they are being held and cuddled and can sense attitudes toward them in other intangible ways. At the beginning, the number of times an infant eats will vary from baby to baby. Most infants will set up a rhythm of eating and sleeping in keeping with their own special needs. One child may sleep quietly for four to five hours between feedings, whereas another may be restless and hungry every three hours. This is one good reason in support of infant-regulated feeding times or a demand schedule. Demand feeding does not mean, as many people think, that babies are to be fed every time they cry. In general, on a demand schedule, the infant is fed every three to five hours. Within that framework the parent can work out a feeding schedule for the infant that fits the adult's time needs as well as the child's nutritional ones. With a little give and take the baby and the rest of the family can settle down to a reasonably regular schedule. There is always a need to recognize individual differences and a flexible attitude toward any family adjustments to having a baby in the house.

At some time during the first 6 months the baby will give up night feedings and begin to take four feedings during the day. As the child grows the digestive system gradually comes to maturity, and by 6 months of age the infant can handle a wide variety of foods without difficulty. Infants develop more sophisticated sucking patterns and swallowing movements by about 3 months of age. To eat

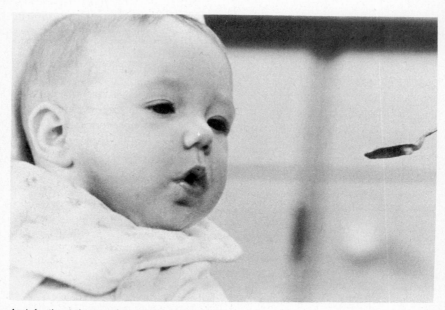

An infant's early experience with solid food.

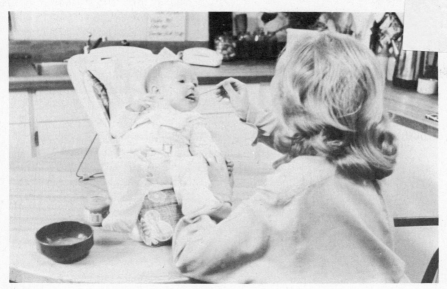

Solid foods can be fun, as well as nutritious.

solid food, infants, however, must learn to use their tongues and move the food in their mouths in a manner vastly different from the motions used in sucking and swallowing fluid milk. Think for a moment about your own tongue and mouth movements when you drink a fluid and then think about how these differ when you eat a more solid food. For an infant it's a whole new learning process! No wonder the feel of a spoon and strained food are puzzling to the infant. An infant will often appear to spit out most of the first strained food offered. This is not necessarily an indication of dislike for the particular food. It just means that the baby does not know what to do with the food. The tongue and lip motions needed to manage solid food in the mouth are not yet perfected, and the first time the food may not get pushed back to where it can be swallowed. Parents (or whoever is feeding the child) can help out by using a small, narrow, shallow spoon that fits easily into the baby's mouth. A small amount of strained, cooked food should be placed on the end of the spoon and then placed in the infant's mouth, far back enough on the tongue to make swallowing easier. The first solid foods should be given when infants are in a pleasant frame of mind and at a time when they can be expected to be reasonably hungry and more accepting of new foods. Babies will vary greatly about the time of greatest receptivity to new foods, and the parent will need to take some time experimenting to find what works best.

THREE MEALS A DAY

By the age of 6 months, the child generally adopts a three-meals-a-day schedule. Sometime between the fifth and the seventh months the infant begins the first chewing movements. This new skill, coupled with the ability to grasp at food and to sit up (either alone or with support), means that infants are ready to finger feed. They are now ready to learn another lesson, one that goes one step beyond swallowing smooth foods from a spoon. At this stage the baby should be given foods that can be easily grasped and are easily chewed. Feeding efforts will be clumsy and amusing at first, but babies will soon be well on their way to becoming competent at this skill.

During the 9–12 month period the child begins to master the more precise delicate pincerlike action of the thumb and forefinger in opposition and can pick up foods with greater ease. Hand-to-mouth movements become more accurate. Solid pieces of food (finger foods) are favorites at this age and picking them up is a fascinating game. Rotary chewing movements are being perfected, and the self-feeding process undergoes refinement. As the child enters the second year of life, the three-meals-a-day schedule will continue and fit easily into the household routine. Children at this age love to eat with other family members, reflecting their blossoming social development. They like people and want to be around them at mealtime. By one year, babies are seriously trying to feed themselves. This intense interest in self-feeding is partially due to a desire to imitate other family members (**1**).

DISCOVERING FOODS

Little by little, over the first year, the child begins to discover many of the colors, textures, shapes, smells, and tastes associated with food. After the first few months of life infants begin to prefer the bright orange of carrots to the bland white of cereal. Finger foods with a little body are more fun than pureed foods. The taste of meat may seem to last longer or appeal more than that of fruit. Every child will experience these new sensations differently, so in the interest of meeting individual needs, babies' diets cannot be rigidly standardized. Every child's food needs will differ. The general size and physical development, bone structure, proportion of bone to the rest of the body, rate of growth, activity level, heredity, and many other conditions determine how much an infant will eat. For each parent, therefore, the task of feeding an infant will be much larger than simply buying and feeding certain foods in specified amounts. The first year, however, should see a gradual transition from a milk diet to a much broader pattern that allows for the daily inclusion of suitable portions of foods selected from each of the following groups: milk and milk products, meat and meat alternates, fruit and vegetables, and breads and cereals.

As he or she grows older the child's growth rate decreases markedly from that of the first year of life. Between 1 and 3 years of age both appetite and food intake decrease accordingly. This apparent disinterest in foods by the toddler sometimes concerns parents. It is, however, a normal stage of development.

Very little research has been done on the nutrition composition and quantities of foods consumed by the toddler. This text cannot possibly supply all the information desired by parents and others involved in feeding infants and

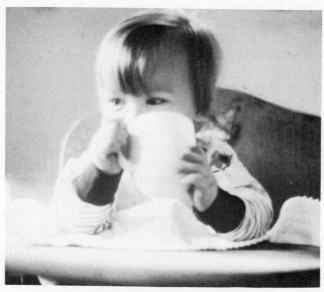

Interest in self-feeding develops at nine to twelve months of age.

young children. The Maternal and Child Health Service has published a useful guide to the proper nutrition and feeding of infants and children under 3 years of age (**5**). It includes sample daily food plans and suggested daily meal plans suitable for the infant and toddler.

INTRODUCING SOLID FOODS

Breast milk supplemented with certain essential nutrients or milk formula enriched with these nutrients can satisfy the nutritional needs of the healthy infant during the first months of life (**6**). Fruit juice, infant cereal, and a variety of strained foods may be introduced into the infant diet as the transition from an all-milk diet to one of adult foods occurs. In this manner the infant becomes accustomed to foods that, along with milk, will provide essential nutrients in later life. If served before 6 months, solid foods should be in a pureed form that aids the infant in swallowing. From 6 months on the child is more adept at chewing and may, therefore, be given firmer foods. By the age of 10 months the infant is capable of eating chopped and soft table foods.

The three major manufacturers of baby foods produce strained and junior foods in a large number of different varieties. The availability of this convenient, relatively inexpensive, and bacteriologically safe commercial food supply has led to a cultural trend in which infants are fed a progressively wider variety of foods at progressively earlier ages. A great deal of discussion and controversy exist concerning the ideal age for the introduction of various types of solid foods into the infant diet (**7**−**10**). Fomon et al., (**7**) feel that breast milk is the preferred food during the first 6 months, with an occasional feeding of formula and that foods other than breast milk or formula probably should not be given the baby during the first 5 to 6 months. The Committee on Foods and Nutrition of the American Academy of Pediatrics suggests that solid foods not be given to infants prior to 3 months of age. Other health professionals suggest 4−5 months as an appropriate time. In this country, though, solid foods are often introduced at a surprisingly early age. By the sixth month of life solid foods already provide a significant portion of calories in many infants' diets. The volume and variety of baby foods fed infants increases so that by the seventh month they supply 35 percent of the child's caloric intake (**11**). By 12 months of age solid foods supply over 50 percent of the caloric intake in some cases, and these solid foods are chosen from an offering of over 550 different items in the market. Commonly stated reasons for the early introduction of solid foods include (1) infants who are not on solid foods have a greater chance of developing anemia; (2) solid foods supply additional required nutrients during the first 3 months of life; and (3) the feeding of solid foods enables the infant to sleep through the night. Scientific research does not support any of these beliefs, however (**12**−**14**).

Fomon (**15**) suggests that if there is a major objection, other than cost, to the early introduction of solid food it may be that the practice is likely to encourage overfeeding and the establishment of unsound food habits. This possibility is discussed later in this chapter. In any case, the transition from a diet consisting exclusively of milk to one eventually consisting of the complete range of adult foods must be suited to the physical and physiological state of development of the child. The following schedule for the addition of solid foods to an infant's diet is a general guide and should be modified according to individual needs.

Age 0−1 months	Supplement the diet with vitamins not provided in breast milk or formula
Age 1−3 months	Begin fruit juice rich in vitamin C or fortified infant juice as a vitamin C source
Age 4 months	Begin strained cereal (rice, oatmeal)
Age 4½−5 months	Begin strained vegetables (peas, squash, carrots, spinach, beets, green beans, etc.). Begin strained fruits (applesauce, bananas, pears, peaches, apricots)
Age 5½−6 months	Begin strained meats (lamb, chicken, veal, beef liver)
Age 7−9 months	Begin finger foods—crackers, toast, zwieback, and bread crusts, or other easy to chew foods. Begin cup feeding

COMMERCIAL BABY FOODS

Infant cereals are generally the first solid food introduced and may be added to the diet when the infant is no longer satisfied with one quart of formula. Commercial cereals are available in single-grain (rice, oatmeal, and barley), mixed grains (wheat, oats, corn—sometimes in combination with barley and soy), and high protein (soy, wheat, and oat flour) forms. Cereals should be introduced in small amounts, beginning with one-half teaspoon mixed in milk or formula, and gradually increasing the serving to one tablespoon. Single-grain cereals should be introduced first, since there is less risk of allergy with these than with mixed cereals. If an allergic reaction does develop it is much easier to identify the type of grain causing the response. Commercially prepared cereals can vary greatly in their nutritive value (Table 8.1). A comprehensive compendium of nutritive values of infant and junior foods may be useful in calculating and estimating nutrient intakes. This type of information is maintained and updated by the USDA (**16**). A useful discussion of the nutrient composition of infant foods is also provided in a recent publication (**17**). The popular cereals with fruit added differ in nutritional value as a group when compared to dry cereal prepared with milk or water. These may provide less of the essential nutrients and more sugar than some of the other cereal preparations. Enriched infant cereals are principal sources of protein, calcium, thiamin, riboflavin, and iron, even after strained foods are introduced into the baby's diet. Studies show, however, that cereal is discontinued earlier than other infant foods (**17**). At 6 months of age, cereal supplies up to 75 percent of calories in the infant's diet. By the age of 1 year, however, less than 1 percent of many children's caloric intake comes from cereals. This is unfortunate, since infant cereal is often the child's major source of dietary iron.

Vegetables may be introduced into the diet around the fourth month. Cooked and pureed vegetables are a good source of vitamins, minerals, and fibrous material in the infant diet. Commercially prepared vegetables are marketed plain or creamed. The latter products contain whole milk solids, modified cornstarch, and sometimes sucrose. The caloric content of these products is generally greater than that of plain vegetables.

Fruits and fruit juices generally are introduced into the diet at approximately the same time as vegetables (4½–5 months). Nutritionists have long observed that if vegetables are introduced before fruits, the baby is likely to accept vegetables more readily than if the fruits are given first. This is because infants, like most people, prefer the sweeter taste of fruits. Fruits, mashed or pureed, supply vitamins, minerals, and natural sugars to the diet. Many commercially prepared fruits and juices are fortified with ascorbic acid. Some of the commercially prepared fruits and juices contain additional sugar, honey, modified tapioca starch, and cornstarch.

Meat and egg yolks are introduced into the diet when the child becomes well established on fruits and vegetables, generally at 5½–6 months of age. Egg yolk is less likely to cause allergic reactions than is egg white and is a good source of iron. It can be hard boiled, sieved, and stirred into vegetables. Canned

TABLE 8.1 AVERAGE COMPOSITION OF SELECTED CEREALS
AND MIXTURES FOR INFANT FEEDING. NUTRIENTS (UNITS PER 100 G)

Product	Energy (kcal)	Protein (g)	Fat (g)	Carbohydrate Total (g)	Fiber (g)	Ash (g)	Calcium[1] (mg)	Phosphorus (mg)	Magnesium (mg)
Cereals, dry									
Barley	365	11.1	3.4	75.3	1.2	3.4	795	439	115
Oatmeal	398	13.6	7.8	69.2	1.2	3.2	733	499	145
Rice	391	7.1	4.9	77.6	0.8	3.6	850	590	206
Mixed cereal	379	12.2	4.4	73.3	1.0	3.3	733	392	100
High protein	362	36.0	5.9	46.7	2.3	5.3	724	607	228
Cereals, with milk[2]									
Barley	111	4.6	3.3	16.3	0.2	1.2	230	150	30
Oatmeal	116	5.0	4.1	15.3	0.2	1.1	220	160	35
Rice	115	3.9	3.6	16.7	0.1	1.2	239	175	45
Mixed cereal	113	4.8	3.5	15.9	0.2	1.1	220	142	27
High protein	111	8.7	3.8	11.6	0.4	1.5	2.8	177	48

Source: Abstracted from *Composition of Foods: Baby Foods—Raw, Processed, Prepared.* Agriculture Handbook No. 8-3. USDA, Science Education Administration, Washington, D.C., 1978 (**16**).
[1]Values based on products containing added nutrients.
[2]Prepared cereal in mixture of 16.4 percent dry cereal and 83.6 percent whole milk.

egg yolks are available on the market, although they are more expensive than those prepared at home. A wide variety of commercially prepared strained meats is available. Meat is also found commercially in soups, dinners, and high meat dinners. The protein content of these products varies, depending on their composition, since water added to strained meats and egg yolks during processing causes a slight reduction in their protein content when compared to the same foods prepared at home (**15**). However, they are a good source of dietary protein.

Fruit desserts and puddings are also available commercially. These all contain sugar and modified cornstarch and/or tapioca starch, so their carbohydrate content is high. The starches are added to prolong the shelf life and improve the consistency of these items. Parents should be aware that the frequent use of baby food containing added sugar or modified starch in place of plainer foods may result in a diet deficient in certain essential nutrients. In addition, the use of sweets at an early age may be habit forming. Studies show that infants do not seem to care whether a food is salted or unsalted (**18**). This, however, is not true of sugar. We have mentioned already that babies appear to prefer sweet fruits to vegetables. Even the smallest infants love sweets and will consume more of a sweeter formula if offered a choice between a sweet formula and a less sweet one (**19**). Serving sugared foods at an early age may, therefore, precondition children to choose sweet foods in preference to others as they begin to make their own food choices. Infants do not require desserts at meals. If desserts are served, the most appropriate choice is fruit.

TABLE 8.1 *(Continued)*

Potassium (mg)	Sodium (mg)	Iron[1] (mg)	Zinc (mg)	Vitamin C (mg)	Carbo-hydrate Vitamin A (R.E.)	Thiamin[1] (mg)	Riboflavin[1] (mg)	B$_6$ (mg)	Folacin (mcg)
395	47	74.8	3.1	2.2	—[3]	2.7	2.7	0.4	29.0
470	33	73.6	3.7	3.2	—	2.9	2.6	0.15	35.3
385	32	73.9	2.0	2.4	—	2.6	2.2	0.48	24.4
437	39	63.2	2.4	2.3	—	2.4	2.7	0.19	42.8
1353	47	73.6	4.4	2.2	—	2.7	2.7	0.48	190.0
192	49	12.3	0.8	1.1	32	0.5	0.6	0.1	8.9
204	46	12.1	0.9	1.3	32	0.5	0.6	0.1	10.0
190	46	12.2	0.6	1.2	32	0.5	0.5	0.1	8.2
199	47	10.4	0.7	1.2	32	0.4	0.6	0.1	11.2
349	49	12.1	1.0	1.1	32	0.5	0.6	0.1	35.4

[3]Indicates lack of reliable data.

Commercially available baby foods should be selected with care, since there are wide variations in the amounts of calories and essential nutrients supplied by each (Table 8.2). The FDA does require that strained and junior foods carry a label listing all ingredients. Because of constant changes in existing knowledge about infant nutrition, food technology, and FDA regulations, published information may not be representative of current marketing practices. The label that provides a list of ingredients, and in many cases nutrition information as well, should serve as a basis to aid concerned parents in the selection of baby foods (Figure 8.1).

Approximately 7 percent of the calories of breast milk, 9–14 percent of the calories of infant formulas, and 20 percent of the calories of whole cow's milk are in the form of protein (**15**). Commercially prepared meat, egg yolk, and high meat dinners supply more than 20 percent of their calories from protein. Less than 7 percent of the calories in commercially prepared fruits, desserts, and puddings are supplied from protein. Commercially prepared vegetables, soups, and dinners provide varying amounts of protein, with values ranging between 7 and 20 percent of the caloric content. It is necessary to take into consideration the protein content as well as the biological value of the different types of protein in baby foods, especially if the infant's diet is limited in protein. An infant fed breast milk or formula generally receives adequate dietary protein from these sources. If more than 25 percent of the calories in the diet are supplied in the form of lower protein infant foods, with less than 75 percent supplied by breast milk, protein intake may

TABLE 8.2 NUTRITIVE VALUE OF SELECTED BABY FOODS[1]

Food	Amount	Percentage of U.S. Recommended Daily Allowance[2]								Food energy (kcal)	Carbohydrate (g)	Fat (g)	Sodium[3] (mg)
		Protein	Vitamin A value	Vitamin C	Thiamin	Riboflavin	Niacin	Calcium	Iron				
Milk, fluid, whole[4]	8 fluid oz	47	23	6	14	68	2	48	1	159	12.0	8.5	122
Commercially-prepared formula without iron added, ready to use	8 fluid oz	20	33	36	28	32	23	22	1[5]	160	16.8	8.6	—[6]
Instant cereal—mixed, dry	½ oz	8	—[6]	—[6]	72	58	36	24	77	52	4.4	0.2	10
Teething biscuits	½ oz	6	—[6]	—[6]	11	10	4	11	2	54	9.1	0.6	66
Strained baby food, commercially prepared:[7]													
Orange juice, strained	3½ oz	2	7	111	10	3	3	2	3	52	11.8	0.3	1
Mixed cereal with apples and bananas	3½ oz	5	—[6]	33[3]	33[8]	33[8]	33[8]	1	33[8]	84	18.9	0.4	70
Beef with beef broth	3½ oz	74	—[6]	8	4	28	32	2	11	112	—[6]	6.5	166
Chicken with chicken broth	3½ oz	73	—[9]	5	4	27	42	5	8	123	0.1	7.8	156
Beef with vegetables (high meat)	3½ oz	32	59	7	8	12	27	2	5	89	5.7	4.8	127

Chicken with vegetables (high meat)	3½ oz	34	50	9	2	8	24	6	6	88	5.8	4.5	130
Chicken noodle dinner	3½ oz	12	32	5	12	8	8	3	3	50	7.4	1.3	111
Macaroni, tomatoes, beef	3½ oz	14	32	4	22	12	12	3	3	71	8.8	2.9	155
Carrots	3½ oz	3	564	15	4	5	5	4	3	35	7.6	0.1	140
Green beans	3½ oz	5	18	14	8	13	4	6	5	29	5.3	0.2	105
Pears	3½ oz	2	—[6]	33[8]	4	3	2	2	2	72	17.2	0.2	6
Applesauce	3½ oz	1	—[6]	8	2	3	1	1	2	82	20.0	0.1	8
Apple dessert	3½ oz	1	1	17	2	5	1	3	1	100	23.0	0.8	16
Fruit dessert	3½ oz	1	11	10	4	2	1	1	2	97	23.6	0.2	36
Vanilla custard	3½ oz	6	7	6	2	15	1	8	2	94	17.9	1.7	95

Source: Reprinted from B. Peterkin and S. Walker, Family Economics Review, 4:3, 1976 (21).

[1] Nutritive values are averages for foods from three major baby food manufacturers, except for fluid whole milk.

[2] Allowance specified for use in nutritional labeling of foods for infants by the FDA. Title 21, Code of Federal Regulations CF2(10–199), 125.1 b. Percentages in this table have not been rounded as required for use on food labels.

[3] Sodium content varies, depending on the amount of salt added.

[4] Derived from nutritive values given in Watt and Merrill (20).

[5] Commercially-prepared formula with iron added provides about 19 percent of the U.S. Recommended Daily Allowance.

[6] Value judged to be insignificant or was not determined by manufacturers.

[7] Values shown for baby foods are for 100 g (approximately 3½ oz) of food. Cans of fruit juice contain 4.2 fluid oz, jars of strained meat contain 3½ oz, and jars of other strained foods contain 4½–4¾ oz.

[8] Products vary widely in content, depending on the amount, if any, of the nutrient added. Value is for product with nutrient added.

[9] Only one of three manufacturers gave a value. It represented 19 percent of the U.S. RDA.

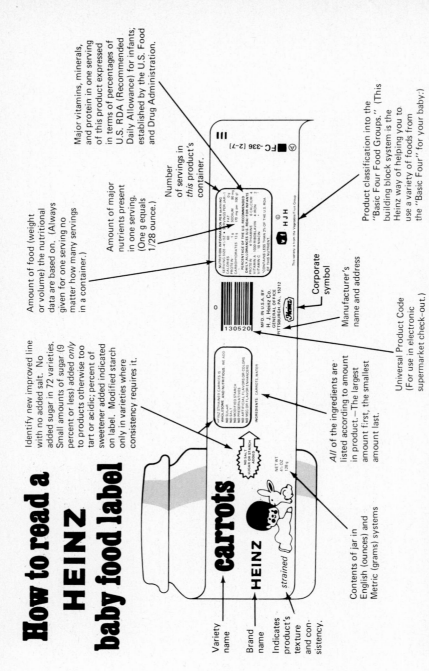

How to read a HEINZ baby food label

Variety name

Brand name

Indicates product's texture and consistency.

Contents of jar in English (ounces) and Metric (grams) systems

All of the ingredients are listed according to amount in product.—The largest amount first, the smallest amount last.

Universal Product Code (For use in electronic supermarket check-out.)

Identify new improved line with no added salt. No added sugar in 72 varieties. Small amounts of sugar (9 percent or less) added *only* to products otherwise too tart or acidic; percent of sweetener added indicated on label. Modified starch only in varieties where consistency requires it.

Amount of food (weight or volume) the nutritional data are based on. (Always given for one serving no matter how many servings in a container.)

Amount of major nutrients present in one serving. (One g equals 1/28 ounce.)

Number of servings in *this* product's container.

Major vitamins, minerals, and protein in one serving of this product expressed in terms of percentages of U.S. RDA (Recommended Daily Allowance) for infants, established by the U.S. Food and Drug Administration.

Product classification into the "Basic Four Food Groups." (This building block system is the Heinz way of helping you to use a variety of foods from the "Basic Four" for your baby.)

Corporate symbol

Manufacturer's name and address

carrots

HEINZ

strained

NO SALT, SUGAR OR STARCH ADDED

NET WT 4½ OZ 128 g

HEINZ STRAINED CARROTS IS WHOLESOME AND NUTRITIOUS. WE ADD
NO SUGAR
NO SALT
NO MODIFIED STARCH
NO PRESERVATIVES
NO ARTIFICIAL FLAVORS OR COLORS
NO MSG OR FLAVOR ENHANCERS

INGREDIENTS: CARROTS, WATER

0   130520

MFD. IN U.S.A. BY
H. J. Heinz Co.
GENERAL OFFICE
PITTSBURGH, PA. 15212

NUTRITION INFORMATION PER SERVING
SERVING SIZE: 4½ OZ. • 1 SERVING PER JAR.
CALORIES   60   FAT   0 g
PROTEIN   0 g   SODIUM   90 mg
CARBOHYDRATES   13 g   (70 mg per 100 g)

PERCENTAGE OF THE U.S. RECOMMENDED
DAILY ALLOWANCES (U.S. RDA) FOR INFANTS
PROTEIN   *   THIAMINE   4   CALCIUM   4
VITAMIN A 1030 RIBOFLAVIN   4   IRON   2
VITAMIN C   *   NIACIN   10
*CONTAINS LESS THAN 2% OF THE U.S. RDA
OF THIS NUTRIENT.

This variety is from the Vegetable/Fruit Group.

▼ⅠHJH

Ⓐ ▉FC-336 [2-7]
ⅠⅠⅠ

Figure 8.1 *How to read a baby food label. (Source: Reproduced with permission from H. J. Heinz Co., Pittsburgh, Pennsylvania.)*

become limiting (Table 8.3). A significant portion of the calories contributed by foods other than breast milk should, therefore, be in the form of cow's milk, infant formula, or protein-rich infant foods rather than the low protein foods. This problem is generally not encountered in infants receiving milk or infant formula which supply a higher protein intake per calorie content than breast milk.

Large amounts of water are used in the commercial preparation of most infant foods. They, therefore, have a higher water content than those prepared at home and generally a lower fat content. Many infant foods provide relatively low percentages of calories from fat when compared with milk or infant formula. When total fat content is low, and in a more highly saturated form than milk formula fat, the supply of essential fatty acids may also be low. Certain commercial baby foods contain vegetable oils, and these products would be expected to provide a greater percentage of unsaturated fatty acids to the diet than products containing fat supplied from animal sources such as meat, whole milk solids, or egg yolk.

Virtually all infant foods with the exception of egg yolks, meat, and high meat dinners are high in carbohydrate content. Many fruits, fruit juices, creamed vegetables, desserts, and puddings contain added sucrose. Lactose, in the form of whole milk solids or nonfat dry milk, is added to many soups, dinners, desserts, and all creamed vegetables. Starch-containing ingredients in the form of wheat, oat, rice, and potato flour, wheat starch, and modified cornstarch and/or tapioca starch are added to dinners, desserts, and creamed vegetables to provide desirable texture and consistency to the product. These starches make up a considerable portion of the total solids and calories in infant foods. Relatively few studies have been conducted to determine the ability of the infant to digest and absorb these starches.

Infant cereals are fortified with iron, but, as has been pointed out already, the use of these cereals generally declines after 5–6 months of age. The higher water content of other commercially prepared infant foods results in a lower iron concentration than similar foods prepared at home. The iron content of certain

TABLE 8.3 INFLUENCE OF LOW-PROTEIN COMMERCIALLY-PREPARED STRAINED FOODS ON PROTEIN INTAKE BY INFANTS RECEIVING VARIOUS MILKS OR FORMULAS

Milk or formula	Protein Intake (gm/100 kcal)	
	Milk or Formula only	75 percent milk or formula, 25 percent low-protein foods[1]
Human milk	1.6	1.4
Commercially prepared formula		
Milk-based, 1.5 gm protein/100 ml	2.2	1.9
Soy isolate based, 2.3 gm protein/100 ml	3.4	2.8
Whole cow milk	5.2	4.1

Source: Reprinted with permission from *Infant Nutrition,* 2nd edition, by S. J. Fomon (**15**). Copyright © 1974 by W. B. Saunders Co., Philadelphia.

[1]Most fruits and desserts. Protein intake calculated on the assumption that the average protein concentration of fruits and desserts is 0.8 gm/100 kcal.

infant foods is shown in Table 8.4, as well as in Table 8.1. Most strained meats provide less than 2 mg of iron per 100 g of food. Liver and egg yolks supply higher amounts. Soups, dinners, vegetables, and fruits supply less than 1 mg of iron per 100 g of food consumed. As discussed later in this chapter, iron-deficiency anemia is a common nutritional disorder among young children. The iron content of the diet is, therefore, of special concern.

Sodium chloride is presently provided in infant foods at a level not to exceed 0.25 percent (**22**). The possible relationship between sodium intake by the infant and the development of hypertension later in life, discussed in a following section in this chapter, has resulted in less salt being added to infant foods. A clear example of this change is shown in a comparison of sodium contents of selected infant foods in the 1963 Agriculture Handbook No. 8 with recent values (Table 8.5). The elimination of added monosodium glutamate is a major source of the reduction.

Some information on the concentrations of other minerals in infant foods is available in the publication *Composition of Foods* (**16**). Mineral content is generally low because of the low total solids content of most infant foods. Most composition tables do not contain much information on the trace element content of baby foods, but some research is now being published in the literature (Table 8.6), and other information is available from the food industry.

TABLE 8.4   IRON CONTENT OF SELECTED
FOODS FED TO INFANTS IN THE UNITED STATES

| | Elemental iron | |
Food	(mg/100 gm of food)	(mg/100 kcal)
Milk or formula		
Human milk	0.05	0.07
Cow milk	0.05	0.07
Iron-fortified formula	0.9−1.3	1.2−1.8
Formula unfortified with iron	<0.05	<0.05
Infant cereals		
Iron-fortified (dry) mixed with milk[1]	7	7
Wet-packed cereal-fruit	5	7
Strained and junior foods		
Meats		
Liver and a few others	4−6	4−6
Most meats	1−2	1−2
Egg yolks	2−3	1.0−1.5
"Dinners"		
High meat	<1	<1
Vegetable-meat	<0.5	<0.5
Vegetables[2]	<0.5	<0.5
Fruits[2]	<0.5	<0.5

Source: Reprinted with permission from *Infant Nutrition*, 2nd edition, by S. J. Fomon (**15**). Copyright © 1974 by W. B. Saunders Co., Philadelphia. Additional data generously provided by Dr. Fomon.
[1]Assuming that one part by weight of dry cereal is mixed with six parts of milk.
[2]A few varieties of vegetables and fruits provide 1−2 mg of iron/100 gm (1−3 mg/100 kcal).

TABLE 8.5 SODIUM IN SELECTED BABY FOODS

Food	Agriculture Handbook No. 8 values (mg/100 g)	Revised values (mg/100 g)
Oatmeal (dry)	437	30
Beans, green	213	88
Beef, strained	228	140
Vegetables and lamb	269	118

Source: Reprinted with permission from R. H. Matthews and M. Y. Workman, *Journal of the American Dietetic Association* 72:27, 1978 (**17**).

TABLE 8.6 TRACE MINERAL CONTENT OF STRAINED BABY FOODS

Variety	Percentage of moisture	Iron	Copper	Zinc	Magnesium	Manganese	Strontium	Cadmium
Precooked dry cereals								
Barley	7	67.20	0.48	2.99	124.00	1.28	1.73	0.11
High protein	6	76.10	1.34	4.86	250.00	3.68	2.18	0.07
Mixed	6	73.00	0.33	2.38	107.00	2.43	1.82	0.08
Oatmeal	6	70.20	0.53	3.64	164.00	4.41	3.78	0.08
Rice	7	67.20	0.38	2.21	236.00	5.54	3.62	0.02
Average	6	70.70	0.61	3.21	176.00	3.47	2.63	0.07
Strained fruits								
Applesauce	84	0.22	0.04	0.03	4.10	0.03	<0.01	<0.01
Apricots with tapioca	86	0.19	0.02	0.05	4.20	0.03	0.02	<0.01
Bananas with tapioca	84	0.18	0.04	0.06	10.00	0.05	0.02	0.01
Pears	83	0.25	0.05	0.07	7.00	0.03	0.03	0.01
Peaches	84	0.19	0.05	0.07	6.40	0.02	0.01	0.01
Plums with tapioca	80	0.16	0.03	0.08	4.00	0.03	0.04	0.01
Prunes with tapioca	84	0.31	0.05	0.09	8.80	0.06	0.06	<0.01
Average	84	0.21	0.04	0.06	6.36	0.04	0.03	0.01
Strained vegetables								
Green beans	91	0.73	0.04	0.25	32.30	0.14	0.22	0.01
Beets	92	0.27	0.07	0.15	15.80	0.15	0.12	0.01
Carrots	94	0.26	0.04	0.15	9.20	0.04	0.14	0.02
Garden vegetables	92	0.91	0.07	0.27	26.90	0.31	0.37	0.02
Mixed vegetables	91	0.39	0.04	0.13	11.70	0.10	0.10	0.02
Peas	88	0.98	0.06	0.33	14.80	0.12	0.08	0.02
Squash	94	0.38	0.06	0.19	13.10	0.08	0.19	0.02
Spinach, creamed	90	1.00	0.06	0.31	55.40	0.41	0.35	0.01
Sweet potatoes	85	0.37	0.08	0.20	14.20	0.24	0.11	0.01
Average	91	0.59	0.06	0.22	21.50	0.18	0.19	0.02
Strained meats and egg yolks								
Beef	82	1.76	0.04	2.43	12.76	0.01	0.03	0.06
Chicken	77	1.26	0.04	1.26	13.52	<0.01	0.04	0.04
Egg yolk	79	2.49	0.07	1.53	6.35	0.04	<0.01	0.04
Ham	78	1.18	0.07	2.42	15.23	<0.01	0.02	0.02

(Continued)

TABLE 8.6 *(Continued)*

	Percentage of Moisture	Iron	Copper	Zinc	Magne-sium	Manga-nese	Stron-tium	Cad-mium
Variety					mg/100 g			
Lamb	80	2.27	0.05	2.98	13.67	0.01	0.01	0.03
Liver	89	6.43	1.71	3.09	13.53	0.21	0.04	0.09
Turkey	79	1.24	0.04	1.86	14.57	<0.01	0.01	0.07
Veal	84	1.03	0.04	2.10	12.96	0.02	<0.01	0.02
Average	81	2.21	0.24	2.21	12.82	0.04	0.02	0.05
Vegetable-and-meat combination dinners								
Beef and egg noodle	89	0.63	0.03	0.37	6.98	0.08	0.03	0.01
Chicken noodle	89	0.36	0.04	0.30	8.96	0.10	0.04	0.01
Vegetables and beef	89	0.37	0.01	0.33	5.39	0.04	0.03	0.01
Vegetables and ham	90	0.27	0.03	0.17	5.04	0.04	0.03	0.01
Macaroni and cheese	86	0.40	0.02	0.36	10.01	0.06	0.02	0.01
Macaroni, tomato, beef, and bacon	89	0.55	0.04	0.31	9.34	0.10	0.02	0.01
Average	89	0.43	0.03	0.31	7.62	0.07	0.03	0.01

Source: Reprinted with permission from S. B. Deeming and C. W. Weber, *Journal of the American Dietetic Association,* 75:149, 1979 (**23**). Copyright © 1979 by the American Dietetic Association. Chicago.

Information on the vitamin A, thiamin, riboflavin, niacin, and ascorbic acid content of commercially prepared infant foods is available from manufacturers and from food composition tables (**16**). In some cases data may also be available on vitamin B_6, vitamin B_{12}, and folacin content. Ascorbic acid is added to fruit juices (50 mg per 126 ml) and to many strained junior fruits (10 mg per 134 gm). Dry cereals and cereals with fruit are the only other infant foods to which vitamins are added in processing. Enriched infant cereals are a good source of niacin, thiamin, and riboflavin. Again, because of the total solids content of most strained and junior foods, the vitamin content is generally lower than that of the corresponding home prepared food.

COMMERCIALLY-PREPARED VERSUS HOME-PREPARED INFANT FOODS

Is it better, from the nutritional standpoint, to feed solid foods such as commercially-prepared infant foods or to prepare these foods in the home? This is a question frequently asked of nutritionists. The infant can be fed nutritiously if home-prepared foods are used in place of commercially-prepared varieties, provided that simple, nourishing foods are prepared under sanitary conditions. Foods prepared for family meals can be pureed for immediate use or quick frozen in small sterilized containers or ice cube trays for later use. Some foods from the family table suitable for infant feeding with proper straining and diluting include cottage cheese, milk custards, fruit juices, ripe bananas, cooked or canned fruit such as peaches, pears, squash, potatoes, and egg yolk.

Fat, sugar, salt, or other seasonings should not be added to food prepared for a family until after the infant's portion has been removed. The lower sodium content of home-prepared vegetables, meats, and meat-vegetable mixtures is generally considered an advantage when fresh or unsalted canned and frozen foods are used in home preparation. Baby foods prepared at home from commercially-canned meat or vegetables often contain more sodium than similar commercially-prepared baby foods.

In 1977 two of the three major baby food manufacturers stopped adding salt to their products (**19**). The third has removed it from vegetables and is considering removing it from other foods. Recently, there has been a reduction in the number of products to which sugar is added. No sugar is added to products other than those considered by baby food manufacturers to be too tart or too acidic for a baby to eat without some sweetener. Two of the major baby food companies will list the percentage of added sweetener on the nutrition label. In no case will this be greater than 9 percent. Of all possible food additives, including monosodium glutamate, artificial flavors and colors, flavor enhancers, preservatives, modified food starches, nitrites, and others, today's baby foods contain only the modified food starches. These products are vacuum packed and do not need preservatives. In 1975 the USDA ordered the removal of nitrates and nitrites from all baby foods. The use of monosodium glutamate in infant foods was banned in 1969. Although they have long been absent from commercial baby food such additives are still present in many adult processed foods, so it is necessary to choose family foods carefully if they are to be fed to an infant.

Modern methods of food processing minimize the destruction of certain nutrients, but in some cases baby foods prepared at home may be more nutritious than those prepared commercially (Table 8.7). As pointed out previously, because of the low total solids content of some commercially prepared baby foods and the addition of starch to many, the concentrations of protein, vitamins, and minerals are usually less than in the corresponding foods prepared at home.

The choice between the use of home-prepared or commercial baby foods is an individual one. The food industry has taken a change for the better with recent reductions in the use of food additives. Many pediatricians and nutritionists would like to see salt removed entirely from all baby foods and sugar reduced to absolute minimum (**19**). Some would like to see modified food starches removed as well. There is no evidence that food starches are harmful, but there is some indication that they may be poorly absorbed by infants (**19**). On the plus side, commercially-prepared baby foods are sanitary, convenient, readily available and time saving. So, in homes where hygienic preparation and storage are inadequate, commercially-prepared baby foods are worth an additional cost in terms of safeguarding the infant's health. Generally, these costs are 30—50 percent more than home-prepared foods, depending on seasonal variation in the price of fresh produce. Commercially-prepared baby foods are a blessing, also, for the working mother who may not have the time to prepare infant foods at home.

TABLE 8.7 NUTRITIVE VALUE OF 100 G (APPROXIMATELY 3½ OZ) OF SELECTED STRAINED BABY FOODS PREPARED COMMERCIALLY AND AT HOME[1]

Food	Percentage of U.S. Recommended Daily Allowance[2] for								Food energy (kcal)	Carbo-hydrate (g)	Fat (g)	Sodium[3] (mg)
	Pro-tein	Vitamin A value	Vitamin C	Thiamin	Ribo-flavin	Niacin	Calcium	Iron				
Orange juice, prepared												
Commercially	2	7	111	10	3	3	2	3	52	11.8	0.3	1
At home (from fresh)	4	13	140	18	5	5	2	2	47	10.5	.3	1
At home (from frozen concentrate)	3	13	129	18	2	4	2	1	45	10.7	.1	1
Beef, prepared												
Commercially (with broth)	74	—[4]	8	4	28	32	2	11	112	—[4]	6.5	166
At home (lean only)	167	1	—[5]	10	38	58	2	25	214	0	9.5	60
Chicken, prepared												
Commercially (with broth)	73	—[6]	5	4	27	42	5	8	123	0.1	7.8	156
At home (fresh only)	166	7	—[5]	12	27	108	2	10	171	0	4.8	75
Carrots, prepared												
Commercially	3	564	15	4	5	5	4	3	35	7.6	0.1	140
At home (from fresh)	4	700	17	10	8	6	6	4	31	7.1	0.2	33
At home (from canned)	3	1000	6	4	5	5	5	5	30	6.7	0.3	236

Green beans, prepared												
Commercially	5	18	14	8	13	4	6	5	29	5.3	0.2	105
At home (from fresh)	6	36	34	14	15	6	8	4	25	5.4	0.2	4
At home (from canned)	6	31	11	6	8	4	4	10	24	5.2	0.2	236
At home (from frozen)	6	39	14	14	15	5	7	5	25	5.7	0.1	1
Pears, prepared												
Commercially	2	—[4]	—[3]	4	3	2	2	2	72	17.2	0.2	6
At home (from fresh)	3	1	3	4	7	1	2	2	61	15.3	0.4	2
Applesauce, prepared												
Commercially	1	—[4]	8	2	3	1	1	2	82	20.0	0.1	8
At home (from fresh)	1	3	6	6	3	1	1	2	54	14.1	0.1	8
At home (from canned applesauce)	1	3	3	4	2	0	1	3	41	10.8	0.2	2

Source: Reprinted from Composition of Foods: Raw, Processed, Prepared, by B. Watt and A. Merrill. Agriculture Handbook No. 8, USDA, 1963 (20).

[1] For commercially prepared foods the costs and nutritive value are averages for foods from three major baby food manufacturers; and for home-prepared foods nutritive values are derived from Watt and Merrill (20).

[2] Allowance specified for use in nutritional labeling of foods for infants by the FDA. Title 21, Code of Federal Regulations CF2(10–199), 125.1 b. Percentages in this table have not been rounded as required for use in food labels.

[3] Products vary widely in content, depending on the amount, if any, of the nutrient added.

[4] Value judged to be insignificant or was not determined by manufacturers.

[5] Insufficient data available to provide a reliable value.

[6] Only one of three manufacturers gave a value. It represented 19 percent of the U.S. Recommended Daily Allowance.

HEALTH PROBLEMS RELATED
TO FOOD INTAKE DURING THE EARLY YEARS

The infant is particularly susceptible to several nutritional problems that affect his or her overall growth, development, and general health. These problems include undernutrition (resulting in growth retardation and iron-deficiency anemia) and overnutrition, leading to obesity, hypertension, and cardiovascular problems. These nutritional problems are discussed in the following sections.

Undernutrition and Related Problems

Two of three children in the world suffer from some type of malnutrition or hunger. The incidence of protein-calorie malnutrition worldwide is highest during infancy. The more serious forms of malnutrition such as kwashiorkor (severe protein deficiency) and marasmus (protein-calorie malnutrition) are most frequently seen in developing countries. Infants in America are not usually so undernourished that they suffer from marasmus or kwashiorkor. They may suffer, though, from several less overt deficiency symptoms.

Underweight Children.   Rates of growth differ significantly between individuals as does the genetic potential for mature body size. Certain children fail to grow at an acceptable rate. The basic problem may not always be a nutritional or physiological one but may be emotional. An emotional difficulty may be the basic barrier to normal growth if there is adequate food available and the child does not consume sufficient amounts to thrive. Many such children require emotional support and social interaction with the parents or another person. In some cases, the eating problem may be the result of tension. Ignoring the emotional problem will not bring a solution. Positive steps are needed to remove or reduce the tension to the point that the child's appetite is restored.

The long-term development of the child who does not grow for a time because of a nutritional problem is dependent on (1) the age at which the feeding problem occurred and (2) the length of the period of deprivation. Children and infants do not grow in height and weight at the same rates, and a steady or normal gain in height is a better index of sound development than is weight gain. Thus children who are growing in height may be generally healthy, even though they are thin and their weight is below normal. Failure to gain in height is a signal of a potential problem.

Malnutrition, severe enough to limit height and weight gain, can also limit organ growth, including that of the brain (**24**). The adverse effects of malnutrition on the development of the fetal central nervous system were discussed in Chapter 4. As discussed previously, the effects of undernutrition will differ according to the stage of development when undernutrition occurs. Figure 8.2 shows the different phases of brain maturation. At birth the human brain is growing at the rate of $1-2$ mg per minute, and the next 12 months represent one of the more critical times in human brain development (**25**). The brain size of those infants who are malnourished during these crucial first months is significantly smaller than the brain

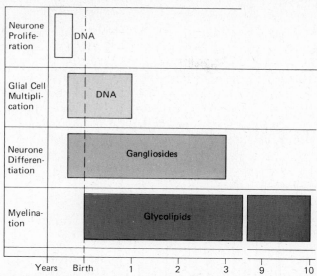

Figure 8.2 *Brain maturation.* (*Source:* Reproduced with permission from N. Herschkowitz in *Nestlé Symposium,* 1975, [**24**]. Copyright © 1975 by Nestlé Products Technical Assistance Co., Ltd., Lausanne, Switzerland.)

size of the well-fed child. Many studies have been conducted to determine the possible influence of undernutrition on brain development and intellectual and psychomotor development in the malnourished infant (**26–28**). The extent of nutritional deprivation necessary to cause faulty brain and intellectual development may actually be less severe than traditionally believed.

Iron-Deficiency Anemia.   Iron-deficiency anemia is the most prevalent nutritional disorder among infants in the United States (**29**). Estimates are that 30 percent of the infants from low-income families and 5 percent of those from upper-income families have hemoglobin values of less than 11 g per 100 ml, indicative of iron-deficiency anemia (**30**). The liver of the full-term healthy infant contains 50–70 mg of iron, most of which was stored during the last 3 months of fetal life. An approximately equal amount is present in the infant's hemoglobin. Normal iron stores at birth are sufficient for the first 3–6 months of life in the full-term infant, and there is generally little need for dietary iron during this period. The infant born before term, however, will have relatively smaller iron stores than those of the normal infant. Those infants at risk for developing iron-deficiency anemia include premature infants, infants born at term with low initial iron stores, and infants suffering from perinatal blood loss. Once the initial iron stores are depleted, an inadequate supply of dietary iron is the most common cause of iron-deficiency anemia. The recommended dietary allowance of 1.5 mg per kilogram of body weight per day takes into account individual variability in iron endowment and absorption. The Committee on Nutrition of the American

Academy of Pediatrics (**29**) recommends an intake of 1 mg per day per kilogram of body weight up to a maximum of 15 mg begun at an appropriate time with respect to initial iron stores to maintain normal hemoglobin values and allow for individual variability in absorption between normal infants. A larger amount of 2 mg per day per kilogram of body weight begun by 2 months of age is recommended for low birth-weight infants, those with low initial hemoglobin values and those who have experienced significant blood loss (**29**). The Committee on Iron Deficiency of the American Medical Association suggests that the desired iron intake be accomplished through the use of foods fortified with iron or medicinal iron in cases of severe iron-deficiency anemia. Human and cow's milk are extremely poor dietary sources of iron, containing only 1.5 and 0.5 mg of iron per liter, respectively. An infant would need to consume 15 quarts (qt) of cow's milk per day to meet the iron requirements during the first year of life. Infant cereals, commercially-prepared formulas, and fluid milk products fortified with reduced iron or iron pyrophosphate during processing are the major sources of iron in the infant diet (Table 8.1). For the most part the early feeding of solid foods does not meet the infant's iron requirements. The fruits, vegetables, and limited amounts of eggs and meat consumed during the first year of life contribute only a relatively small proportion of the total iron requirement. Some studies indicate that parents do not consciously choose iron-rich foods for the infant during the second 6 months of life (**31, 32**). Also, iron-enriched formula, which gives an average iron intake of 50 percent of the RDA during the early months, is generally not fed past the age of 6 months. The feeding of iron-enriched cereal will meet an infant's iron requirements during the second 6 months. However, if both these sources of iron are gradually discontinued after 6 months and if no food containing sufficient iron is fed in place of them, the infant of 12 months may only be getting one-half the required intake of iron. Parents should, therefore, pay particular attention to the source and amount of iron in the infant diet.

Overnutrition and Related Problems

Undernutrition of infants is a major health problem in many areas of the world. In the United States health professionals are becoming increasingly aware of malnutrition associated with overconsumption. Overnutrition during early infancy may play a role in the development of certain pathological conditions that do not become evident until much later in life. Conditions such as coronary heart disease, hypertension, and obesity are now suspected to have their origin in infancy as a consequence of imbalanced dietary composition or poor food habits. The increasing incidence of these conditions indicates the need to improve food habits in the early years.

Cardiovascular Disease.   Morbidity and mortality from cardiovascular disease is a major public health problem in the United States. Pathological studies show evidence of the development of atherosclerosis as early as the teen years. If this is indeed prevalent, then intervention should begin much earlier. Studies on adults show that a high serum cholesterol concentration is a significant risk factor in the development of cardiovascular disease. A 15—20 percent reduction in plasma cholesterol has been observed in adults on a diet low in cholesterol and saturated fat. At the present time it is not clear whether serum lipid levels in the adult can be predicted from estimated levels during infancy and childhood, nor is the long-term effect of dietary changes made during infancy known. A great deal of controversy exists, though, about whether dietary intervention reducing saturated fat and cholesterol content of the diet should occur in infancy (**33, 34**). The Inter-Society Commission for Heart Disease Resources advises a reduction in the fat and cholesterol content of the diet for all age groups (**35**). The Committee on Nutrition of the American Academy of Pediatrics, however, stresses that dietary intervention of this type is still in the experimental stages and recommends against dietary changes for all children (**33**). There is no concrete evidence showing that prevention or decreased severity of cardiovascular disease can be achieved by limiting intake of cholesterol early in life. It is too early to draw conclusions and make recommendations for intake based on present available knowledge of cholesterol metabolism in the infant (**36**). The Committee on Nutrition (**33**), therefore, advises against drastic reductions in saturated fat and cholesterol intake of infants until more is known about the possible beneficial or adverse effects. Dietary intervention would be warranted in special circumstances when a child exhibits an extremely high serum cholesterol level or when a family history of cardiovascular disorders may indicate a need for a more restrictive diet. Hereditary hypercholesterolemia can be detected early by infant screening (**37, 38**). Also, a family history of coronary heart disease should alert the physician to the possibility that the condition could occur in an infant. Placing a normal infant on a skim milk diet to avoid saturated fat intake would not be justifiable (**39, 40**), since such a diet carried to extremes could result in a deficiency of essential fatty acid intake. For those at risk for coronary heart disease, the use of skim milk is an important measure for the reduction of cholesterol and saturated fat intake. However, a general recommendation to restrict milk fat in infant feeding does not appear desirable now (**40**), and in no case should a parent place a child on a low fat diet without first consulting a doctor.

Within the past few years, questions have been raised about the role of high-density lipoproteins (HDL) in cardiovascular disease. Recent research suggests that HDL protects the individual by preventing the buildup of cholesterol deposits in the arteries (**41**). At the present time, though, little evidence exists to explain the relationship between HDL and heart attacks, particularly the role of HDL in the young infant and child.

Obesity. One of the major changes in infant feeding practices during the past 70 years has been the decline in breast-feeding and the corresponding increase in artificial feeding. This has been accompanied by the introduction of solid foods to infants at an increasingly early age. Around the turn of the century physicians noted that infants fed solely on milk from birth to the age of 1 year did not achieve favorable growth rates or optimal levels of health. The subsequent trend toward the earlier introduction of solid foods into the infant diet proved beneficial in terms of growth and health and the trend accelerated. In the United States today few infants depend solely on breast milk as a nutrient source even as long as 2 months. The majority receive solid foods much before 3 months of age and some as early as 2 weeks (**42−44**). By the age of 6 months the infant is often consuming a wide variety of solid foods.

Few topics evoke more confusion and emotionalism than the relationship between infant feeding practices and concurrent and subsequent obesity (**45**). Nutritionists now see a possible relationship existing between early feeding patterns and the development of obesity. One effect, therefore, of the early introduction of solid foods into the infant diet is the increasing incidence of a major infant nutrition problem in this country, that of infantile obesity.

Recent information emphasizes the critical nature of the first few months of life in establishing long-term patterns of body build (**46−48**). Juvenile or early onset obesity is characterized by an increase in the number of fat cells as well as an increase in cell size. So those infants who become obese before age 1 show a significantly greater number of fat cells than their nonobese counterparts. Figure 8.3 illustrates fat cell development from 24 weeks of gestation to 1 year of age. At 28 weeks of gestation, the mean diameter of fat cells is about 40 micrometers. At term the value has increased to 65 and at the age of six months has reached 110 micrometers. Between 28 and 40 weeks of gestation the fetus increases its total body fat content tenfold. Fat cell volume, however, increases only fourfold during this same period. The most appreciable fat cell multiplication, therefore, appears to occur during the last trimester of gestation. During the first 6 months of life, the increase in body fat appears to be due to an increase in fat cell size rather than cell number. Health professionals need more research, aided by knowledge of the exact age and manner in which cell number is affected by overfeeding, to provide a more rational basis for dietary control of obesity during early growth and development. An increase in fat cell number at any age appears to be permanent, and cannot be reversed with caloric restriction. Most infants who develop greater than normal fat cell numbers remain overweight as they grow older (**42, 50, 51**). A rapid weight gain during the first 6 months of life may serve as a good indicator of adult obesity.

Obesity is difficult to determine in the young child. Significant differences in the percentiles of height and weight on the growth charts, however, do suggest a tendency toward or the beginning of obesity. For example, a child whose height is in the thirtieth percentile and whose weight is in the ninetieth percentile for normal growth may be heading toward obesity (**52**).

Pediatricians and nutritionists are in a position to minimize infant and adult obesity and its accompanying complications through the proper guidance of parents in infant feeding practices. By controlling the infant's weight increase in the first year of life it may be possible to reduce the number of children who ultimately become obese. Some control over food intakes, particularly of the high-energy, low-nutrient foods, may be advisable to prevent obesity during childhood and adulthood. Effective intervention at an early age could, therefore, make a significant contribution toward obesity control in the entire population.

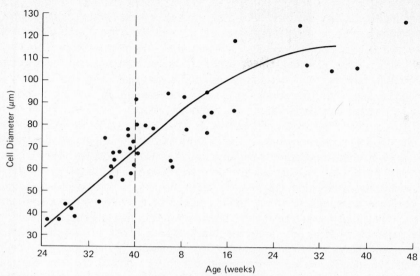

Figure 8.3 *Mean diameter of fat cells of human adipose tissue from 24 weeks fetal life to 48 weeks. (Source:* Reproduced with permission from D. Gairdner, *Proceedings of the Nutrition Society,* 33:121, 1974. Copyright © 1974 by the Syndics of the Cambridge University Press. Reprinted by permission from Cambridge University Press, New York.)

Basic to the whole issue of prevention and management of infantile obesity is sound education of the parents. Parents should have some understanding of the nutritive values of different foods used in infant feeding, the approximate amounts of each nutrient needed at different phases of growth, and the feeding behavior of infants at different ages. The diet should also satisfy the caloric requirements for normal growth. Appetite, too, can generally be used as a guide to healthy food intake.

Biological rhythms exist in infancy which must be respected if healthy eating patterns are to develop. Since the infant's self-regulation is more accurate with breast-feeding, infants who are breast-fed appear less likely to become obese than bottle-fed infants (**53**). Bottle feeding is believed to be a factor in overfeeding because the amount of milk consumed can be easily seen, so parents often encourage an infant to finish all the formula in the bottle even after he or she may have reached the point of satisfaction (**54**). The breast-fed child, though, ceases to nurse when satisfied. Therefore, it would be wise to encourage breast-feeding, discourage the early feeding of solid foods, and routinely check weight and length measurements for the infant from a family with a history of obesity.

Hypertension.   The evidence from studies with young animals and adult humans indicates a possible relationship between the sodium content of the diet and the development of hypertension. This has led to an increased concern about the high sodium content of infant diets as a predisposing factor to adult hypertension (**9, 55**). In the 1960s most commercial infant foods, except for fruits, contained a salt concentration, added by processors, ranging from 5 to more than 100 times that of the original natural product. Infants who received a diet of milk and commercial baby foods, often consumed 50–60 mEq of sodium per day. This amount is far in excess of the 2.6 mEq per day estimated to meet the needs of the rapidly growing infant for the expansion of extracellular fluid, replacement of obligatory losses, and the deposition of exchangeable sodium in the bone and the 8 mEq per day established to provide a margin of safety.

The total daily intake of sodium is approximately 5–10 mEq for the breast-fed infant who consumes no other food. Studies show that the appetite for salt appears to be an acquired taste that can adapt itself readily to the salt level of the diet. The addition of extra salt to infant foods does not necessarily increase the acceptability of the food (**18**). Furthermore, the infant's functionally immature kidney may be unable to handle the increased renal solute load imposed by a high sodium diet in which solid foods replace milk, increasing electrolyte levels in the diet and simultaneously decreasing the total amount of fluid available for their excretion. The amount of salt added to commercial baby foods has been drastically reduced, but the concerned parent who wishes to know the salt content of certain infant foods should read the labels carefully.

NUTRITIONAL MANAGEMENT OF THE LOW BIRTH-WEIGHT INFANT

The ability of an infant to adapt effectively to the extrauterine environment is related to the degree of physiological and biochemical maturity at birth. As pointed out in Chapter 4, low birth-weight occurs frequently in infants born in both developing and developed countries. Fortunately, increasing numbers of small-for-date and premature infants are surviving as a result of improved perinatal care (**56**). A special nutritional approach, however, is required for these infants (**56–65**). Because of early cessation, or poor placental transfer of nutrient supply, these infants' nutrient stores are low compared to those of full-term, mature infants. Those born at less than 32–34 weeks of gestation have limited sucking and swallowing reflexes and immature gastrointestinal systems. Also, certain enzymes do not attain maximum activity until 8–9 months of gestational age. The infant's digestive ability may be adequate in relation to protein and carbohydrate but is generally limited with regard to fat. The metabolic capacity of the liver is reduced. The immature renal anatomy and function limits the body's ability to regulate water and electrolyte excretion. In addition to these limitations the low birth-weight infant has an increased requirement for most of the essential nutrients because of an extremely rapid growth rate.

Traditionally, the feeding of premature infants was delayed until 48–72 hours after birth largely because of the hazards associated with aspiration. This practice persisted through the 1950s in the United States, and arguments are still put forth in favor of late feeding. The present theory, however, is that early feeding is desirable (**57**). Even now the best time to start feeding is not certain. The survival time in days for low birth-weight infants (Table 8.8) fed water only

TABLE 8.8 CALCULATED SURVIVAL TIMES IN DAYS FOR
PREMATURE AND FULL-TERM INFANTS AND ADULTS WITH
INTAKES OF WATER ONLY OR DEXTROSE SOLUTION
(CONCENTRATION OF 100 G DEXTROSE/L. GIVEN AT 75 ML/KG
BODY WEIGHT PER DAY FOR INFANTS 3 L PER DAY FOR ADULTS)

	Water only	Dextrose solution
Small premature infant	4	11
Large premature infant	12	30
Full-term infant	35	80
Adult	90	350

Source: Reprinted with permission from W. C. Heird, J. M. Driscoll, Jr., J. N. Schullinger, B. Grebin, and R. W. Winters. *Journal of Pediatrics,* 80:351–372, 1972 (**66**). Copyright © 1972 by C. V. Mosby Co., St. Louis, Missouri.

illustrates the urgent need to introduce adequate nutrition as soon after birth as possible. The problems associated with aspiration and oral feedings are very real, but the need for fluid and calories by these infants is urgent.

At term, the normal infant has adequate liver glycogen stores which can be converted to glucose and used for energy (**67**). Fat depots are formed late in the gestational period. During the neonatal period demands on these energy stores increase rapidly because of increased caloric requirements for muscular energy and the need to maintain a constant internal thermal environment by adjusting the metabolic rate. Low birth-weight infants demonstrate greater energy needs because of a higher metabolic rate per unit of body weight, the result of greater heat loss caused by insufficient subcutaneous fat insulation. Neonatal starvation of such infants can cause hypoglycemia and result in immediate and long term tissue damage, especially to the central nervous system. Delayed feedings are associated with increased serum free fatty acids, ketonuria, and decreased liver glycogen stores. With earlier feedings weight loss after birth is decreased, lost weight is regained earlier, and blood glucose levels are higher.

Larger infants weighing 2000 g or more, with no respiratory distress or gastrointestinal abnormalities and with good sucking reflexes, may take their first feedings by bottle within 6–12 hours after birth. With certain precautions these infants may also be breast-fed. Breast-feeding may be attempted with infants of approximately 36 weeks of gestational age or when a similar level of maturity is reached. Human milk, however, is inadequate in protein and minerals for the low birth-weight infant, and breast-feeding is best supplemented with one or two bottle feedings. In such situations nutritionists most often recommend soy isolate formulas supplemented with skim milk powder to give a final concentration of 100 kcal per 100 ml.

Infants weighing 1500–2000 g with no evidence of distress or abnormalities and showing an ability to suck may be given 5–15 ml of distilled water by nipple four to six hours after birth. If the water is accepted and retained, 5–15 ml of a 10 percent glucose solution may be given at three-hour intervals for two feedings. Then equal parts of a 10 percent glucose solution and formula supplying 100 kcal per 100 ml may be given at three-hour intervals, increasing the size of the feeding by 3–5 ml each day and gradually replacing the glucose solution with formula.

Intravenous administration of fluid should begin the first day of life to those infants weighing less than 1500 g at birth or larger infants suffering from respiratory distress, disease, or lacking the ability to suck. This fluid should be supplied initially in the amount of 60 ml per kilogram of body weight per day and increased by 10–20 ml per kilogram per day to a total intake of 120 ml per kilogram per day. Each 100 ml of fluid should contain 10 g of glucose, 2 mEq of sodium, and 2 mEq of potassium. With the beginning of nasogastric tube feedings, the amount of fluid administered intravenously is decreased (Figure 8.4). Initial nasogastric feedings should supply 2–3 ml of distilled water per kilogram of body weight. Distilled water is gradually replaced with 2–4 ml of a 5 percent glucose solution in water. At 3–24-hour intervals feeding volume can be increased by 2–4 ml until the infant is actively sucking at feeding times or is consuming 60–75 ml per kilogram per day. The infant's individual feedings should not exceed 30 ml in volume. After the third to fourth feeding, formulas providing 100 kcal per 100 ml may be substituted for the glucose solution. Such a formula generally contains vegetable oils and a protein content similar to that of human milk. Formula to reach a level of 100–150 ml per kilogram of body weight should be fed by the seventh to tenth day to meet the child's protein requirements. This amount provides adequate fluid in the diet and calories to support growth (Table 8.9). For the very small infant this level of intake must be built up gradually.

Commercially available formulas are not always entirely satisfactory to meet

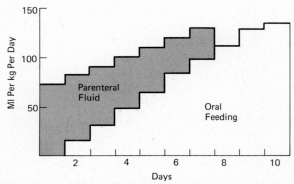

Figure 8.4 *Scheme for combining parenteral and oral feeding of low birth weight infants unable to nurse. (Source:* Reproduced with permission from S. G. Babson, *Journal of Pediatrics* 79:694–701, 1971. Copyright © 1971 by C. V. Mosby Co., St. Louis, Missouri.)

TABLE 8.9 SAMPLE CALORIE REQUIREMENT FOR A GROWING PREMATURE INFANT

	Kcal/kg day
Resting expenditure	50
Intermittent activity	15
Occasional cold stress	10
Specific dynamic action	8
Fecal loss	12
Growth	25
	120

Source: Reprinted with permission from *Infant Nutrition—Feeding the Infant, Building the Man* by L. A. Barness. Wyeth Laboratories, New York, 1972 (**69**).

the needs of the low birth-weight infant (**15**). Formulas must provide adequate nutrient intake without providing an unnecessarily high renal solute load. Ideally, formulas should supply approximately 80−100 kcal per 100 ml, with 11 percent of the calories in the form of protein (2.8 g protein/100 kcal), 50 percent in the form of fat, and the remainder in the form of carbohydrate. One-half to two-thirds of the carbohydrate should be supplied as lactose, with the rest as corn syrup solids. Fat, calcium, and phosphorus should be readily available from such formulas.

The low birth-weight infant has increased requirements for calories per unit of body weight, related to its more rapid growth rate. The guidelines for estimating requirements of low birth-weight infants for initial maintenance and subsequent growth are shown in Table 8.10. Depending on the degree of intrauterine growth

TABLE 8.10 RANGE IN FEEDING REQUIREMENTS OF LOW BIRTH-WEIGHT INFANTS PER KILOGRAM OF BODY WEIGHT

Requirements	First week of life	Active growth period
Water (ml)	60−130	120−150
Calories (gm)	50−100	110−140
Protein		3−4
Glucose		10−15
Fat		5−7
Electrolytes (mEq)		
Sodium	0.5−2	1.5−3.0
Potassium	0.5−2 (after 24 hours)	2.0−3.0
Chloride	0.5−2	1.5−3.0
Mineral (mEq)		
Calcium		4−6
Phosphorus		2−4
Magnesium		0.5−1.0

Source: Reprinted with permission from S. G. Babson, *Journal of Pediatrics,* 79:694, 1971 (**68**). Copyright © 1971 by C. V. Mosby Co., St. Louis, Missouri.

retardation and maturity at birth, the infant's calorie requirements during the active growth period range from 110 to 140 kcal per kilogram of body weight per day. Formulas supplying calories in a concentration similar to that of human milk (65 kcal/100 ml) may have to be fed in volumes exceeding the infant's gastric capacity to meet its calorie requirements. Formulas supplying 80–100 kcal per 100 ml are more acceptable. Calorie concentrations higher than this produce increased solute loads and may provide insufficient water for renal excretion. Some nutritionists feel that a calorie density of even 80–100 kcal is too high and that it may have some adverse effects, even though it results in more rapid weight gain.

An optimal protein intake for the premature infant is not defined yet by nutritionists (**14**). Low birth-weight infants have lower plasma protein levels than mature infants at birth, with the lowest weight infants having the lowest blood protein levels. Initial protein levels tend to decrease during the first 6–8 weeks of the neonatal period. Attempts to overcome this tendency or to promote growth by feeding a high protein diet are often harmful because of the infant's biological immaturity. Protein requirements for low birth-weight infants have been estimated from determinations of the chemical composition of weight gain in the fetus and weight gain of low birth-weight infants fed measured amounts of protein. Such studies show that infants weighing at least 2000 g require 2.2 g of protein per 100 kcal. Protein requirements for full-term infants are set at 20 percent above the estimated requirements. An advisable protein intake for the low birth-weight infant should be set at 30 percent above estimated requirements (**15**). Advisable intakes are, therefore, 2.8 g of protein per 100 kcal for infants weighing 1500–2500 g and 2.1 g per 100 kcal for those weighing 2500–3500 g. For infants weighing less than 1500 g the advisable protein intake is 2.2 g, the same as the estimated requirement (**15**). Because of increased renal solute load, intakes greater than this may be potentially harmful, causing blood urea nitrogen to increase excessively and producing protein intoxication (**70, 71**).

Recent reports show that low birth-weight infants may have increased requirements for the amino acid cystine (**69, 72**). The amino acid requirements of premature infants are shown in Table 8.11.

Premature infants absorb medium chain triglycerides well (**69**). Vegetable oils supplying polyunsaturated fatty acids are generally fed to low birth-weight infants to promote intestinal absorption. Fifty percent of the child's calorie requirements may be fed in the form of fat.

Up to 40 percent of the calories in an infant's diet may be fed in the form of carbohydrate. However, if disaccharide intolerance develops, these should be removed from the diet.

No minimal daily requirements for vitamins have been established for low birth-weight infants. Therefore, vitamins should be supplied in amounts meeting the requirements of normal full-term infants. Vitamins supplied in a formula developed for normal infants meet the daily requirements of the low birth-weight infant only if the formula is consumed in amounts of 1 l per day. Low birth-weight infants do not normally consume this much formula, and some suffer vitamin

TABLE 8.11 MINIMUM DAILY REQUIREMENT OF AMINO ACIDS FOR PREMATURE INFANTS

	Mg/kg
Histidine	32
Isoleucine	90
Leucine	150
Lysine	105
Methionine	65
Cystine	50
Phenylalanine	90
Threonine	60
Tryptophan	22
Valine	93

Source: Reprinted with permission from *Textbook of Pediatrics* by W. Nelson (**73**). Copyright © 1969 by W. B. Saunders Co., Philadelphia.

deficiencies as a result (**69**). Certain vitamin supplements in addition to those in the formula should be given, beginning the third to fifth day following birth.

Hemorrhagic disease of the newborn, associated with a vitamin K deficiency, is more prevalent in low birth-weight infants than in normal infants. One to two milligrams of vitamin K injected intramuscularly at birth, however, protects against the development of hemorrhagic disease. Low birth-weight infants may demonstrate increased requirements for vitamins A and D because of poor fat absorption and greater growth needs. To fill this need, 1500 IU (300 R.E.) of vitamin A and 400 IU (10 mcg) of vitamin D may be given daily (**69**). An increased need for ascorbic acid is seen in some low birth-weight infants who may be given 50 mg per day, beginning with the second week of life. The amount is dependent on the protein content of the diet and may be increased to 100 mg per day as dietary protein content increases. Some low birth-weight infants develop an anemia responsive to vitamin E given at 6–10 weeks of age (**69, 74, 75**). Such anemia is most common if infants are receiving large amounts of dietary linoleic acid or excessive iron. The anemia can be prevented by the administration of 50 mg of D-α-tocopherol per day or the feeding of a formula with a desirable vitamin E : polyunsaturated fatty acid ratio. A value of 0.6 is considered necessary to prevent hemolytic anemia (**69**). Once the anemia has developed it responds to 1 g of vitamin E given over a seven- to ten-day period.

Iron-deficiency anemia is characteristic of low birth-weight infants around 12 weeks of age when blood cells begin to increase rapidly. The American Academy of Pediatrics recommends that low birth-weight infants receive 2 mg of iron in the form of ferrous sulfate per kilogram of body weight per day, beginning as early as 2 months of age (**69**). Excessive amounts of iron, 8 mg per day or more, are associated with the development of hemolytic anemia described previously (**69**). The risk of hemolytic anemia is greater in the presence of a vitamin E deficiency, and iron may serve as a cofactor catalyzing the oxidative breakdown of red cell lipids. No antioxidant effect to offset this process is available when a state of vitamin E deficiency exists.

The nutritional problems of low birth-weight infants are not completely understood (**14**). Significant advances have been made in recent years, but more precisely defined nutritional requirements are needed for these babies in relation to their physiologic maturity. Because of the considerable variation in size and degree of maturity of these infants at birth, a careful evaluation is necessary to determine appropriate diet and feeding methods to meet individual needs.

SUMMARY

Breast milk or commercially available formulas provide excellent nutrition to the infant during the first months of life. As the child grows, though, a milk diet alone can no longer meet all nutritional requirements. The physiological changes that occur with growth allow for the inclusion of a greater variety of foods in the diet, and semisolid foods are generally introduced about the third month or even earlier in some instances. A great deal of controversy, however, surrounds the problem of how and when to first introduce solid foods into the infant diet.

Health professionals are becoming increasingly aware of the significance of nutrition during infancy in the development of certain pathological conditions (hypertension, obesity, cardiovascular disease) that may not become apparent until later life. Certain consequences of infant feeding on the child's physical and mental makeup may be irreversible. At present health professionals can only speculate about the influence of certain types of infant diets on the genesis of various disease conditions and need to continue research in these areas. Findings from such research programs could lead to preventative health measures in the form of good nutrition practices begun in infancy.

STUDY QUESTIONS AND
TOPICS FOR INDIVIDUAL INVESTIGATION

1. The content of a specific essential nutrient may be ten times greater in one commercially available infant cereal than in another. Choose several different cereals available on the market. Look at the nutrition labels on each. How do the cereals differ in content of calories, protein, carbohydrate, fat, vitamins, and minerals? Which one (or ones) do you feel is the best buy nutritionally?
2. Strained cereals with fruit are becoming increasingly popular. How do these differ in nutritional properties from the dry cereals after the latter have been diluted with milk or water and are ready to feed? Read the labels on different brands of strained cereal with fruit and compare them with one another and with the dry cereals. Pay particular attention to calories, protein, calcium, iron, niacin, thiamin, riboflavin, ascorbic acid, and vitamin B_6. Would you buy dry cereal or strained cereal with fruit for your infant if you were a parent? Do different brands differ in nutrient content?
3. Visit your local supermarket or arrange to have baby food products brought to class. Compare several strained meat, soup, dinner, and high-meat dinner products. How much meat, vegetables, and "filler" does each contain? Do certain products represent a better buy nutritionally?
4. The question of the use of home-prepared versus commercially-prepared infant foods comes up often. Suppose that you are a nutrition educator who has been asked that question. How will you answer? What are the advantages and disadvantages associated with both food sources? Would you advocate one choice over the other? Explain.
5. You have been asked to develop a nutrition education tool for use in group or individual teaching situations in the area of infant nutrition. You have decided

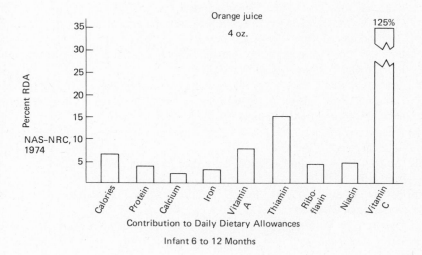

Orange juice
4 oz.

Contribution to Daily Dietary Allowances

Infant 6 to 12 Months

to prepare a series of flash cards similar to the nutrition comparison cards for teens and adults developed by the National Dairy Council. These cards will be a graphic presentation of selected nutrients and caloric values of goods commonly eaten by infants. Choose foods common to your community. On a separate 8 × 11 in. card print the name and serving size of each food. For most strained foods a serving size of four tablespoons can be used. Draw bar graphs representing the percentage of the recommended dietary allowance (for a 6−12 month-old child) for eight nutrients and calories that are contributed by each food. Color code each nutrient. Display the cards with the actual food product in an exhibit. An example of a card for orange juice is shown.

6. Every mother with a newborn infant will soon face the concerns of when and how to introduce solid foods into the diet. What advice would you give to a parent asking you about such matters? Why do nutritionists tend to recommend later rather than earlier introduction of solid foods?

REFERENCES

1. Gesell, A., and F. Ilg. *Feeding Behavior of Infants.* Lippincott, Philadelphia, 1937.
2. Ardran, G., F. Kemp, and J. Lind. A cineradiographic study of breast feeding. *British Journal of Radiology,* 31:156, 1958.
3. Ardran, G., F. Kemp, and J. Lind. A cineradiographic study of bottle feeding. *British Journal of Radiology,* 31:11, 1958.
4. Subtelny, J. Examination of current philosophies associated with swallowing behavior. *American Journal of Orthodontics,* 51:161, 1965.
5. Maternal and Child Health Service and Committee on Infant and Preschool Child, American Academy of Pediatrics. *Nutrition and Feeding of Infants and Children Under Three in Group Day Care.* DHEW Publication No. (Health Services and Mental Health Administration) 72−5606. U.S. Government Printing Office, Washington, D.C., 1971.
6. Jelliffe, D., and E. Jelliffe. Duration of breast feeding. *Lancet,* 1:752, 1975.
7. Fomon, S. J., L. J. Filer, Jr., T. A. Anderson, and E. K. Ziegler. Recommendations for feeding normal infants. *Pediatrics,* 63:52, 1979.
8. Pipes, P. When should semisolid foods be fed to infants? *Journal of Nutrition Education,* 9:57, 1977.
9. National Dairy Council. Current concepts in infant nutrition. *Dairy Council Digest,* 47:7, 1976.
10. Harris, L., and J. Chan. Infant feeding practices. *American Journal of Diseases of Children,* 117:483, 1969.
11. Fomon, S. J. What are infants fed in the United States? *Pediatrics,* 56:350, 1975.

12. Beal, V. Termination of night feeding in infancy. *Journal of Pediatrics,* 75:690, 1969.

13. Guthrie, H. Effect of early feeding of solid foods on nutritive intake of infants. *Pediatrics,* 38:879, 1966.

14. Roe, D. Concepts of neonatal malnutrition. *New York State Journal of Medicine,* 70:420, 1970.

15. Fomon, S. J. *Infant nutrition,* 2nd ed. Saunders, Philadelphia, 1974.

16. U.S. Department of Agriculture. *Composition of Foods: Baby Foods–Raw, Processed, Prepared.* Agriculture Handbook No. 8–3. USDA Science and Education Administration, Washington, D.C., 1978.

17. Matthews, R. H., and M. Y. Workman. Nutrient content of selected baby foods. *Journal of the American Dietetic Association,* 72:27, 1978.

18. Fomon, S. J., L. Thomas, and L. Filer. Acceptance of unsalted strained foods by normal infants. *Journal of Pediatrics,* 76:242, 1970.

19. Mayer, J. Baby foods grow up. *Family Health/Today's Health,* October:36, 1977.

20. Watt, B., and A. Merrill. *Composition of Foods—Raw, Processed, Prepared.* Agriculture Handbook of U.S. Department of Agriculture, Washington, D.C., 1963.

21. Peterkin, B., and S. Walker. Food for the baby—cost and nutritive value considerations. *Family Economics Review,* 4:3, 1976.

22. Filer, L. J. Subcommittee on Safety and Suitability of MSG and Other Substances in Baby Foods. Food Protection Committee, Food and Nutrition Board, National Academy of Science—National Research Council. Salt in infant foods. *Nutrition Reviews,* 29:27, 1971.

23. Deeming, S. B., and C. W. Weber. Trace minerals in commercially prepared baby foods. *Journal of the American Dietetic Association,* 75:149, 1979.

24. Herschkowitz, N. Influence de l'alimentation sur le metabolisme cerebral. Symposium Nestle, 1975, p. 143.

25. Dobbing, J. The later growth of the brain and its vulnerability. *Pediatrics,* 53:2, 1974.

26. Frisch, R. E. Present status of the supposition that malnutrition causes permanent mental retardation. *American Journal of Clinical Nutrition,* 23:189, 1970.

27. Barnes, R. H. Introductory remarks. Points of concern with current interpretations of the effects of early malnutrition on mental development. *Bibliography of Nutrition and Dietetics,* 17:1, 1972.

28. Subcommittee on Nutrition, Brain Development and Behavior of the Committee on International Nutritional Programs: *The Relationship of Nutrition to Brain Development and Behavior.* National Academy of Sciences-National Research Council, Washington, D.C., 1973.

29. Committee on Nutrition, American Academy of Pediatrics. Iron balance and requirements in infancy. *Pediatrics,* 43:134, 1969.

30. Filer, L. J. About iron. In: *Infant Nutrition—Feeding the Infant, Building the Man.* Wyeth Laboratories, Medcom, Inc., New York, 1972.

31. Purvis, G. What nutrients do our infants really get? *Nutrition Today,* 8:28, 1973.

32. Lovric, V., A. Lammi, and J. Friend. Nutrition, iron intake and haematological status in healthy children. *Medical Journal of Australia,* 1:11, 1972.

33. Committee on Nutrition, American Academy of Pediatrics. Childhood diet and coronary heart disease. *Pediatrics,* 49:305, 1972.

34. Drash, A. Atherosclerosis, cholesterol, and the pediatrician. *Journal of Pediatrics,* 80:693, 1972.

35. Fredrickson, D. Factors in childhood that influence the development of atherosclerosis and hypertension. *American Journal of Clinical Nutrition,* 25:221, 1972.

36. Monkeberg, F. Fats in infant nutrition. *Annales Nestle,* 28:62, 1972.

37. Tsang, R., R. Fallat, and C. Glueck. Cholesterol at birth and age 1: comparison of normal and hypercholesterolemic neonates. *Pediatrics,* 53:458, 1974.

38. Tsang, R., C. Glueck, R. Fallat, and M. Mellius. Neonatal familial hypercholesterolemia. *American Journal of the Diseases of Children,* 129:83, 1975.

39. Fomon, S. J. Nutrition in infancy. In: *Infant Nutrition—Feeding the Infant, Building the Man.* Wyeth Laboratories, Medcom, Inc., New York, 1972.

40. Fomon, S. J., and E. E. Ziegler. Skim milk in infant feeding. DHEW Publication No. (HSA) 77–5102. U.S. Government Printing Office, Washington, D.C., August 1977.

41. Marx, J. L. The HDL: the good cholesterol carriers? *Science,* 205:677, 1977.

42. Shukla, A., H. Forsyth, C. Anderson, and A. Marwah. Infantile overnutrition in the first year of life: a field study in Dudley, Worcestershire. *British Journal of Medicine,* 4:507, 1972.

43. Taitz, L. Infantile overnutrition among artificially fed infants in the Sheffield Region. *British Medical Journal,* 1:315, 1971.

44. Oates, R. Infant feeding practices. *British Medical Journal,* 2:762, 1973.

45. Himes, J. H. Infant feeding practices and obesity. *Journal of the American Dietetic Association,* 75:122, 1979.

46. Hirsch, J., and J. Knittle. Cellularity of obese and non-obese human adipose tissue. *Federation Proceedings,* 29:1516, 1970.

47. Brook, C. Evidence for a sensitive period in adipose-cell replication in man. *Lancet,* 2:624, 1972.

48. Milner, R. Nutrition and growth of the fetus and newborn infant. *Nutrition,* 27:404, 1973.

49. Gairdner, D. The effect of diet on the development of the adipose organ. *Proceedings, Nutrition Society,* 33:119, 1974.

50. Charney, E., H. Goodman, M. McBridge, B. Lyon, and R. Pratt. Childhood antecedents of adult obesity. *New England Journal of Medicine,* 296:6, 1976.

51. Eid, E. Follow-up study of physical growth of children who had excessive weight gain in the first six months of life. *British Medical Journal,* 2:74, 1970.

52. Mitchell, H. S., H. J. Rynborgen, L. Anderson, and M. O. Dibble. *Nutrition in*

Health and Disease, 16th ed. Lippincott, Philadelphia, 1976.

53. Hall, B. Changing composition of human milk and early development of appetite control. *Lancet,* 1:779, 1975.

54. Dwyer, J., and J. Mayer. *Overfeeding and Obesity in Infants and Children.* S. Karger, Basel, Switzerland 1973, p. 123.

55. Guthrie, H. Infant feeding practices—a predisposing factor in hypertension? *American Journal of Clinical Nutrition,* 21:863, 1968.

56. Shaw, J. Malnutrition in very low birth weight, pre-term infants. *Proceedings, Nutrition Society,* 33:103, 1974.

57. Wu, P., P. Teilmann, M. Gabler, M. Vaughn, and J. Metcalf. "Early" versus "late" feeding of low birth weight neonates: effect on serum bilirubin, blood sugar, and responses to glucagon and epinephrine tolerance tests. *Pediatrics,* 39:733, 1967.

58. Krauss, A., and P. Auld. Metabolic requirements of low birth weight infants. *Journal of Pediatrics,* 75:952, 1969.

59. Lavy, U., M. Silverberg, and M. Davidson. Role of bile acids in fat absorption in low birth weight infants. *Pediatric Research,* 5:387, 1971.

60. Benda, G., and S. Babson. Peripheral intravenous alimentation of the small premature infant. *Journal of Pediatrics,* 79:494, 1971.

61. Ziegler, E., and S. J. Fomon. Fluid intake, renal solute load, and water balance in infancy. *Journal of Pediatrics,* 78:561, 1971.

62. Ghadimi, H., K. Arulanantham, and M. Rathi. Evaluation of nutritional management of the low birth weight newborn. *American Journal of Clinical Nutrition,* 26:473, 1973.

63. Heird, D. Improved methods of non-oral neonatal feeding: a commentary. *Journal of Pediatrics,* 82:963, 1973.

64. Dallman, P. Iron, vitamin E, and folate in the preterm infant. *Journal of Pediatrics,* 85:742, 1974.

65. Rickard, K., and E. Gresham. Nutritional considerations for the newborn requiring intensive care. *Journal of the American Dietetics Association,* 66:592, 1975.

66. Heird, W. C., J. M. Driscoll, Jr., J. N. Schullinger, B. Grebin, and R. W. Winters. Intravenous alimentation in pediatric patients. *Journal of Pediatrics,* 80:351, 1972.

67. Melichar, V., and M. Novak. Energy metabolism in the human fetus and newborn. In: *Utilization of Nutrients During Postnatal Development,* eds. P. Hahn and O. Koldovsky. Pergamon Press, London, 1966.

68. Babson, S. Feeding the low birth weight infant. *Journal of Pediatrics,* 79:694, 1971.

69. Barness, L. Feeding the premature infant. In: *Infant Nutrition—Feeding the Infant, Building the Man.* Wyeth Laboratories, Medcom, Inc., New York, 1972.

70. Snyderman, S., L. Holt, P. Norton, and S. Phansalkar. Protein requirement of the premature infant. 2. Influence of protein intake on free amino acid content of plasma and red cells. *American Journal of Clinical Nutrition,* 23:890, 1970.

71. Valman, H., R. Brown, T. Palmer, V. Oberholzer, and B. Levin. Protein intake and plasma amino acids of infants of low birth weight. *British Medical Journal,* 4:789, 1971.

72. Sturman, J., G. Gaull, and N. Raiha. Absence of cystathionase in human fetal liver: Is cystine essential? *Science,* 169:74, 1970.

73. Nelson, W. *Textbook of Pediatrics*. Saunders, Philadelphia, 1969.

74. Melhorn, D., and S. Gnoss. Vitamin E dependent anemia in the premature infant. 1. Effects of large doses of medicinal iron. *Journal of Pediatrics,* 79:569, 1971.

75. Melhorn, D., and S. Gnoss. Vitamin E dependent anemia in the premature infant. 2. Relationships between gestational age and absorption of vitamin E. *Journal of Pediatrics,* 79:581, 1971.

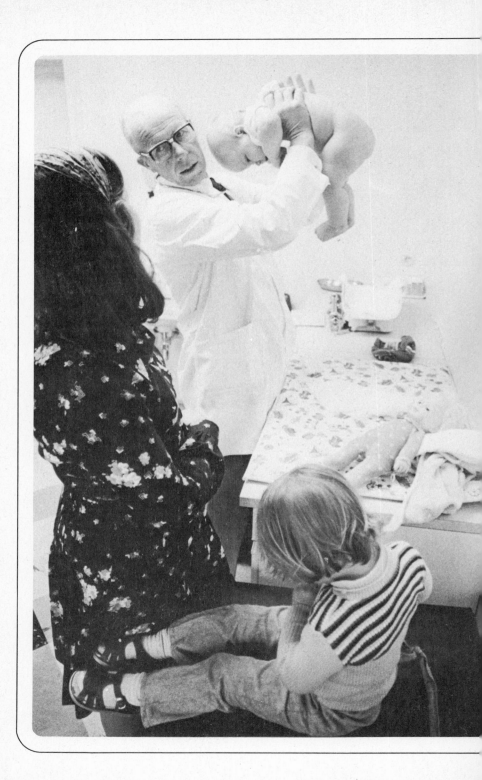

CHAPTER 9

NUTRITIONAL PROBLEMS IN THE INFANT AND CHILD

Many infants at birth have metabolic and physical difficulties which imply serious problems for their future normal growth and development. Although the numbers of children involved may be a small percentage of the total births, the effects of these maladies create serious complications in the lives of the individuals and their families. This chapter discusses the more commonly occurring problems, particularly those that can be partially remedied with dietary modifications and controls. The presentation does not cover the wide range of metabolic and medical problems confronting limited numbers of infants. Neither does this section present sufficient details for physicians and dietitians to use as a guide for nutritional therapy. We recommend texts on therapeutic nutrition and diet manuals from established centers of medicine for that purpose.

Infants and children with metabolic and other problems require diets that provide the essential nutrients to support normal growth and development whenever possible. Although modifications are necessary to alleviate the evidence of the problem, a normal intake of nutrients should be maintained as much as possible. The long-range goal is to maintain normal development, even while treating the problem, particularly those problems of long duration and with lasting effects on the child.

Food intake will likely become a real problem if the child is to be on a modified diet for a long time. In many instances, the dietary habits of the entire family must be altered to meet the emotional needs of the afflicted child.

Children who are ill tend to regress to an earlier stage of development, so sound treatment for the youngster will require both physiological and psychological support from the parents and siblings. Furthermore, the treatment may be very expensive. Special diet formulas, medications, frequent visits to the physician, short stays in the hospital for tests and checks, purchase of uncommon and less available foods, transportation, and so on, are all costly and place an extra burden on the entire family. The family must learn quickly to cope with these difficulties and problems.

GENERAL NUTRITIONAL GUIDELINES

Energy and Protein

Sufficient amounts of energy and protein must be provided to support normal growth. The following table (Table 9.1) provides reasonable goals, but the intake may require adjustments, especially in energy intake, for each individual (**1**).

The protein must be from a good quality source, since it must provide all the essential amino acids, as well as adequate total protein. This poses particularly difficult problems when the metabolic offender is one of the essential amino acids. Moreover, excess protein can also present a problem, since protein in amounts of 4–5 g/per kilogram per day may prove hazardous to the young child. The immature liver and kidney of the infant may be overloaded with those amounts of protein. Dehydration may result because of the volume of fluids required to excrete the end products of protein metabolism (**2**).

Fats

The breast-fed infant consumes approximately 50 percent of his or her total energy intake from fats. In the commonly prescribed infant formulas fats supply from 35–45 percent of the total energy intake. In certain dietary problems, linoleic acid, the essential fatty acid, must be added to the diet. For example, when medium chain triglycerides are used with infants with malabsorption problems, small amounts of corn oil are added to provide linoleic acid. In other maladies, such as the hyperlipoproteinemias, the source of dietary fat and the cholesterol intake must be controlled closely (**2**).

TABLE 9.1 GUIDELINE FOR ESTIMATING ENERGY AND PROTEIN NEEDS OF INFANTS AND CHILDREN

Age (years)	Energy (kcal)	Protein (g)
0.0–0.5	115/kg	2.2/kg
0.5–1.0	105/kg	2.0 g/kg
1–3	900–1800	23
4–6	1300–2300	30
7–10	1650–3300	34

Source: Food and Nutrition Board, *Recommended Dietary Allowances,* 9th edition, National Academy of Sciences, 1980 (**1**).

Carbohydrate

The source and level of carbohydrate may be modified for several metabolic problems. Usually, carbohydrates supply 45–50 percent of the total energy intake (**2**).

Vitamins and minerals

Careful monitoring of special formulas and diets is essential to insure adequate intakes of vitamins and minerals. Supplements may be necessary in many cases (**2**).

Electrolytes

The levels of sodium and potassium are critical in several metabolic aberrations, as well as in the normal individual. Oral supplements may be necessary in conditions involving excessive fluid and electrolyte losses and in kidney and heart diseases.

Fluids

Except in those cases when it is necessary medically to limit intake, the child should consume normal amounts of fluid. The following table (Table 9.2) presents a guideline for fluid intake (**3**).

SPECIAL FORMULAS AND SUPPLEMENTS

Several commercial sources provide a wide variety of special formulas and supplements. The following table gives information about some of those that are

TABLE 9.2 RANGE OF AVERAGE DAILY FLUID REQUIREMENTS FOR INFANTS AND CHILDREN UNDER ORDINARY CONDITIONS

Age	Average body weight (kg)	Fluid/kg (ml)
3 days	3.0	80–100
10 days	3.2	125–150
3 months	5.4	140–160
6 months	7.3	130–155
9 months	8.6	125–145
1 year	9.5	120–135
2 years	11.8	115–125
4 years	16.2	100–110
6 years	20.0	90–100
10 years	28.7	70–85
14 years	45.0	50–60
18 years	54.0	40–50

Source: Reprinted with permission from *Textbook of Pediatrics*, 10th edition, by V. C. Vaughan, R. J. McKay, and W. E. Nelson (**3**). Copyright © 1977 by W. B. Saunders Co., Philadelphia.

available (Table 9.3). The reader, however, should recognize that the formulas and supplements change continuously. The manufacturer will provide the most recent information on request. The information is also available with the product.

MALABSORPTION SYNDROMES

Several metabolic diseases have their onset during infancy and affect the digestion, absorption, or transport of food components. Dietary modifications are necessary to relieve painful symptoms in several of these diseases.

Cystic Fibrosis

This inherited disease occurs in approximately 1 per 1500 live births. The mucous and sweat glands are affected, with the mucous glands secreting a very thick mucous and the sweat glands producing sweat higher in salt than normal (**4**).

   The thick mucous presents serious problems, since the air passages in the lungs can become clogged, resulting in labored breathing. The mucous may fill the pancreatic duct, thus preventing the secretion of the pancreatic digestive enzymes. Malabsorption and fatty stools are prevalent problems in these people.

   The etiology of the disease is not clearly understood. Infants are usually given formulas higher in protein (approximately 24 percent of the total calories from protein) and lower in fat (about 30 percent of total calories) than normal. The source of fat may be either long chain or medium chain triglycerides (**5**). Foods with a high fat content are avoided for older children (**6**).

   Persons with cystic fibrosis may survive to an age of 20 or 30 years, but many perish during infancy.

Sucrase-Isomaltase Deficiency

This is a rare inherited disease in which the body is deficient in the enzymes sucrase and isomaltase. *Isomaltase* is the enzyme that hydrolyzes the 1,6 linkage in amylopectin. The infant is treated with formulas free of sucrose and starch or by being fed breast milk. As growth and development occur, the infant can tolerate small amounts of starch (**7**).

Glucose-Galactose Malabsorption

The active transport of glucose and galactose through the intestine is impaired in this rare, inherited disease. Fructose can be tolerated, but almost all other carbohydrate must be excluded from the diet. A limited tolerance for carbohydrate however, is achieved with age (**8**).

Celiac Sprue

Celiac sprue (gluten-induced enteropathy, Celiac Disease, nontropical sprue) is a malabsorption syndrome found in both children and adults. The disease is characterized by steatorrhea and the passage of two or three stools each day. The fecal excretions are foamy, light-colored, bulky, and very foul smelling. They

TABLE 9.3 EXAMPLES OF SPECIAL FORMULAS[1,2]

Product and Producer	Protein	Carbohydrate	Fat	Comments	Uses
Soy-Based					
Lactose Free:					
Soylac, Loma Linda Foods, Riverside, Ca. 92515	Soy, plus methionine	Corn syrup and other sources	Soybean oil	Available as powdered formula, concentrated liquid, and ready-to-serve formula. Based on water extract of whole soybean	Allergies to cow's milk, substitute for human milk
1-Soylac, Loma Linda Foods, Riverside, Ca. 92515	Soy isolate, plus methionine	Sucrose	Soy oil	Free of corn and milk; cholesterol free	Allergic infants; substitute for cow's and human milk
Isomil, Ross Laboratories, Columbus, Ohio 43216	Soy isolate	Corn syrup; sucrose; modified cornstarch	Soy and coconut oil	Concentrate or ready to serve	Lactose intolerance; allergies to cow's milk; diarrhea
Prosobee, Mead-Johnson Laboratories, Evansville, Ind. 47721	Soy isolate, plus methionine	Sucrose; corn syrup	Soy oil	Concentrated liquid or ready to serve	Allergies to milk; lactose intolerance
Nonsoy, Lactose Free:					
MBF (Meat-Base Formula) Gerber Products Co., Fremont, Mich. 49412	Beethearts	Sucrose; tapioca starch	Sesame oil primarily	Concentrated as purchased	Allergies to milk; galactosemia; glycogen-storage disease
Nutramingen, Mead-Johnson Laboratories	Enzyme hydrolyzed casein; charcoal treated	Sucrose; tapioca starch	Corn oil	Powdered concentrate; liquid for use in hospitals	Allergies to milk; diarrhea; galactosemia
Progestimil, Mead-Johnson Laboratories	Enzyme hydrolyzate of casein, plus added cystine, tyrosine, and tryptophan	Glucose polymers	Medium chain triglycerides and corn oil	Concentrated powder	Diarrhea; allergies; malabsorption problems; cystic fibrosis; others

(Continued)

297

TABLE 9.3 (Continued)

Product and Producer	Protein	Carbohydrates	Fat	Comments	Used
Other Special Formulas:					
Enfamil Premature Formula, Mead-Johnson Laboratories	Skim milk	Sucrose; lactose	Medium chain triglyceride; corn oil; coconut oil	Formula for hospital use only	Special formula for low birth-weight infants
Lofenalac, Mead-Johnson Laboratories	Casein hydrolyzate processed to remove most of phenylalanine; amino acids added	Corn syrup; tapioca syrup	Corn oil	Powdered for dilution with water	Phenylketonuria
Portagen, Mead-Johnson Laboratories	Sodium caseinate	Corn syrup; sucrose	Corn oil; medium chain triglycerides	Powdered for dilution with water	Fat malabsorption
Probana, Mead-Johnson Laboratories	Whole and skim milk; casein hydrolyzate	Banana powder; dextrose; lactose	Corn oil	Powdered for dilution; fluid hospital use	Cystic fibrosis; (for steatorrhea; gluten induced enteropathy
Similac PM 60/40, Ross Laboratories	Demineralized, delactosed whey solids; sodium caseinate	Lactose	Coconut oil; corn oil	Ready-to-feed powder for dilution	Problem eaters; hypocalcemia; renal, digestive, cardiovascular problems to provide low levels of minerals and protein.
MSUD Diet Powder; Product 3200AB; Product 3200K; Product 80056, Mead-Johnson Laboratories	Varies with formula				Disease: tyrosinemia; homocystinuria, other amino acid disorders

¹Based on information provided to the authors by producers. Each product has added amounts of vitamins and minerals to meet the needs of the infant.
²Many other special formulas and products are available.

contain a high percentage of fat and calcium soaps as a result of poor digestion in the intestinal tract (**9**).

Infants and children are typically pot bellied, suffer from significant weight loss, muscle wasting, anorexia, and anemia. The anemia is a reflection of poor absorption of iron and folic acid. Poor use of calcium is also a factor and may result in tetany, bone pain, and even fractures. The body does not utilize fat-soluble vitamins well.

Gluten in certain cereal grains is a toxic substance to the affected individuals (**9**). Gluten in wheat, rye, and oats presents a problem; however, rice and corn can be tolerated. The specific offending substance is glutamine when bound to a peptide during digestion of the protein molecule. Glutamine is present in high concentrations in the cereal proteins. The disease can be controlled through the use of gluten-free diets, but this presents difficulties because of the wide use of cereal proteins in the food supply.

Lactose Intolerance and Malabsorption

Lactose malabsorption is a reduced use of lactose because of lowered lactase activity (**10**). It is characterized by abdominal pain, diarrhea, bloating, and impaired glucose tolerance.

Lactose intolerance or a low level of lactase activity affects a high percentage, 60–90 percent, of the non-Caucasian population of the world. From 5–15 percent of all Caucasians have low levels of lactase (**11, 12**). In the United States, from 6–19 percent of the white population and from 72–75 percent of the black population suffer from the disease (**13, 14**).

Congenital lactase deficiency is a rare problem that becomes evident soon after birth (**15**). In the normal infant lactase is present at a low level during fetal development. The enzyme level increases by a factor of 2 or 3 just prior to birth (**11**). Premature infants may be intolerant of milk for the first few days after birth. Full-term infants may have soft stools if consuming breast milk, which contains 8 percent lactose, but the consumption of cow's milk, with only 4 percent lactose, does not cause the same response (**16**). Intolerance can be quite serious in the affected infants and often leads to death. In those children, neither breast milk nor cow's milk can be tolerated and lactose-free formulas must be substituted. All foods containing lactose, including milk, cheese, breads made with milk, and so on, should be excluded from the diet of these infants and children (**11**). Calcium supplements are therefore necessary to meet growth needs when milk and milk products are excluded from the diet.

Lactose intolerance may appear early in life, particularly among black children (**17**). Severe abdominal pain, cramping, and diarrhea are common in lactose intolerant persons. The primary cause of the pain is the increased volume of water in the intestines as a consequence of the osmotic effects of lactose (**18**). Also, bacterial action on lactose produces carbon dioxide and other gases. Lactose intolerance can be diagnosed clinically by measuring lactase activity and by a glucose tolerance test. Blood glucose levels fail to rise in persons intolerant of lactose following the ingestion of a 50 g load of lactose by an adult or 2 g per kilogram of body weight by children.

Most persons seem to be able to tolerate small quantities of milk without experiencing the severe symptoms of intolerance (**18**). The introduction of milk and milk products to areas with a history of lactose intolerance, however, should be done with care (**19**). Small quantities of milk, though, can be consumed satisfactorily by persons with positive lactose intolerance tests. Thus the introduction of small amounts of milk is suggested rather than the consumption of large quantities that may result in a serious problem.

ALLERGIES

An *allergy* is an adverse physiological reaction in various tissues resulting from the interaction of an antigen with an antibody or with a lymphoid cell. Tissues usually involved are skin, mucous membranes, and the vascular endothelium.

Antibodies are immunoglobulins, the most common one being immunoglobulin E (IgE). Numerous allergic reactions are attributed to IgE antibodies, and there is a significant, familial incidence that serves as an aid in diagnosis.

Foods are a common cause but are by no means the only cause of allergic reactions. Other causative agents include pollens, dust, animal hair, cosmetics, drugs, and vaccines. The foods that commonly cause allergies are milk, eggs, wheat, oranges, fish, shellfish, tomatoes, strawberries, and chocolate. Although these foods vary widely in protein content, the protein component is generally the causative factor (**20, 21**).

In infants and children, the most common symptoms are eczema, asthma, and rhinitis. These may occur in adults, also. Any allergy may influence a person's general health and nutritional status. Children are particularly susceptible, and growth and development can be seriously affected because of a depressed appetite. Careful testing and the elimination of foods can lead to the determination of the cause, but the procedures are lengthy, complicated and stressful (**21**). Infants and young children may be placed on formulas such as MullSoy or Neo-MullSoy while foods are added to the diet one at a time to isolate the allergy-producing agent.

The more common food-based allergies are discussed briefly in the following sections.

Milk Allergy

Allergic reactions to cow's milk usually appear in children under 2 years of age (**22**), and the lactoglobulin fraction of milk protein is the most common causative factor. Treatment consists of feeding milk-free formulas, usually soy protein based, and removing all solid foods having milk as an ingredient (**21**). The child undergoing this treatment will require supplements of calcium and riboflavin. In most cases, the tolerance for milk increases with age, thus the controls need not be so stringent with older persons.

Wheat Allergy

Wheat is another common problem (**22**). The major difficulty in treatment is the selection of foods without wheat.

Desensitizing the Allergic Person

Desensitization is a process through which the person is guided to remove the allergic reaction from the system. The process usually follows a period of complete avoidance of the food causing the problem. Small, even minute, amounts of the food are added back to the diet and increased gradually until the food can be tolerated.

INBORN ERRORS OF METABOLISM

Numerous inborn or inherited errors of metabolism may adversely affect the growth, development, or general health of the infant and child. The following table presents a partial listing of inborn errors (Table 9.4). The more common prevalent diseases are discussed in the following sections.

Diabetes Mellitus

Diabetes may be regarded as an inborn error of metabolism, although there is some disagreement about this classification (**23**). The susceptibility to diabetes is conditioned by genetic factors, but the onset of the disease is a clear reflection of environmental factors.

Diabetes is a complex and widespread metabolic disorder. Indeed, the U.S. Public Health Service estimates that 2.3 percent of the population has diabetes (**2**). This figure of 2 percent, or approximately 3.5−4 million people, is

TABLE 9.4   PARTIAL LISTING OF INBORN ERRORS OF METABOLISM

Carbohydrate Metabolism:	Amino Acid Metabolism:
Diabetes Mellitus	Familial goiter
Pentosuria	Phenylketonuria
Fructose intolerance	Tyrosinosis
Glycogen storage diseases	Alcaptonuria
Galactose disorders	Albinism
Primary hyperoxaluria	Histidinemia
Lipid Metabolism:	Proline disorders
	Hydroxylproline disorders
Familial lipoprotein deficiency	Urea cycle
Familial lecithin	Hyperlysinemia
Familial hyperlipoproteinemia	Homocystinuria
Tay-Sachs Disease	Cystathionuria
Gangliosides	Maple Syrup Urine Disease
Fabrey's Disease	**Purine and Pyrimidines:**
Sulfatide lipidosis	
Gaucher's Disease	Gout
Krabbe's Disease	Lesch-Nyham syndrome
Metals:	Xanthuria
Wilson's Disease	
Hemachromatosis	

generally accepted by medical and health authorities. Diabetes occurs in all age groups but is much more predominant in those above 45 years of age (**24**).

Health professionals see two types of diabetes in their patients. Growth onset diabetes occurs in children from birth to 14 years of age but is rare in infants below 1 year. Onset of the disease is usually sudden. It is generally preceded by weight loss, and the person is frequently in a state of "ketoacidosis" on diagnosis. The insulin deficiency is usually severe, and both insulin and dietary control are necessary for successful treatment. Maturity onset diabetes usually occurs in persons over 40 years of age and more frequently in those above 55 years. Onset is gradual. Diet and exercise are the major influences on the development of diabetes in the person predisposed to diabetes or those likely to experience the maturity onset type. Mild diabetes during pregnancy results in increased fetal wastage and manifests itself further through hypertrophy of the fetal Islet of Langerhans. Metabolic changes during pregnancy bring out the existence of latent diabetes in the mother (**2**), and only in recent years have pregnant women with diabetes been able to carry the fetus to term successfully.

The basic defect in diabetes is the absolute or relative lack of insulin which leads to an abnormal carbohydrate metabolism. Insulin controls glucose metabolism by mediating the movement of glucose from the extracellular spaces to the cells; amino acids are affected similarly. When insulin is lacking, glycogen synthesis is restricted and there is an increased synthesis of glucose through gluconeogenesis. The process of glucose synthesis proceeds as the result of increased protein degradation, accompanied by a decreased cellular uptake of the amino acids. Lipolysis or the breakdown of body fat is increased, and fatty acids become the major source of fuel for the tricarboxylic acid cycle (TCA cycle) or for the generation of energy.

An excess of acetyl coenzyme A occurs as the TCA cycle becomes short of other necessary substances. When this happens, cholesterol and ketone bodies are synthesized in the liver. They are excreted (ketonuria) as the quantity of these substances exceeds the capacity of other tissues to metabolize them. The production of glucose exceeds the capacity of the renal tubules for reabsorption, and glucose is excreted in the urine. Since glucose requires water for excretion, the volume of urine increases and the body loses water and sodium.

The demand on body fluids is further magnified because body protein is being catabolized and the amino acids are being used for gluconeogenesis. There is an increase in urea excretion. As cellular protein is catabolized, cellular potassium is lost. Both potassium and urea require water for excretion from the body. Further, the ketone bodies require water for excretion. Cellular dehydration occurs with an increased hydrogen ion concentration in the blood. The net effect can be circulatory failure. The sequence of events is outlined in Figure 9.1.

The onset is abrupt in juvenile diabetes (**2**). Ketoacidosis is accompanied by nausea, vomiting, and lethargy. The initial signal of onset is two to three weeks prior to severe symptoms when the patient suffers weight loss, polydipsia, polyphagia, and polyuria. The most commonly used screening method for persons suspected of having diabetes is the glucose tolerance test. The test

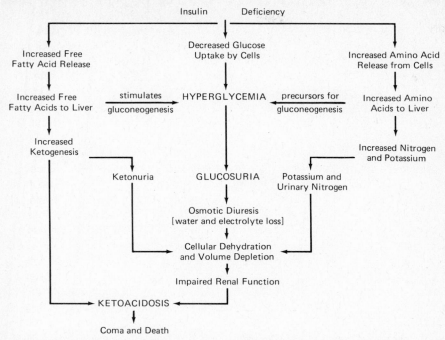

Figure 9.1 *Metabolic consequences of insulin deficiency.* (*Source:* Reproduced with permission from *Metabolic and Endocrine Physiology,* 3rd edition, by J. Tepperman. Copyright © 1973 by Year Book Medical Publishers, Inc., Chicago.)

evaluates the return to a normal plasma glucose concentration following a dose of glucose. A comparison of the response of a normal individual and a diabetic is demonstrated in Figure 9.2.

The U.S. Public Health Service uses a point system based on blood glucose levels to interpret glucose tolerance tests (Table 9.5).

The treatment of diabetes is aimed at preventing hyperglycemia and glycogen wastage, preventing hypoglycemia when using insulin, and fostering normal growth and development of the child (**2**). Control of weight is the goal in adults. The maintenance of normal levels of blood lipids is also an objective of treatment in both children and adults. Extensive materials are available on diabetes, "dietary exchanges" (foods that may be substituted for each other in meeting specified dietary goals), the action of insulin, the forms of oral agents, and other aspects of the disease. These are beyond the scope of this publication but are recommended for the professional concerned with a diabetic.

Galactosemia

This disorder of galactose metabolism involves the failure to convert galactose to glucose, with a subsequent rise in galactose levels in cells, blood, and urine. The enzyme, galactose-l-phosphate uridyl transferase, is defective or missing, and

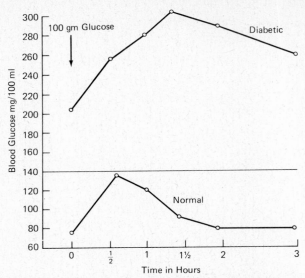

Figure 9.2 *Results of glucose tolerance tests in a normal person and a diabetic.* (*Source:* Reproduced with permission from *Nutrition in Health and Disease,* 16th edition, by H. S. Mitchell, H. J. Rynbergen, L. Anderson, and M. V. Dibble. Copyright © 1976 by J. B. Lippincott Co., Philadelphia.)

TABLE 9.5 CRITERIA AND INTERPRETATION OF GLUCOSE TOLERANCE TESTS BY U.S. PUBLIC HEALTH SERVICE

	Whole blood	Serum or plasma	Points[1]
	mg glucose/100 ml		
Fasting	100	130	1.0
1 hour	170	195	0.5
2 hours	120	140	0.5
3 hours	110	130	1.0

Source: U.S. Public Health Service.
[1]Two or more points is definitely indicative of diabetes; one point is possibly indicative of diabetes.

there is an accumulation of galactose-l-phosphate and of phosphate in cells (**25**). The following schematic diagram shows the general metabolic scheme for galactose metabolism, including the defective site (Figure 9.3).

The result of the disease is progressive damage to the central nervous system, the liver, renal tubules, and the lens of the eye. Cataracts may develop, even in a fetus, because the lens can convert galactose to galactitol, and excessive amounts of galactose will be shunted via that pathway if there is a blockage in the normal pathway (**31**).

Galactosemia is suspected in infants with prolonged neonatal jaundice,

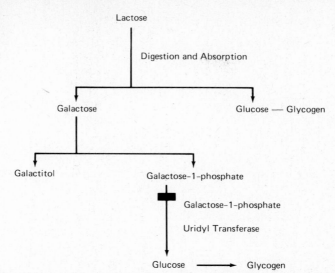

Figure 9.3 *General scheme for galactose metabolism and blockage of normal metabolism.*

cataracts, and nonglucose reducing substances in the urine (**26**). The disease is an autosomal recessive trait, thus siblings have a one in four risk of being affected. The usual tests for diagnosing the disease are measurements of blood and urine levels of galactose or the activity of the enzyme. A sample of cord blood at birth may be used for screening purposes.

Dietary control involves the rigorous exclusion of galactose from the diet, thus all milk and milk products must be avoided (**26**). The control aims at keeping urinary galactose levels below 10 mg per 100 ml and the level of galactose-l-phosphate in the red blood cell below 3 mg per 100 ml. Food plans for individuals with this disorder have been devised based on the diabetic exchange list.

Glycogen Storage Diseases

At least eight different abnormalities related to glycogen storage have been identified by nutritionists. Several different enzymes that are involved in glycogen synthesis and degradation may be deficient. The diseases may manifest themselves in a variety of clinical symptoms and in disorders of the liver, heart, muscle, and skeleton. For example, the liver and heart can be grossly enlarged, and there can be failure to grow. In some cases, the symptoms are similar to those associated with diabetes. In many cases, death occurs within two years (**26**).

Phenylketonuria

Phenylketonuria is a defect in normal phenylalanine metabolism as the result of the absence of phenylalanine hydroxylase (Figure 9.4). The defect occurs in approximately 1 per 10,000 births (**27**). In those individuals, phenylpyruvic acid accumulates in blood and tissues and is excreted in the urine. The buildup of

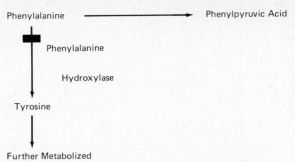

Figure 9.4 *Partial metabolic routes of phenylalanine and tyrosine.*

phenylpyruvic acid impairs normal brain development and causes severe mental retardation. Diagnosis and the initiation of treatment are necessary during the first few days of life. Most hospitals, accordingly, routinely screen newborn babies for phenylketonuria using the Guthrie test for blood levels of phenylalanine (**28**). All states except one use this test that has proved to be sensitive and reliable (**29**).

Treatment and control of phenylketonuria are difficult and critical. Phenylalanine is an essential amino acid and is necessary for normal growth and development of the infant and child. The intake of phenylalanine must be controlled closely during the early years of life and perhaps beyond (**30**). To do this, continual monitoring of blood levels is necessary to maintain a phenylalanine concentration between 2.0 and 8.0 mg per 100 ml. Diets must be planned and adjusted to allow as much phenylalanine as possible and still retain serum levels within acceptable ranges. A general guideline for intakes of phenylalanine ranges from 40 to 100 mg per kilogram body weight per day for infants and as low as 15 mg per kilogram per day for 6-year-old children. The following table (Table 9.6) showing average nutrient contents of food groups provides a useful guide in planning dietaries for phenylketonurics (**31**).

Foods with high protein contents must be avoided generally because of the high phenylalanine content. The child's protein needs can be met by feeding special formulas, though. The most common one is Lofenalac, a hydrolyzate of casein from which phenylalanine has been removed. The hydrolyzate is fortified with minerals, vitamins, carbohydrate, fat, and any amino acids destroyed in processing (**32**). The protein hydrolyzate is less well utilized than an intact protein, so an excess protein level is needed to maintain growth. Combinations of Lofenalac with added milk and mixtures of the formula with cow's milk are used to maintain the desired blood levels and to provide intake of phenylalanine (**33**).

Tyrosinemia

The inborn error, neonatal tyrosinemia, is present in from 1 to 3 percent of all newborn children. Nutritionists see two types of the disease (**34**). Type I is hereditary and is characterized by modular cirrhosis of the liver, defects in the renal tubules, and hypophosphatemic rickets. Most patients suffering this defi-

TABLE 9.6 AVERAGE NUTRIENT CONTENT OF SERVING LISTS FOR PHENYLALANINE-RESTRICTED DIETS

List	Phenylalanine (mg)	Protein (g)	Energy (kcal)
Vegetables, strained and junior	15	0.5	20
Table foods (adult)	15	0.5	10
Fruits, strained and junior	15	0.6	150
Table foods and juices (adult)	15	0.6	70
Bread and cereals	30	0.6	30
Fats	5	0.1	60

When analyses were not available, the phenylalanine content was calculated on the following basis:

Breads and cereals	Phenylalanine 5 percent of protein
Fat	Phenylalanine 5 percent of protein
Fruits	Phenylalanine 2.6 percent of protein
Vegetables	Phenylalanine 3.3 percent of protein

Source: Reproduced with permission from *Dietary Management of Inherited Metabolic Diseases,* by P. B. Acosta and L. J. Elsas (**31**). Copyright © 1976 by ACELU Publishers, Atlanta, Georgia.

ciency fail to respond to therapy. Type II or hypertyrosinemia, however, will improve with therapy. The basic impairment is the absence of either tyrosine amino transferase or parahydroxylphenylpyruvic acid oxidase (Figure 9.5). Tyrosine accumulates in the presence of a metabolic block.

Treatment is designed to restrict tyrosine and phenylalanine in the diet to maintain blood plasma levels of tyrosine in the range of 1.5−6.5 mg per 100 ml (**31**). Careful monitoring is then essential in the infant or until plasma tyrosine levels are stabilized. The guidelines for intakes of affected children are summarized in Table 9.7. A recent report recommends that treatment of type I in the acute phase should include restriction of methionine as well as phenylalanine and tyrosine (**35**). Monitoring of plasma levels of methionine is also recommended.

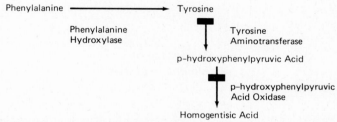

Figure 9.5 *Partial scheme of tyrosine metabolism showing metabolic defects involved in tyrosinemia.*

TABLE 9.7 RECOMMENDED PHENYLALANINE, TYROSINE,
PROTEIN, AND ENERGY INTAKE BY NORMAL AND TYROSINEMIC CHILDREN[1]

Age	Phenylalanine (mg/kg)	Tyrosine (mg/kg)	Protein (g/kg)	Energy kcal/kg
0−3 months				
Tyrosinemic	60−80	60−80	4.4	120
4−6 months				
Tyrosinemic	58−75	61−82	3.3	115
7−12 months				
Tyrosinemic	42	42	2.2	110
1−3 years				
Tyrosinemic	25−85	25−85	23 Total[2]	1300 Total
4−8 years				
Tyrosinemic	22−50	8−50	30 Total	1800 Total
9−10 years				
Tyrosinemic	25	25	36 Total	2400 Total
13−14 years				
Tyrosinemic	1026 Total	523 Total	44 Total	2400−2800 Total

Source: Reproduced with permission from *Dietary Management of Inherited Metabolic Diseases,* by P. B. Acosta and L. J. Elsas (**31**). Copyright © 1976 by ACELU Publishers, Atlanta, Georgia.
[1]Total phenylalanine and tyrosine must be considered.
[2]Total represents entire daily intake rather than amount per kg.

Homocystinuria

Homocystinuria is an inborn error involving several defects in methionine metabolism. The traditional defect is an impaired cystathionine synthase (Figure 9.6), but other problems in binding of cofactors, such as pyridoxal phosphate or methylcobalamine, may be the error (**36**).

Homocystine accumulates and leads to symptoms such as mental retardation, friable fair hair, and osteoporosis. The presence of homocystine in the plasma or urine is used as a diagnostic tool (**37**).

Treatment consists of the exclusion of excess methionine from the diet and the provision of cystine in a pure form. Other remedies include the additions of vitamin B_6, in an effort to improve the utilization of methionine, or supplementary vitamin B_{12}. When neither vitamin B_6 nor B_{12} is effective, the individual is placed on the methionine restricted diet (**37**).

General guidelines for the ranges of methionine in different classes of foods are as shown here:

	Percentage of Methionine in Protein
Vegetables	0.67−1.42
Fruits	0.62
Breads and cereals	1.33
Fats	2.00

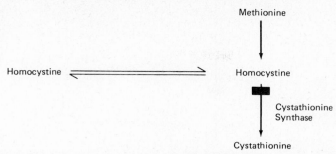

Methionine

Homocystine ⇌ Homocystine

Cystathionine
Synthase

Cystathionine

Figure 9.6 Partial metabolic pathway of methionine indicating the usual blockage or defect.

As with all other metabolic disorders, growth and development of the infant and child are major considerations, although dietary control is essential. Guidelines for intakes of critical nutrients to treat the defect are summarized in Table 9.8 (**31**). Special formulas are also available for control of methionine intake.

Maple Syrup Urine Disease

This inherited disorder of leucine, isoleucine, and valine metabolism is known also as branched chain alpha ketoaciduria (**38**). The disease occurs because of an impairment of branched chain alpha ketoacid dehydrogenase activity. The metabolic block is illustrated using leucine (Figure 9.7).

This disease, an autosomal recessive trait, is characterized by high concentrations of the branched chain amino acids in blood and urine, degeneration of the nerve function, and excretion of urine having the odor of burnt sugar (basis of the name). In the newborn infant, the disease manifests itself through poor sucking, irregular respiration, rigidity alternating with flaccidity, progressive loss of mors reflex, and seizures. Detection and treatment are essential during the

TABLE 9.8 SUGGESTED METHIONINE, PROTEIN, AND ENERGY FOR USE IN TREATMENT OF HOMOCYSTINURIA

Age (years)	Methionine (mg/kg)	Protein (g/kg)	Energy (kcal/kg)
0–0.5	42	2.00[1]/4.4[2]	120
0.6–1.0	20	1.50/2.5	110
1–3	10–23	1.25/25 Total[3]	1300 Total
4–6	10–18	1.00/30 Total	1800 Total
7–10	10–13	1.00/35 Total	2400 Total

Source: Reproduced with permission from *Dietary Management of Inherited Metabolic Diseases,* by P. B. Acosta and L. J. Elsas (**31**). Copyright © 1976 by ACELU Publishers, Atlanta, Georgia.
[1]Protein suggested is to be used when Isomil is used.
[2]Greater amounts of protein may be offered when Methionaid or 3200K is used.
[3]Total refers to entire daily intake rather than on a per kg basis.

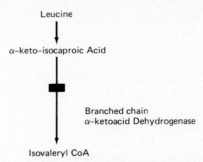

Figure 9.7 *Illustration of the metabolic block in Maple Syrup Urine Disease; similar defects occur for isoleucine and valine.*

first week of life, since those who survive without treatment show retardation in both physical and mental development (**39**).

This disease is treated through diets low in the branched chain amino acids. The guidelines for intakes are summarized in Table 9.9. Some patients are helped by high doses, 100 mg of thiamin per day, but the dietary control of the amino acids is also essential for recovery. Plasma concentrations of the amino acids between 2 and 5 mg per 100 ml serve as an index for monitoring the treatment (**31**).

Gout

Gout or tophic arthritis is an inborn error of purine metabolism and is characterized by an increased blood level of uric acid and the deposition of crystals in the joints and soft tissues. The fingers and toes are particularly susceptible to

TABLE 9.9   PROTEIN, ISOLEUCINE, LEUCINE, VALINE, AND ENERGY
RECOMMENDED FOR CHILDREN WITH BRANCHED CHAIN KETOACIDURIA

Age	Isoleucine	Leucine (mg/kg)	Valine	Protein (g/kg)	Energy (kcal/kg)
<3 months	70	161	93	2.2[1]/4.4[2]	120
3−6 months	70	161	93	2.2/3.3	115
6−9 months				2.0/2.5	110
9−11 months				2.0/2.5	105
1−3 years				25 Total[3]	1300 Total
4−6 years				30 Total	1800 Total
7−10 years	30	45	33	35 Total	2400 Total

Source: Reproduced with permission from *Dietary Management of Inherited Metabolic Diseases,* by P. B. Acosta and L. J. Elsas (**31**). Copyright © 1976 by ACELU Publishers, Atlanta, Georgia.
NOTE: There is no data available on amino acid needs for ages 7 months to about 10 years. Plasma levels of branched chain amino acids should be used to determine amounts to offer in the diet.
[1]Amounts to use with gelatin amino acid mix.
[2]Amounts to use with MSUDAid or pure amino acids.
[3]Total refers to entire daily intake rather than amount per kg.

crystal deposits. Children are affected occasionally, but most victims are males over 30 years of age. Gout rarely occurs in women.

An overproduction and/or an underexcretion of uric acid is the metabolic error. Gout is usually present when blood levels of uric acid exceed 6 mg per 100 ml in males and 5.5 mg per 100 ml in women. Normal levels of uric acid range from 2.5 to 5 mg per 100 ml of blood (**31**).

Familial Hyperlipoproteinemia

Primary familial hyperlipoproteinemia (HLP) is a heritable group of diseases characterized by increased concentrations of cholesterol and triglycerides in blood plasma (**40**). Hyperlipoproteinemias are usually defined in terms of plasma concentrations of cholesterol and triglycerides. An example of normal ranges of cholesterol and triglyceride concentrations, representing slightly over 500 subjects, is summarized in the following table (Table 9.10). Reliable data must be gathered for any particular group, and values obtained from normal persons are not necessarily indicative of good health. Cholesterol and triglyceride levels are useful in detecting hyperlipoproteinemia since over 95 percent of those with HLP have high blood levels of these lipids.

Most of the heritable HLPs are one of five types that are classified on quantitative terms, with the exception of type III (Table 9.11).

The basic metabolic defects are not known at this time, and the classification is based primarily on lipoprotein fractions of the plasma. Recognized differences do exist, however, that provide the basis for dietary treatment and control measures (**41**).

Type I or Lipase Deficient Hyperchylomicronemia. The basic problem involves the deficit in the removal of chylomicrons resulting from a depressed plasma lipoprotein lipase and lowered activity of the enzyme in tissues. The

---

TABLE 9.10 PLASMA LIPID
CONCENTRATIONS OF NORMAL SUBJECTS

| Age (years) | mg/100 ml[1] | |
	Cholesterol	Triglyceride
0–19	175 (120–230)	65 (10–140)
20–29	180 (120–240)	70 (10–140)
30–39	205 (140–270)	75 (10–150)
40–49	225 (150–310)	85 (10–160)
50–59	245 (160–330)	95 (10–190)

Source: Reprinted with permission from D. S. Frederickson and R. I. Levy in *The Metabolic Basis of Inherited Disease,* 4th edition, eds. J. B. Stanbury, J. B. Wyngaarden, and D. S. Frederickson (**40**). Copyright © 1978 by McGraw-Hill Book Co., New York.

[1]Values represent mean and 90 percent limits and are derived from 511 subjects (279 males; 237 females).

TABLE 9.11 ABNORMAL LIPOPROTEIN PATTERNS IN FAMILIAL HYPERLIPOPROTEINEMIA

Type	Definitive lipoprotein abnormalities[1]	Appearance of plasma[2]	Usual changes in lipid concentrations[3]
I.	1. Chylomicrons present and markedly increased 2. VLDL, LDL, HDL normal or decreased	Cream layer on top, clear below	C↑, TG↑ (C/TG < 0.2)
II.	1. LDL increased[4] 2. VLDL normal (Type IIa)[5]; or VLDL increased (Type IIb)[5]	Usually clear, may be slightly turbid	C↑, TG normal or ↑ (C/TG usually >1.5)
III.	1. Presence of β-VLDL ("floating beta," LDL of abnormal lipid composition)	Usually turbid, often with faint cream layer	C↑, TG↑ (C/TG variable, often = 1)
IV.	1. VLDL increased 2. Chylomicrons "absent" 3. LDL not increased	Usually turbid; no cream layer	C↑ or normal, TG↑ (C/TG variable)
V.	1. Chylomicrons present 2. VLDL increased	Cream layer on top, turbid below	C↑, TG↑ (C/TG usually >0.15 and <0.6)

Source: Reprinted with permission from D. S. Frederickson and R. I. Levy in *The Metabolic Basis of Inherited Disease*, 4th edition, eds. J. B. Stanbury, J. B. Wyngaarden, and D. S. Frederickson (**40**). Copyright © 1978 McGraw-Hill, New York. Used with permission of McGraw-Hill Book Company.
[1]VLDL, very low-density lipoproteins; LDL, low-density lipoproteins; HDL, high-density lipoproteins.
[2]After standing at 4° C for 18 hours or more.
[3]C, cholesterol; TG, triglycerides.
[4]"Increased" implies in excess of whatever cutoff limit is used.
[5]The classification scheme is as follows:
   Type IIa = VLDL normal
   Type IIb = VLDL ↑.

problem asserts itself as soon as the infant consumes fat. Symptoms include abdominal pain and xanthomas of an eruptive nature. The disorder is found in Caucasians, Chinese, and blacks but is the rarest of the HLP types.

Lipoprotein lipase is one of several lipases found in the body. The enzyme hydrolyzes the ester bonds of glycerides in the chylomicrons. The *chylomicrons* are a collection of triglycerides formed from fatty acids of 12 carbons or longer chain length. Chylomicrons move through lymph and enter the plasma through the thoracic duct.

Treatment consists of placing the patient on a restricted fat diet and using medium chain triglyceride sources that do not form chylomicrons (**41**). The plasma triglyceride levels may be up to 4000 mg per 100 ml and drop to about 300 mg per 100 ml on a nearly fat-free diet. Values of 1000–2000 mg per 100 ml are commonly present during treatment.

Type II or Familial Hyperbetalipoproteinemia. This abnormality is an inherited increase in the plasma concentration of low-density lipoproteins (LDL) or

β-lipoproteins, but the basic defect is not really known. There are actually two different phenotypes that differ in usual ranges of plasma levels of cholesterol, triglycerides, and low-density lipoproteins. Primary symptoms of the disease include the appearance of xanthomas, usually prior to 10 years of age, in areas such as the palms, knees, and buttocks (Figure 9.8). In addition, the incidence of ischemic heart disease is much higher in affected persons, particularly males. The malady may be described as primitive ischemic heart disease (**42**).

Dietary treatment is dependent primarily on diets high in polyunsaturated fat and low in saturated fats and cholesterol (**41**). The caloric guidelines are for from 8 to 15 percent of the total calories to be provided as unsaturated fat, much of this in the form of linoleic acid. Less than 5 percent of the total calories should come from saturated fat. Cholesterol intake should be less than 250 mg per day. Most patients respond to this regime, and plasma cholesterol concentrations decline 15 to 30 percent in two to five weeks. The usual pretreatment levels of cholesterol and triglycerides may range up to 600 mg and 500 mg per 100 ml plasma, respectively.

Type III or "Broad Beta" Disease.   This is an uncommon disorder usually not detected until maturity. The disease is characterized by the presence of very low-density lipoproteins (VLDL) with an abnormal composition in the plasma. LDLs contain a high level of glycerides. Individuals with the disorder have hypercholesterolemia and hypertriglyceridemia that vary with changes in body weight.

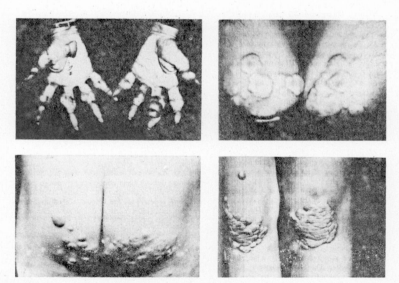

Figure 9.8 Xanthomas commonly observed in type II hypercholesterolemia. These examples are observed on palms, elbows, buttocks, and knees. (Source: Reproduced with permission from D. S. Frederickson and R. I. Levy in *The Metabolic Basis of Inherited Disease,* 3rd edition, eds. J. B. Stanbury, J. G. Wyngaarden, and D. S. Frederickson. Copyright © 1978 by McGraw-Hill Book Co., New York.)

Nutritionists usually see a good response to a dietary treatment aimed at weight reduction for the patient suffering from the disease. Fat and carbohydrate each provide approximately 40 percent of the total energy in this diet (**43**).

Type IV or Familial Hyperpre-β-Lipoproteinemia.   This is a disorder in which the body apparently has a limited capacity to remove VLDL from the plasma. The treatment is aimed at weight reduction and carbohydrate restriction (**44**).

Type V or Familial Hyperpre-β-Lipoproteinemia and Hyperchylomicro-nemia.   This type is similar to type IV. The excess of VLDL is associated with reduced clearance of dietary fat, and the problems become worse when the individual is obese. Children rarely are affected with this disease. Dietary treatment and control involve avoiding excess carbohydrate and fat (**45**).

CARDIAC DISEASE

Infants and young children may be afflicted with cardiac problems. Sometimes the problem is congenital in origin. Although the defect can often be corrected with surgery, the affected infant does present special problems until he or she is old enough for corrective surgery.

These infants frequently tire very easily and require more rest than do normal youngsters. During the feeding period, the mother or other attendant should be careful that the need to rest is not mistaken for normal relaxation after an adequate intake of milk. Otherwise, the child may not receive enough nourishment. Children afflicted with cardiac disease do not grow at a normal rate. In some cases, special formulas are used in which the caloric density is raised to about 100 kcal per 100 ml as compared to a usual density of about 65−70 kcal per 100 ml. Other nutrient supplements may be essential when the infant consumes a lower quantity of food.

HANDICAPPING CONDITIONS

Approximately 125,000 infants are born each year with handicaps or disabling diseases (**46**). The more common diseases are cerebral palsy, Down's syndrome, and paraplegia which result from injuries or defects. Almost all these infants present unique nutritional problems because of their difficulties in consuming adequate amounts of food from inherent handicaps in sucking, chewing, or swallowing food. A summary of feeding problems associated with various handicapping conditions is given in Table 9.12 (**2**).

Generally, infants with handicaps do not mature as rapidly as or to the full extent of the normal child. Deviations from normal growth and development appear most pronounced in children with Down's syndrome. Those with cerebral palsy and multiple congenital abnormalities are also underdeveloped (**47, 48**). Children with minimal brain damage and mental retardation, however, have the

TABLE 9.12 HANDICAPPING CONDITIONS AND FEEDING DISABILITIES

Handicapping conditions	Feeding Disabilities				
	Inability to suck, close lips	Inability to bite, chew, swallow	Poor grasp	Poor hand-mouth coordination	Poor trunk and upper extremities control
Cerebral vascular accident					
With facial paralysis	+	+		+	
With hemiplegia on dominant side	+	+	+	+	+
Cerebal palsy					
Athetoid type	+	+	+	+	+
Ataxic type		+ −		+	+
Spastic type				+ −	+
Traumatic spinal cord Injury					
Paraplegia					
Quadraplegia			+	+	+
Muscular dystrophy					
Duchenne's			+	+	+
Fascio-scapular-humeral	+ +	+	+	+	+
Multiple sclerosis	+	+	+	+	+
Parkinson's Disease	+	+	+	+	+
Myasthenia gravis			+	+	+
Rheumatoid arthritis			+	+	+ −
Severe and profound Mental Retardation	+	+	+	+	+

Source: Reprinted with permission from *Nutrition in Health and Disease,* 16th edition, by H. S. Mitchell, H. J. Rynbergen, L. Anderson, and M. V. Dibble (**2**). Copyright © 1976 by J. B. Lippincott Co. Philadelphia.
  +Moderate
  + +Severe.
  + −Varies.

potential to achieve normal physical development. The most frequent nutritional problems, aside from general development, are underweight or obesity. In most cases, the basic cause of the abnormal weight can be traced to activity levels, both excessive and insufficient, poor personal relationships with the guardian or mother, and inappropriate care (**49**).

Treatment must be on an individual basis, with the goal of achieving adequate nutrient intake in spite of the handicapping condition. This means devising methods and approaches to improve food intake, conquering the obstacles to physical coordination, and appropriate control of both exercise and food intake (**50**). Health professionals have developed strategies for improving and developing the feeding skills of the handicapped child (Table 9.13).

TABLE 9.13 SUGGESTED STRATEGIES FOR DEVELOPING FEEDING SKILLS

Areas of concern

1. Inability to suck, chew and swallow

   Suck: —Use cold substances around lips to stimulate sucking
   —Use a cloth soaked with water for the child to suck
   —Try different types of nipples
   —As child begins to improve in ability, change to nipple with smaller holes

   Chew: —Place a small amount of food between back teeth and move jaw up and down. A mirror may help demonstrate and point out various body parts
   —Wash with tongue—place foods such as peanut butter on lips to allow tongue to be used. Gradual change from pureed foods to solid foods (sprinkle crackers in soup, etc.)

   Swallow (swallowing easiest when mouth closed):
   —Close jaw and lips of child together
   —Stroke throat upward under chin
   —Offer next bite of food only after child swallows
   —Demonstrate—let child feel you swallow

2. Inability to grasp; hand-mouth coordination

   (i) To assist grasping coordination:
   —Allow child to finger food
   —Guide child in exploring mouth
   —Cut food into small pieces
   —Place your hand over child's hand and help him or her grasp spoon
   —Use adaptive equipment (plastic spoon, etc.)
   —Make sure bowl is stabilized (suction, tape)
   —Use plates with high straight sides or build higher edge using aluminum foil

   (ii) Develop activities that will help child with coordination:
   —Pour sand, and the like
   —Play with ball
   —Push-pull objects
   —Study body parts with child

   (iii) Visually impaired:
   —Place meats and vegetables consistently in same area of plate so that child can find

3. Caloric problems: overweight/underweight
   Obtain medical examination and evaluate growth
   Provide variety of foods

   Overweight: —Cut down snacks and high-caloric foods
   —Refrain from rewarding with food
   —Increase exercise and leisure-time activities

   Underweight: —Increase number of meals per day
   —Include high-caloric foods, especially liquid supplements
   —Proper exercise is important

TABLE 9.13   *(Continued)*

Areas of concern

4. Lack of nutrition education: work with families
   - Stress importance of proper nutrition for all family members
   - Teach proper feeding environment (good eating habits, eating positions)
   - Provide nutrition instruction materials

Source: Reprinted with permission from S. Calvert and F. Davies, *Dietetic Currents* 4:(3) May/June, 1977 (**50**). Copyright © 1977 by Ross Laboratories, Columbus, Ohio.

HYPERBILIRUBINEMIA

The levels of bilirubin in the newborn infant are usually much higher than in the older child and adult. Bilirubin is produced at rates two or three times higher in infants than in adults when differences in weight are considered. These high levels of bilirubin increase the risk of damage to cells and the central nervous system of the child (**51**). For many years the problem in young infants was treated by exchange transfusion or changing of the blood. Many infants, however, are now treated by phototherapy or by placing the infant in light. The infant may be undressed to expose more of the body to the light source, but the child's eyes should be protected. This procedure, discovered almost by accident, brings about a reduction in the bilirubin levels and a disappearance of the jaundice or yellow color of the skin, present because of the high levels of bilirubin (**51**).

SUMMARY

A small percentage of children are born with metabolic and/or physical difficulties which have serious implications for their future normal growth and development. Many of these problems are treated in part through dietary modifications and controls. The long-range goal of any dietary treatment is to maintain normal development in the child, at least as far as is possible. Physiological and psychological support for both the infant and family are of prime importance. The long-term effect on growth and development of the child will depend to a large extent on the age at which the feeding problem occurred and the length of the period of nutrient deprivation.

Several malabsorption syndromes have their onset during infancy and affect digestion, absorption, and/or transport of food components. Dietary modifications are necessary to *relieve* some of the symptoms associated with these disorders. These disorders include cystic fibrosis, sucrase-isomaltase deficiency, glucose-galactose malabsorption, celiac sprue, and lactose intolerance.

Foods such as milk, eggs, wheat, fish, strawberries, chocolate, and others are commonly involved in allergic reactions in some people. Food allergies can influence the general health and nutritional status of an individual. Children, particularly, are susceptible, and normal growth and development may be seriously affected.

Numerous inborn errors of metabolism affect growth, development, and the general health of infants and children. These include diabetes, phenylketonuria, tyrosinemia, and the hyperlipoproteinemias. These conditions are all characterized by some defect in nutrient metabolism and the accumulation of the nutrient or an abnormal metabolite in the system. Diagnosis and initiation of treatment is necessary during the first few days of life. Carbohydrate, protein, amino acid, and/or lipid metabolism can be a problem in these disorders. Dietary treatment is, therefore, aimed at controlling the intake of the specific nutrient affected to maintain levels in the system in a safe range and/or to reduce the possibility of accumulation of undesirable metabolites of these nutrients in the system. Special formulas have been developed for use with infants and children suffering from certain inborn errors of metabolism.

Approximately 125,000 infants are born in the United States each year who are classified as developmentally delayed. These children present unique nutritional problems. They may not mature as rapidly as or to the full extent of the normal child. Deviations from normal growth and development appear most pronounced in children with Down's syndrome. Those with cerebral palsy and multiple congenital abnormalities are also underdeveloped. In addition to abnormal growth patterns that affect nutrient requirements, many of these children exhibit feeding disabilities that affect nutrient intake. These include the inability to suck, bite, chew, or swallow, poor grasp, and poor hand-to-mouth coordination. Treatment of these children must be on an individual basis, and innovative approaches to improve and develop the feeding skills of these children must be developed. As in other areas of nutrition, there is a need for more research on the specific nutritional needs of the developmentally delayed child.

STUDY QUESTIONS AND
TOPICS FOR INDIVIDUAL INVESTIGATION

1. Special formulas have been developed for use with infants who suffer from certain metabolic disorders. Visit a supermarket in your area. What formulas are available for infants and children with special dietary needs? Discuss the economic aspects of using these special formula diets.
2. Choose one inborn error of metabolism, for example, phenylketonuria, tyrosinemia, Maple Syrup Urine Disease, HLP, and so on. What is the basic metabolic defect involved? What modifications in dietary intake would need to be made to treat the disorder successfully?
3. There may be several handicapped children in your local school district. If possible try to locate several handicapped children. Develop a questionnaire that would allow you to evaluate these children's nutritional health. What is the average height, weight? Does growth compare favorably with that of classmates or growth charts for this age group? Do a food history or 24-hour recall of food intake for the handicapped children. How does the nutrient intake of these children compare with that of their classmates or recommended dietary intakes for this age group?
4. This chapter has pointed out several physical difficulties related to feeding the handicapped child. If possible, try to talk with the mother of a handicapped child and find out what special feeding problems her child has. How has this woman tried to help her child improve or develop feeding skills? What resources in the community has she been able to turn to for help? Does she see a need for additional research and/or aid to parents in the area of nutritional needs of the handicapped child?
5. Home preparation of breads, cakes, cookies, and pastry is often necessary to eliminate wheat, eggs, or milk from the diets of children who are allergic to one or more of these foods. If you know a family that has a child with a food allergy ask what foods have they eliminated from the child's diet? Is it difficult to meet the special dietary needs with many of the foods available in the local supermarket? Does the family do much home preparation of foods to satisfy the needs of the individual with the food allergy? What sources does the family use for nutrition information and help in food preparation for this special diet?

REFERENCES

1. Food and Nutrition Board. *Recommended Dietary Allowances,* 9th ed. National Academy of Sciences, Washington, D.C., 1979.
2. Mitchell, H. S., H. J. Rynborgen, L. Anderson, and M. V. Dibble. *Nutrition in Health and Disease,* 16th ed. Lippincott, Philadelphia, 1976.

3. Vaughan, V. C., R. J. McKay, and W. E. Nelson. *Textbook of Pediatrics,* 10th ed. Saunders, Philadelphia, 1975.

4. di Sant' Agnose, P. A. The pancreas. In: *Textbook of Pediatrics,* 10th ed., eds. V. C. Vaughan, R. J. McKay, and W. E. Nelson. Saunders, Philadelphia, 1975.

5. Berry, H. K., F. W. Kellogg, and M. M. Hunt. Dietary supplement and nutrition in children with cystic fibrosis. *American Journal of the Diseases of Children,* 129:165, 1975.

6. Partin, J. C., J. S. Partin, and W. K. Schubert. Micronodular cirrhosis in β-lipoproteinemia: possible exacerbation by medium chain triglycerides (MCT) feeding. *Pediatric Research.* (Abstract), 8:384, 1974.

7. Donaldson, R. M., Jr., and J. D. Gryboski. Carbohydrate intolerance. In: *Gastrointestinal Disease—Pathophysiology-Diagnosis-Management,* eds. M. H. Sleisenger and J. S. Fordtran. Saunders, Philadelphia, 1973.

8. Sleisenger, M. H., and J. S. Fordtran, eds. *Gastrointestinal Disease— Pathophysiology-Diagnosis-Management.* Saunders, Philadelphia, 1973.

9. Goodhart, R. S., and M. E. Shils, eds., *Modern Nutrition in Health and Disease,* 5th ed. Lea & Febiger, Philadelphia, 1973.

10. Dahlquist, A. Specificity of the human intestinal disaccharidases and implications for hereditary disaccharide intolerance. *Journal of Clinical Investigation,* 41:463, 1962.

11. Bayless, T. M., and N. L. Christopher. Disaccharidase deficiency. *American Journal of Clinical Nutrition,* 22:181, 1969.

12. Gilat, T., R. Kuhn, E. Gelman, and O. Mizrahy. Lactose deficiency in Jewish communities in Israel. *American Journal of Digestive Diseases,* 15:895, 1970.

13. Bayless, T. M., and N. S. Rosenswieg. A racial difference in incidence of lactase deficiency. *Journal of the American Medical Association,* 197:968, 1966.

14. Littman, A., and J. B. Hammond. Diarrhea in adults caused by deficiency in intestinal disaccharidases. *Gastroenterology,* 48:237, 1965.

15. Holzel, A., V. Schwartz, and K. W. Sutcliffe. Defective lactose absorption causing malnutrition in infancy. *Lancet,* 1:1126, 1969.

16. Haemmerli, U. P., and H. Kistler. Disaccharide malabsorption. Disease-a-month. Year Book Medical Publishers, Chicago, 1966.

17. Huang, S. S., and T. M. Bayless. Lactose intolerance in healthy children. *New England Journal of Medicine,* 276:1283, 1967.

18. Stephenson, L. C., and M. C. Latham. Lactose intolerance and milk consumption. The reaction of tolerance to symptoms. *American Journal of Clinical Nutrition,* 27:296, 1974.

19. Protein Advisory Group. Milk Intolerance—Nutritional Implications. United Nations System, Document 1, 27/9, 1972.

20. Fontana, V. J., and M. B. Strauss. Allergy and diet. In: *Modern Nutrition in Health and Disease,* 5th ed., eds. R. S. Goodhart and M. E. Shils. Lea & Febiger, Philadelphia, 1973.

21. Robinson, C. H., and M. R. Lawler. *Normal and Therapeutic Nutrition,* 15th ed. Macmillan, New York, 1977.

22. Visakorpi, J. K., and P. Immonen. Intolerance to cow's milk and wheat gluten in the primary malabsorption syndrome in infancy. *Acta Paediatrics Scandinavica,* 56:49, 1967.

23. Tattersall, R. B., and S. Fajans. A difference between the inheritance of classical juvenile onset and maturity onset type diabetes of young people. *Diabetes,* 24:44, 1975.

24. Tepperman, J. *Metabolic and Endocrine Physiology,* 3rd ed. Year Book Medical Publishers, Chicago, 1973.

25. Segal, S. Disorders of Galactose Metabolism. In: *Metabolic Basis of Inherited Disease,* 4th ed., eds. J. B. Stanbury, J. B. Wyngaarden, and D. S. Frederickson. McGraw-Hill, New York, 1978.

26. Wong, P. W., and R. Y. Hsia. Inborn Errors of Metabolism. In: *Modern Nutrition in Health and Disease,* 5th ed., eds. R. S. Goodhart and M. E. Shils. Lea & Febiger, Philadelphia, 1973.

27. Guthrie, R., and S. Whitney. Phenylketonuria detection in the newborn infant as a routine hospital procedure. Children's Bureau Publication No. 419, Washington D.C., 1964.

28. Menkes, J. H. Metabolic diseases of the nervous system. In: *Pediatrics,* ed. J. Brennerman. Harper & Row, New York, 1971.

29. Mammes, P. Newborn screening for metabolic disorders. *Clinics in Perinatology,* 3:231, 1976.

30. Acosta, P. B., G. E. Schaeffler, E. Wenz, and R. Koch. PKU—a guide to management. California State Department of Public Health, Berkeley, 1972.

31. Acosta, P. B., and L. J. Elsas. Dietary management of inherited metabolic diseases: phenylketonuria, galactosemia, tyrosinemia, homocystinuria, Maple Syrup Urine Disease. Emory University School of Medicine, Atlanta, Ga., 1976.

32. Wenz, E. A comparison of Lofenalac, Albumaid and Aminogram. Report of the 4th Nutrition Conference, Stateline, Nev., 1972.

33. Acosta, P. B., E. Wenz, and M. Williamson. Methods of dietary inception in infants with PKU. *Journal of the American Dietetic Association,* 72:164, 1978.

34. Buist, N. R. M., N. G. Kennaway, and J. H. Fellman. Disorders of tyrosine metabolism. In: *Heritable Disorders of Amino Acid Metabolism,* ed. W. L. Nyham. Wiley, New York, 1974.

35. Michals, K., R. Matalon, and P. W. K. Wong. Dietary treatment of tyrosinemia type I. *Journal of the American Dietetic Association,* 73:507, 1978.

36. Levy, H. L., S. H. Mudd, J. D. Schulman, P. M. Dreyfus, and R. H. Abeles. A derangement in B_{12} metabolism associated with homocystinemia, aptathioniemia and methylmalonic aciduria. *American Journal of Medicine,* 48:390, 1970.

37. Perry, T. L. Homocystinuria. In: *Heritable Disorders of Amino Acid Metabolism,* ed. W. L. Nyham. Wiley, New York, 1974.

38. Westall, R. G., J. Dancis, and S. Miller. Maple Syrup Urine Disease—a new molecular disease. *American Journal of Diseases of Children,* 94:571, 1957.

39. Snyderman, S. E. Maple Syrup Urine Disease. In: *Heritable Disorders of*

Amino Acid Metabolism, ed. W. L. Nyham. Wiley, New York, 1974.

40. Frederickson, D. S., and R. I. Levy. Familial hyperlipoproteinemia. In: *The Metabolic Bases of Inherited Disease,* 4th ed., eds. J. B. Stanbury, J. G. Wyngaarden, and D. S. Frederickson. McGraw-Hill, New York, 1978.

41. Khachadurian, A. K. Hyperlipoproteinemia. *Dietetic Currents* (Ross Laboratories, Columbus, Ohio), 4:19, 1977.

42. Slack, J. Risks of ischaemic heart disease in familial hyperlipoproteinaemic states. *Lancet,* 2:1380, 1969.

43. Levy, R. I., and N. Ernst. Diet, Hyperlipidemia and Atherosclerosis. In: *Heritable Disorders of Amino Acid Metabolism,* ed. W. L. Nyham. Wiley, New York, 1974.

44. Antonis, A., and I. Bersohn. The influence of diet on serum triglycerides. *Lancet,* 1:3, 1961.

45. Fernandes, J., and N. A. Pikaar. Hyperlipidemia in children with liver glycogen disease. *American Journal of Clinical Nutrition,* 22:617, 1969.

46. President's Committee on Mental Retardation. Mental Retardation—The Known and Unknown. U.S. Government Printing Office, Washington, D.C., 1976.

47. Pryor, H., and H. Thelander. Growth deviations in handicapped children. *Clinical Pediatrics,* 6:501, 1967.

48. Mosier, H., H. Grossman, and H. Dingman. Physical growth in mental defectives. *Pediatrics,* 36:465, 1965.

49. Hammar, S., and K. Bernard. Mentally retarded adolescents: review of characteristics and problems of 44, noninstitutionalized retardates. *Pediatrics,* 38:845, 1966.

50. Calvert, S., and F. Davies. Nutrition of children with handicapping conditions. *Dietetic Currents* (Ross Laboratories, Columbus, Ohio), 4:13, 1977.

51. Seligman, J. W. Recent and changing concepts of hyperbilirubinemia and its management in the newborn. *Pediatric Clinics of North America,* 24:509, 1977.

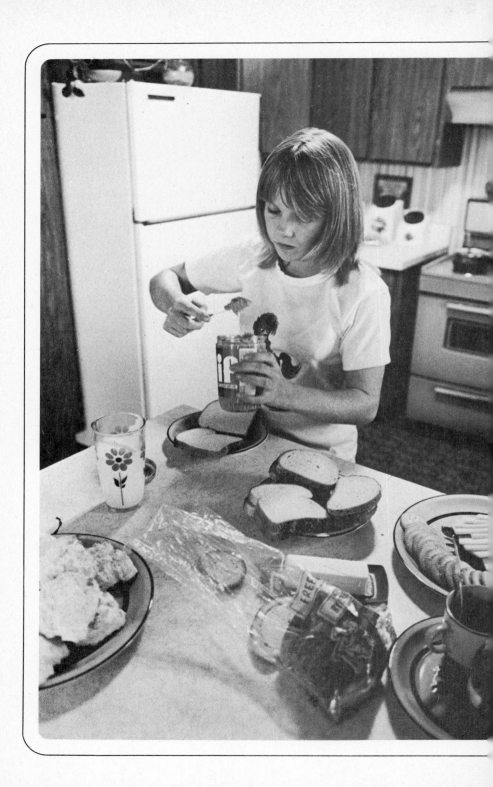

CHAPTER 10

NUTRITION DURING CHILDHOOD AND ADOLESCENCE

The period from early childhood or weaning to maturity is a highly critical time in the growth and development of the youngster. The child's diet during these growing years can affect the whole pattern of life. During the period from late infancy to maturity, the child is exposed to tremendous stresses that affect individual growth and development. The youngster experiences a period of transition from a diet composed almost exclusively of milk or formula to one composed of the wide variety of foods consumed in the adult diet.

In many parts of the world the child may be exposed to poor nutrition, parasites, infection, and inadequate health care during these critical years. In those areas of the world, children often develop deficiency diseases such as kwashiorkor, marasmus, blindness, goiter, beri-beri, and other nutrition-related maladies following weaning. In such developing countries, most deaths occur during the ages of 1−4 years (1). Thousands of youngsters die each year as a result of malnutrition, and hundreds of thousands fail to attain their full physical and mental capacity because of this problem.

Even in affluent nations children often do not achieve their full physical and mental potential because of inadequate nutrient intake in early childhood. As the youngster's diet more and more reflects the influence of family food habits and customs, sufficient attention may not be given to the specific nutrient needs of the actively growing child. Nutrition needs for growth may not be met and problems can result. In developed countries such problems will most likely be subclinical in nature and may go undetected, but the long-term health of these children may well be affected. They may fail to achieve in school and may not perform as well in other childhood activities. One wonders often how much human potential has been lost because of marginal nutrition during these critical years of growth and development.

GROWTH PATTERNS DURING CHILDHOOD

Growth during the childhood years is not a steady process and occurs in periods of tremendous spurts followed by periods of relative inactivity. Human growth occurs in three distinct stages: (1) infantile growth, characterized by initial rapid growth which then slows but continues until approximately age 4; (2) juvenile or childhood growth, in which the growth rate is relatively constant and slow, covering the period from about 4 years of age to the time of puberty; and (3) adolescent growth, with an initial rapid growth phase at puberty which diminishes until maturity (**2**).

The rapid weight gain, characteristic of the immediate postnatal months, decreases to an average of 2−3 kg per year during the mid-childhood years, with little difference between the sexes until girls enter their adolescent spurt. Boys begin this rapid growth time about two years later. The growth changes during adolescence are striking. Body weight nearly doubles during the adolescent growth spurt, and the child adds approximately 15 percent of his or her adult height. At peak velocity the average adolescent girl gains 8.3 kg in weight and 8.3 cm in height per year. Corresponding values for adolescent boys are a mean peak velocity of 9.0 kg and 9.4 cm per year (**3**). Females begin their adolescent growth spurt between the tenth and twelfth years. The mean male growth spurt begins 1½−2 years later, with maximum growth occurring usually somewhere between the fourteenth and fifteenth years. Females attain their ultimate height by ages 16−18, three years ahead of the male. Males are taller than females on the average because they enter adolescence later, thus gaining 5−6 cm in these two extra years of normal growth. They also grow more than girls during the actual growth spurt.

Some changes in body composition during growth provide information about the accumulation of nutrients and serve as a basis for estimating the child's nutritional needs at this time. Macy and Kelly (**4**) provide, through their classic research, data on the chemical composition of the body during growth. During the years from 4 to 12, or until puberty, the percentage of water, fat, and lean body mass does not change, but the increase in body size can provide an idea of the amount of fat, protein, and fluids being accumulated.

Studies of body composition changes during adolescence reveal distinct differences between the sexes. In general, males deposit proportionately more lean body tissue and skeletal mass, whereas females deposit proportionately more fat. Fat deposition in males does increase during adolescence, but it is modest and at 180 cm of height fat mass in the male averages 9 kg (**3**). Girls deposit proportionately more fat tissue and at 180 cm in height average 20 kg of adipose tissue (**3**).

NUTRITIONAL NEEDS DURING GROWTH

Since nutritional needs are usually related to body size, the requirements for nutrients per unit of body size are greater during periods of rapid growth. Growth charts (Figures 6.9–6.16) are a good index of the periods of rapid growth, although each individual child will have a different growth curve.

The Recommended Dietary Allowances (**5**) for nutrients is the guide referred to most frequently when information is needed about general nutritional needs. The recommended allowances for the growing period are summarized in Table 10.1. Certain considerations are important to understanding the basis of the allowances and to knowing how to meet the nutritional needs of growing children. These considerations are the basis of the following section.

From the standpoint of nutrition, important features are associated with the growth pattern from early childhood through adolescence. The growth pattern, which is characterized by periods of relatively stable growth as well as growth spurts, affects individual nutrient requirements at any specific age in the developing child. The magnitude of the growth spurt differs between the sexes as does age of onset and duration. Too, nutritional status throughout childhood may affect the initiation of adolescence through its effect on childhood growth. A failure to meet nutrient needs at the time of adolescence may adversely influence subsequent growth and result in a smaller size at maturity.

The child's nutritional requirements increase in relation to rapid growth and tissue deposition. The human grows more rapidly during adolescence than at any other time except during the first year of life; yet little information is available on the role of nutrition during this phase of development. Information on the nutritional needs of adolescents and RDAs are derived largely from dietary histories and nutritional surveys or by extrapolation from the nutrient requirements of other age groups. Adolescence is a nutritionally vulnerable period, and nutritious food practices must be maintained throughout adolescence for several reasons. These include the fact that the body is still growing and forming, that the emotional stress associated with maturing may affect nutrient absorption and utilization, and that good food practices developed in childhood and adolescence will be carried over into a healthful adulthood (**6**). Because of the lack of research that has been done on this age group studies need to be conducted to determine the specific nutrient requirements of adolescents. In 1980, the FNB published the following revised guidelines for nutrient requirements throughout childhood and adolescence.

Energy

The total energy needs of the growing child are the sum of energy used for basal metabolism, activity, losses in excreta and specific dynamic action, and the amount of energy deposited in new tissue. Based on unit of weight, these total energy needs decline throughout growth. The recommended allowance declines

TABLE 10.1 RECOMMENDED DAILY ALLOWANCES FOR KEY NUTRIENTS FROM INFANCY TO MATURITY

	Children (Ages)			Males (Ages)			Females (Ages)		
	1–3	4–6	7–10	11–14	15–18	19–22	11–14	15–18	19–22
Weight (kg)	13	20	28	45	66	70	46	55	55
(lb)	29	44	62	99	145	154	101	120	120
Height (cm)	90	112	132	157	176	177	157	163	163
(in.)	35	44	52	62	69	70	62	64	64
Energy (with	1300	1700	2400	2700	2800	2900	2200	2100	2100
range [kcal])[1]	(900–1800)	(1300–2300)	(1650–3300)	(2000–3100)	(2100–3900)	(2500–3300)	(1500–3000)	(1200–3000)	(1700–2500)
(MJ)	5.5	7.1	10.1	11.3	11.8	12.2	9.2	8.8	8.8
Protein (g)	23	30	34	45	56	56	46	46	44
Vitamin A (mcg R.E.)[2]	400	500	700	1000	1000	1000	800	800	800
Vitamin D (mcg)[3]	10	10	10	10	10	7.5	10	10	7.5
Vitamin E (mg αT.E.)[4]	5	6	7	8	10	10	8	8	8
Ascorbic acid (mg)	45	45	45	50	60	60	50	60	60
Folacin (mcg)	100	200	300	400	400	400	400	400	400

Niacin (mg N.E.)[5]	9	11	16	18	18	19	15	14	14
Riboflavin (mg)	0.8	1.0	1.4	1.6	1.7	1.7	1.3	1.3	1.3
Thiamin (mg)	0.7	0.9	1.2	1.4	1.4	1.5	1.1	1.1	1.1
Vitamin B$_6$ (mg)	0.9	1.3	1.6	1.8	2.0	2.2	1.8	2.0	2.0
Vitamin B$_{12}$ (mcg)	2.0	2.5	3.0	3.0	3.0	3.0	3.0	3.0	3.0
Calcium (mg)	800	800	800	1200	1200	800	1200	1200	800
Phosphorus (mg)	800	800	800	1200	1200	800	1200	1200	800
Iodine (mcg)	70	90	120	150	150	150	150	150	150
Iron (mg)	15	10	10	18	18	10	18	18	18
Magnesium (mg)	150	200	250	350	400	350	300	300	300
Zinc (mg)	10	10	15	15	15	15	15	15	15

Source: From Food and Nutrition Board, *Recommended Dietary Allowances*, 9th edition. National Academy of Sciences, Washington, 1980 (**5**).

[1] Energy allowances for children through age 18 are based on median energy intakes of children followed in longitudinal growth studies. The values in parentheses are tenth and ninetieth percentiles of energy intake to indicate the range of energy consumption among children of these ages.

[2] 1 R.E. = 1 mcg retinol or 6 mcg β carotene.

[3] As cholecalciferol. 10 mcg cholecalciferol = 400 IU vitamin D.

[4] α tocopherol equivalents. 1 mg D-α-tocopherol = 1 αT.E.

[5] 1 N.E. (niacin equivalent) = 1 mg niacin or 60 mg dietary tryptophan.

from approximately 115 kcal per kilogram of body weight at birth, to 105 kcal per kilogram at 1 year of age, to 88 kcal per kilogram at 10 years, and to about 60 and 48 kcal per kilogram for the adolescent male and female, respectively (**5**). The total energy needs, however, generally increase with age because of the increasing body size (Table 10.1).

The energy content of foods is calculated using the well-known Atwater energy conversion factors based on food composition. Recently, the joule, a measure of energy used in movement, has begun to appear in nutrition literature. The following (Table 10.2) provides a comparison and a basis for conversion.

The following examines briefly the various components of total energy needs during growth.

Basal metabolism, a major component of energy requirements throughout life, is highest during the first year or two of life, decreases in early childhood, increases again slightly at puberty, and then decreases throughout the remainder of life (Figure 10.1). Although basal metabolism is usually expressed in terms of surface area to indicate the loss of heat or energy, the formulas for surface area are based on height and weight. Thus expressions of basal metabolism may be on the basis of body weight. Table 10.3 contains the standard used as a source of information on basal metabolic rates or energy used daily for basal purposes.

Energy used for activity is a major variable in predicting the energy needs for children and adolescents. These expenditures of energy vary widely among different children, thus children's individual needs must be acknowledged. General expenditures of energy are illustrated for growing boys in Figure 10.2 and for girls in Figure 10.3.

Losses of energy through excretion and specific dynamic action are fairly constant. Approximately 8–10 percent of the intake is excreted, although the nature of the diet obviously will make a difference. Persons consuming a mixed diet will lose about 6 percent of the energy consumed through the specific dynamic effect of foods. This loss represents heat expended from food consump-

TABLE 10.2   ENERGY EXPRESSED IN KILOCALORIES AND JOULES FOR FOOD COMPONENTS AND ALCOHOL

Source	Kcal[1]/g	KJ[2]/g
Carbohydrate	4	17
Protein	4	17
Fat	9	38
Alcohol	7	30

[1]Kilocalorie—amount of heat necessary to raise 1 kg of water from 15 to 16° C; 1 kcal = 4184 J.
[2]Kilojoule—energy used when 1 kg is moved 1 meter (m) by 1 newton (n); kilojoule = kilocalorie × 4.2.

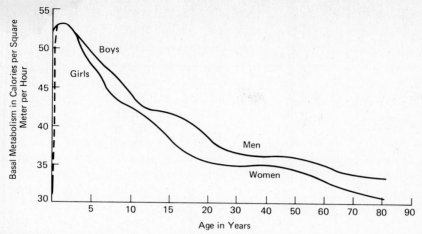

Figure 10.1 Effect of age on basal metabolism. A graphic representation of the Fleisch standards for the basal metabolic rate in humans. (*Source:* Reproduced with permission from *Comparative Nutrition of Man and Domestic Animals,* Vol. 1, by H. H. Mitchell. Copyright © 1962 by Academic Press, New York.)

TABLE 10.3 BASAL METABOLIC RATES ACCORDING TO WEIGHT AND SEX

Body weight (kg)	Kcal per 24 Hours	
	Males	Females
3.0	150	136
4.0	210	205
5.0	270	274
6.0	330	336
7.0	390	395
8.0	445	448
9.0	495	496
10.0	545	541
11.0	590	582
12.0	625	620
13.0	665	655
14.0	700	687
15.0	725	718
16.0	750	747
17.0	780	775
18.0	810	802
19.0	840	827
20.0	870	852
22.0	910	898
24.0	980	942
26.0	1070	984
28.0	1100	1025
30.0	1140	1063

(Continued)

TABLE 10.3	(Continued)	
Body weight (kg)	Kcal per 24 Hours	
	Males	Females
32.0	1190	1101
34.0	1230	1137
36.0	1270	1173
38.0	1305	1207
40.0	1340	1241
42.0	1370	1274
44.0	1400	1306
46.0	1430	1338
48.0	1460	1369
50.0	1485	1399
52.0	1505	1429
54.0	1555	1458
56.0	1580	1487
58.0	1600	1516
60.0	1630	1544
62.0	1660	1572
64.0	1690	1599
66.0	1725	1626
68.0	1765	1653
70.0	1785	1679
72.0	1815	1705
74.0	1845	1731
76.0	1870	1756
78.0	1900	1781
80.0	—	1805
82.0	—	1830
84.0	2000	1855

Source: Reprinted from FAO/WHO *Energy and Protein Requirements,* World Health Organization Technical Report Series No. 522, 1973 (**7**).

tion and is energy, measured as heat, that is not available for use by the body.

Energy needs for growth alone, or for the building of new tissues, are variable because of the dynamic process of growth and represent energy storage in the body. General guides indicate that early in life, growth accounts for about 20–40 kcal of energy stored per kilogram of body weight. At the age of approximately 1 year, growth represents between 5 and 15 kcal per kilogram per day. A general decline follows throughout the years of growth and development, except during the adolescent growth period when energy stores increase (**8**).

Figures 10.2 and 10.3 reveal the changes in total energy needs of growing males and females. These figures also indicate approximate distribution of energy

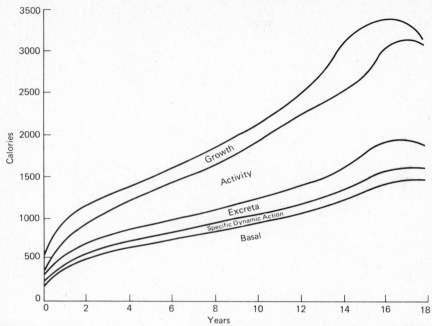

Figure 10.2 *Average total energy uses of boys of average size. (Source:* Reproduced with permission from *Diseases of Infancy and Childhood,* 11th edition, by E. L. Holt, Jr., and R. McIntosh. Copyright © 1941 by Appleton-Century-Crofts, Inc., New York.)

for basal metabolism, losses of energy in excreta, and specific dynamic action; uses of energy for activity; and deposition of energy as growth. Total energy needs or intakes are suggested in such guidelines as the recommended allowances (Table 10.1) and by the FAO/WHO (Table 10.4).

Providing adequate energy intakes for children in a nutritionally desirable manner may pose a difficult problem for parents and health professionals. Active, growing children and teenagers consume large amounts of food to meet their energy needs. Therefore, reasonable guidelines to follow would be the consumption of a variety of foods and avoidance of empty calorie foods or those that may provide energy but are low in essential nutrients. As mentioned before, the establishment of sound eating practices is necessary early in the life of the growing child (see Chapter 6).

Protein and Amino Acids

Adequate intakes of total protein and the essential amino acids are obviously essential for normal growth and development. The growth allowance for protein has been calculated from growth rates and body composition and then adjusted for efficiency of protein utilization. An estimation of net protein needs, or the amount of protein that should be retained, is summarized in Table 10.5. The growth increment, or the amount of protein needed for growth alone, is a relatively small part of the total need for protein. There is, however, significant storage of protein in new tissue during the growth period. A figure generally used in

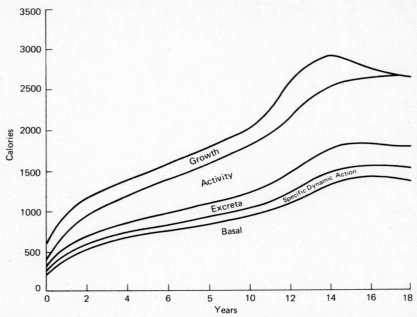

Figure 10.3 Average daily energy uses of girls of average size. (*Source:* Reproduced with permission from *Diseases of Infancy and Childhood,* 11th edition, by E. L. Holt, Jr., and R. McIntosh. Copyright © 1941 by Appleton-Century-Crofts, Inc., New York.)

TABLE 10.4 ENERGY REQUIREMENTS OF CHILDREN AND ADOLESCENTS

Age (years)	Body weight (kg)	Energy per kg per day (kcal)	Energy per kg per day (kJ)[1]	Energy per person per day (kcal)	Energy per person per day (mJ)[2]
Children					
<1	7.3	112	470	820	3.4
1–3	13.4	101	424	1360	5.7
4–6	20.2	91	382	1830	7.6
7–9	28.1	78	326	2190	9.2
Male adolescents					
10–12	36.9	71	297	2600	10.9
13–15	51.3	57	238	2900	12.1
16–19	62.9	49	205	3070	12.8
Female adolescents					
10–12	38.0	62	259	2350	9.8
13–15	49.9	50	209	2490	10.4
16–19	54.4	43	179	2310	9.7
Adult man (moderately active)	65.0	46	192	3000	12.6
Adult woman (moderately active)	55.0	40	167	2200	9.2

Source: Reprinted from FAO/WHO, *Energy and Protein Requirements,* World Health Organization Technical Report Series No. 522, 1973 (**7**).
[1]kJ is kilojoule or 0.239 kcal.
[2]mJ is megajoule or 239 kcal.

calculating protein needs for growth is 0.3 g of nitrogen or 1.88 g of protein daily. This average figure is in the range of values calculated by Mitchell (Table 10.5).

Amino acids are required for the synthesis of protein in the building of tissues and in meeting the needs of the child for tissue maintenance. Good quality protein, or those foods that provide the essential amino acids in desired amounts and proportions, are important during the rapid growth periods. The recommended allowances are based on the assumption that the proteins consumed will be utilized at 70 percent efficiency. Parents and menu planners for feeding programs must recognize the need for adequate amounts of this good quality protein.

Amino acid needs during growth have received only minor attention (**11, 12, 13**) from nutritionists. Estimates of amino acid needs for preadolescent girls, ages 7−9, and boys, ages 10−12, provide some indication of these needs during growth (Table 10.6). The information was obtained in nitrogen balance studies conducted over relatively short periods of time but represents the best estimates presently available. Some obvious discrepancies exist, suggesting the need for further research in this area of human nutrition (**13**).

Since the recognition of widespread protein deficiency problems in many parts of the world, the public is concerned that growing children may not obtain sufficient amounts of protein. The recommended allowance (Table 10.1) gives a realistic guideline for these intakes of protein, as do the guidelines assembled by the FAO Expert Committee (**7**).

Getting enough protein and the essential amino acids will not be a problem for most growing children who consume a variety of foods, including the

TABLE 10.5 NET PROTEIN REQUIREMENTS OF BOYS

| Age (years) | Body weight (kg) | Daily gain in body weight (gm) | Protein in gain[1] (mg) | Net Protein Required per Day | | |
				Main-tenance[2] (gm)	Growth (gm)	Total (gm)
1	10.6	13.9	2502	8.16	2.50	10.66
2	13.7	8.9	1602	9.62	1.60	11.22
3	16.0	5.9	1062	10.47	1.06	11.53
4	17.6	4.5	810	10.99	0.81	11.80
5	19.1	4.3	774	11.39	0.77	12.16
8	27.5	7.6	1368	13.71	1.37	15.08
10	33.3	10.5	1890	16.41	1.89	18.30
12	39.5	12.3	2214	17.55	2.21	19.76
15	55.0	11.3	2034	18.17	2.03	20.20
17	62.6	8.8	1584	22.22	1.58	23.80
19	66.0	3.9	702	22.11	0.70	22.81

Source: Reprinted with permission from *Comparative Nutrition of Man and Domestic Animals*, Vol. 1, by H. H. Mitchell (**2**). Copyright © 1962 by Academic Press, New York.
[1]Assuming 18 percent protein in gains in body weight.
[2]Estimated at 12.5 mg protein per basal calorie (Smuts, 1935).

TABLE 10.6 ESTIMATED ESSENTIAL
AMINO ACID NEEDS OF PREADOLESCENT CHILDREN

Amino acid	Girls (7–9 years)	Boys (10–12 years)
Isoleucine	24	30
Leucine	45	45
Lysine	29	60
Methionine, plus cystine	21	27
Phenylalanine	58	27
Threonine	20	35
Tryptophan	4.9	3.7
Valine	31	33

Source: Reprinted with permission from R. P. Abernathy, M. Speirs, R. W. Engel and M. E. Moore, *American Journal of Clinical Nutrition 19*, 407, 1966 (**11**). Copyright © 1966 by the American Society for Clinical Nutrition, Bethesda, Maryland.

well-known sources of protein such as meats, milk, eggs, poultry, cheese, fish, and legumes. Adequate intakes, however, may be a problem for children reared in families that are vegetarians or cannot afford the more expensive protein-rich foods. A series of studies (**14**) on preadolescent girls demonstrated the possibility of obtaining adequate levels of essential amino acids and protein from plant sources. Although care must be exercised in menu planning when the child receives all protein from plant sources, the protein needs for growth can be met with such a diet.

Fat-Soluble Vitamins

Meeting the recommended allowances for vitamins A, D, E, and K usually presents no particular problems, although vitamin A is cited as one of the nutrients often in short supply in the diets of growing children (**15–16**).

In many parts of the world, diets are seriously deficient in vitamin A, and thousands of children are permanently blinded as a result. Intakes of from 400 to 1000 R.E. are therefore recommended during the growing years (Table 10.1). Care, however, must be exercised when giving supplements of this nutrient, since consumption of 2000 R.E. above the usual dietary level may be toxic (**5**). Vitamin A is provided by a variety of foods, with the richest sources being the dark green leafy vegetables and deep yellow and orange vegetables and fruits and organ meats. These foods are usually not favorite foods of growing children, and special efforts may be necessary to encourage young boys and girls to eat them.

Vitamin D is necessary to promote adequate calcification and growth of the skeleton. Vitamin D may be available to the body through the irradiation of sterols in the skin from exposure to the ultraviolet rays of the sun. The growing child, however, cannot depend entirely on this source. Major food sources are animal products, such as milk, eggs, and fish-liver oils. Vegetables are poor sources. Vitamin D is now also added to milk, infant cereals, bread, breakfast cereals, margarine, and other foods. Monitoring or checking intakes seems a good idea, because of the constantly changing concentrations of the vitamin that are added to foods. Monitoring is also useful to avoid excess intakes that can be toxic.

Neither vitamin E nor vitamin K present problems for the growing child. Deficiencies are rarely seen, except in persons with malabsorption syndromes and in premature infants.

Water-Soluble Vitamins

The water-soluble vitamins do at times cause problems for the growing child. The general functions were discussed in Chapter 1, and reference to sources of the vitamins may be found in a wide range of food composition tables and in general or introductory nutrition texts (**17, 18**).

Vitamin C is often lacking in the diet (**15, 16**) because children do not readily consume those foods that are good sources. Thiamin and riboflavin are related to energy intake, and thus intakes should be increased as the child grows, becomes active, and uses more energy. Consumption of foods that contain adequate amounts of the water-soluble vitamins, as opposed to empty calorie foods, is important to the child's health.

Minerals

Many of the inorganic or mineral nutrients do not cause particular problems, and most growing children apparently consume adequate amounts. Certain minerals, however, are worthy of attention.

Calcium is of particular importance because of its role in the development of the teeth and bones. Growing children may need much more calcium per unit of body weight than adults. The RDA for calcium is 800 mg per day for children up to 10 years of age and 1200 mg for those 10−18 years. Considerable amounts of calcium are deposited in the tissues, primarily the skeleton, during the growing period. An estimate of the calcium content of the body and the daily gain in calcium is given in Table 10.7.

The RDA for calcium has been the focus of controversy for several years, since nutritionists recognize that many population groups consume much less than the recommended intake (in the range of 400−500 mg daily) without apparent problems. The long-term effects of either high or low calcium intakes are not at all clear. The role of a high intake of calcium during the growing period as insurance against osteoporosis in old age is an open question. In addition, evidence that high protein intakes may lead to loss of calcium raises still other questions about the relationship of dietary calcium and protein. The numerous facets of calcium metabolism and human requirements were reviewed by Irwin and Kienholz (**19**).

Nutritionists generally recommend intakes of phosphorus that are equivalent to calcium intakes. We have not identified deficiency of phosphorus in the human because of the presence of this nutrient in almost all foods. Phosphorus, calcium, and vitamin D are closely interrelated in the formation of sound teeth and bones, as well as in the utilization of the two mineral elements. When intakes of vitamin D are adequate the body can tolerate wide variations in the ratios of calcium and phosphorus, even during the growth period.

Iron is one of the most critical nutrients during growth, and an iron deficiency represents the major cause of anemia throughout the world. Based on

TABLE 10.7   CALCIUM CONTENT AND
CALCIUM ACCRETION DURING GROWTH OF BOYS

Age (years)	Body weight (kg)	Calcium content of body[1] (gm)	Daily Accretion of Calcium		
			Total[2] (mg)	Per kg body weight (mg)	Percentage of calcium content of gains
1	10.6	100	160	16.3	1.15
2	13.7	147	105	7.6	1.18
3	16.0	179	70	4.2	1.19
4	17.6	201	53	2.9	1.18
5	19.1	219	50	2.5	1.16
8	27.5	297	105	4.0	1.38
10	33.3	396	167	5.1	1.59
12	39.5	539	223	5.4	1.81
15	55.0	806	249	4.6	2.20
17	62.6	973	196	3.2	2.23
19	66.0	1073	63	1.0	1.62
		Averages	131	5.2	1.52

Source: Reprinted with permission from *Comparative Nutrition of Man and Domestic Animals,* Vol. 1, by H. H. Mitchell (**2**). Copyright © 1962 by Academic Press, New York.
[1]Calculated from an equation developed by Mitchell (**2**).
[2]Calculated from the differential form of the equation in Mitchell's book.

commonly accepted criteria for iron deficiency, up to 15 percent of those children 12–17 who were studied in a U.S. survey (**16**) were deficient in the mineral (Table 10.8).

Major factors influencing iron nutriture are (1) the amount and availability of iron in the diet, (2) the rate of growth, and (3) the loss of iron.

The utilization of iron varies from about 1 percent in certain plant foods to about 15 percent in meats. Current iron nutriture also influences the rate of absorption. Generally, iron utilization increases with body needs, thus a child with low iron stores or an anemic child will utilize a higher percentage of iron than a similar child with adequate iron stores.

Considerable iron is stored during the growth period. Nutritionists estimate that for each kilogram of body weight gain, boys require 42 mg of iron and girls 31 mg of iron. The difference between the sexes reflects the larger gain in muscle mass and blood volume by boys (**20**).

Normal losses of iron through the intestinal tract range from 0.5–1.0 mg daily. The adolescent female loses an additional 0.5 mg of iron daily during menstruation.

The RDA for iron intakes have generally increased during recent updating of nutrient guidelines. During early childhood, the suggested intake is now 15 mg per day, and during the adolescent years, the recommended intake is 18 mg per day (**5**). Since iron deficiency is found frequently during growth, particularly between the ages of 10–18 years, the iron status of individuals should be evaluated during periods of rapid growth and on attainment of sexual maturation.

TABLE 10.8 PREVALENCE OF IRON DEFICIENCY IN PERSONS AGE 12–17 YEARS

	Boys			Girls		
	Criterion for low value	Mean value	Percent with low values	Criterion for low value	Mean value	Percent with low values
Hematocrit	40	43.1	15.5	36	40.7	2.4
Hemoglobin	13	14.8	7.4	11.5	13.7	1.9
Serum iron	60	112.5	2.8	40	102.1	1.1
Transferrin saturation	20	33.6	7.7	15	29.1	5.3

Source: Reprinted from S. Abraham, F. W. Lowenstein and C. L. Johnson, U.S. Department of Health, Education and Welfare, DHEW Publication No. (HRA) 74-1219-1, 1974 (**16**).

Consuming sufficient amounts of iron can present a problem during growth. The difficulty is twofold: (1) The American diet does not contain many rich sources of iron, and (2) most growing children do not like those foods that are rich sources. Liver is one of the best sources, yet children generally regard liver as one of their less favorite foods. Other good iron sources include beef, eggs, spinach, lima beans, broccoli, raisins, and certain fruits. Many nutritionists agree that it is unlikely that the adolescent female will consume 18 mg per day, the recommended intake, if the energy intake remains at about the recommended level. The pros and cons of increasing iron fortification of staple foods were discussed in Chapter 1.

Careful attention must be given to the iron needs of the adolescent. A recent report (**21**) points out that iron deficiency is more common in adolescent males than was previously thought and that iron intakes may need to be increased during the periods of rapid growth. Iron supplements and even therapeutic dosages of iron may be necessary for certain individual children (**21**).

In recent years zinc has been recognized as a possible critical nutrient in the diets of growing children (**22**). The RDA for zinc ranges from 10 to 15 mg daily during the growing years (Table 10.1). The estimated average intakes of zinc range from 5 mg in young children to approximately 13 mg in 10–13-year-olds. Recent studies suggest, though, that zinc intakes of 7 mg per day will meet the requirements of preadolescent children (**23**). The RDA will apparently meet the needs during growth, but since there are reports of zinc deficiency, it is suggested that adequate zinc intakes not be taken for granted (**24**). Children from low-income families, for instance, and those consuming diets primarily of plant origin may have difficulty obtaining sufficient zinc. In addition to the naturally low zinc content of plants, other plant components such as phytates tend to bind zinc and render it unavailable to the human.

Fluorine has been recognized within the past few years as an essential nutrient for humans. Numerous epidemiological studies confirm the importance of fluoride in lowering the incidence of dental caries in growing children. Although public opinion runs against fluoridation of water supplies in many communities, dental caries can be prevented or the incidence lowered when the water supply provides approximately 1 ppm fluoride. Since dental problems are of major consequence in the United States, fluoridation of water supplies with appropriate levels seems clearly to be a sound health practice. The role of fluorine and the importance of sound dental health are discussed in detail in Chapter 11.

EVALUATION OF NUTRIENT INTAKES AND NUTRITIONAL STATUS

Nutritionists, dietitians, physicians, public health personnel, school food service personnel, parents, and others may become involved with the assessment of nutrient intakes of either individual children or groups of growing children. An evaluation of a child's nutrient intake usually begins with a record of food consumption, and this may take several forms:

1. *Food Consumption Recall.* Using this format, an individual will "recall" the kind and amounts of food consumed over a 24-hour period at some time prior to the actual recording. This method is often referred to as a "24-hour recall." Food models and other devices may be used to assist the person in estimating amounts of foods consumed.
2. *Food Record.* This format requires an individual to keep a record of foods consumed (at the time they are consumed) for a specified time, usually five to seven days.
3. *Weighed Food Intake.* Here, food is weighed or measured by the person or by an attendant during a given time period. This method can give a very accurate and complete record of the food consumed by the person. This method is the basis for controlled studies in metabolic units in nutrition research centers and hospitals.
4. *Diet History.* A *diet history* is an attempt to determine the kinds of foods consumed over a long period of time. This approach is useful in determining food habits of individuals or groups but is not very helpful as a basis for evaluating nutritional health over a short period. Information about types of food, usual consumption patterns, and general likes and dislikes may be obtained through this approach.

Calculation of Nutrient Intakes

Records of food intakes or histories of food habits will normally be followed with a calculation of nutrient intake. Food composition tables are used as a basis for calculating these nutrient intakes. Most food composition tables, such as those in introductory nutrition textbooks, are based on data summarized by the USDA. The standard reference is USDA Handbook No. 8 (**25**), now being updated and available in sections representing major groups of foods. USDA Publication No. 456 (**26**), a compendium of nutrient content in common units, is available also. The nutritional content data are also available on computer cards and tapes. Many universities, as well as the USDA, can make computer analysis of dietary records. Other food composition tables are available through FAO/WHO. These data are likely more appropriate for evaluating diets or food intakes in parts of the world other than North America.

Assessment of Nutrient Intake Data

The RDAs (Table 10.1) are the most commonly used standards in evaluating nutrient intake. Therefore, use of the RDA as a guideline seems appropriate if the user understands its basis, and potential use. Groups or individuals may be classified as having "poor" diets when the intake of one or more individual nutrients falls below the level of two-thirds of the RDA. This conclusion can be misleading, however. In many cases, both the RDA values and food composition tables are based on very scanty information. Furthermore, food intake data may be fraught with errors. The combination of these error-prone approaches is useful only in obtaining guidelines concerning potential nutritional problems.

A standard for the interpretation of nutrient intake data was prepared for the Ten-State Nutrition Survey in the United States (**15**). This standard was based on the RDA and FAO guidelines and provides a more realistic basis than does the use of the RDA alone, since it recognizes and considers actual conditions under which people reside (Table 10.9).

TABLE 10.9 GUIDE TO INTERPRETATION OF NUTRIENT INTAKE DATA

Kcal Standards[1]		Protein Standards[2]	
Age	(kcal/kg) Body weight	Age	(gm protein/kg) Body weight
0−1 month	120	0−11 months	2.2
2−5 months	110	12−23 months	1.9
6−11 months	100	24−47 months	1.7
12−23 months	90	48−71 months	1.5
24−47 months	86	6−9 years	1.3
48−71 months	82	10−16 years	1.2
6−7 years	82	17−19 years	1.1
8−9 years	82	20 years and over	1.0
10−12 years		**Calcium Standards[3]**	
Male	68		
Female	64	Age	Mg/day
13−16 years		0−11 months	550
Male	60	12−71 months	450
Female	48	6−9 years	450
17−19 years		10−12 years	650
Male	44	13−16 years	650
Female	35	17−19 years	550
20−29 years		Adults	400
Male	40		
Female	35	**Vitamin A Standards[4]**	
30−39 years		Age	IU
Male	38		
Female	33	0−1 month	1500
40−49 years		2−5 months	1500
		(Continued)	

TABLE 10.9 *(Continued)*

Kcal Standards[1]			Vitamin A Standards[4]	
Age	(kcal/kg) Body weight		Age	IU
Male	37		6–11 months	1500
Female	31		12–23 months	2000
50–59 years			24–47 months	2000
Male	36		48–71 months	2000
Female	30		6–7 years	2500
60–69 years			8–9 years	2500
Male	34		10–12 years	2500
Female	29		12 years	3500
70 years				
Male	34			
Female	29			

Vitamin C Standards (ascorbic acid)

All age groups	30 mg/day

Vitamin B Standards

Age	Thia-min	Ribo-flavin	Nia-cin
For all age groups, including adults	0.4 mg/ 1000 kcal	0.55 mg/ 1000 kcal	6.6 mg/ 1000 kcal

Iron Standards

Age	Mg/day
0–11 months	10
12–47 months	15
48–71 months	10
6–9 years	10
10–12 years	
Male	10
Female	18
13–19 years	
Male	18
Female	18
20 years and over	
Male	10
Female (to 55)	18
Female (55 on)	10

Source: Reprinted from U.S. Department of Health, Education and Welfare, DHEW Publication No. (HRA) 74-1219-1, 1974 (**16**).
[1]For second and third trimesters of pregnancy, increase basic standard 200 kcal. For lactating, increase basic standard 1000 kcal.
[2]For second and third trimesters of pregnancy, increase basic standard 20 gm. For lactating, increase basic standard 25 gm.
[3]For third trimester of pregnancy, increase standard 400 mg. For lactating, increase standard 500 mg.
[4]For lactating, increase standard 1000 IU.

BIOCHEMICAL EVALUATION OF NUTRITIONAL STATUS

The nutritional health of individuals can be assessed by measuring blood and urine levels of nutrients and metabolites. The guidelines established for the Ten-State Nutrition Survey are useful in evaluating the intakes of these key nutrients (Table 10.10). These guides provide for the evaluation of iron status using hemoglobin, hematocrit, serum iron, and transferrin saturation values; folacin, based on the concentration of folacin in red blood cells and in blood serum; protein, based on serum protein and serum albumin; vitamin C, as reflected in serum levels of the vitamin; vitamin A, using as indicators plasma levels of vitamin A and/or carotene; thiamin, as reflected in the urinary excretion of thiamin and based on creatinine excretion; riboflavin, using the same basis as thiamin; and iodine, based on urinary excretion per gram of creatinine excretion.

On the basis of a specific measure, an individual's nutritional status for that nutrient can be classified as acceptable, low, or deficient. Changes in diets may then be recommended to alleviate or correct the difficulty, based on knowing the problem or potential problem nutrients, and the pattern of food intake. An evaluation of growing children, particularly those from risk groups or those suspected of having poor nutrition, can be useful in correcting nutrition problems prior to any long term adverse effects on the health of the child. In addition to the biochemical indices of nutritional status, a medical history should be obtained to evaluate more effectively the status of any child appearing to suffer from a nutritional deficiency as indicated by these parameters.

TABLE 10.10 GUIDELINES FOR CLASSIFICATION AND INTERPRETATION OF GROUP BLOOD AND URINE DATA COLLECTED AS PART OF THE TEN-STATE NUTRITION SURVEY

| | CLASSIFICATION CATEGORY | | |
| | Less than Acceptable | | |
Determination	Deficient	Low	Acceptable[1]
Hemoglobin, g/100 ml			
6–23 months	<9.0	9.0–9.9	≥10.0
2–5 years	<10	10.0–10.9	≥11.0
6–12 years	<10	10.0–11.4	≥11.5
13–16 years, male	<12	12.0–12.9	≥13.0
13–16 years, female	<10	10.0–11.4	≥11.5
16 years, male	<12	12.0–13.9	≥14.0
16 years, female	<10	10.0–11.9	≥12.0
Pregnant, second trimester	<9.5	9.5–10.9	≥11.0
Pregnant, third trimester	<9.0	9.0–10.4	≥10.5
Hematocrit, percentage			
6–23 months	<28	28–30	≥31
2–5 years	<30	30–33	≥34
6–12 years	<30	30–35	≥36
13–16 years, male	<37	37–39	≥40
13–16 years, female	<31	31–35	≥36
16 years, male and older	<37	37–43	≥44

(Continued)

TABLE 10.10   *(Continued)*

| | CLASSIFICATION CATEGORY | | |
| | Less than Acceptable | | |
Determination	Deficient	Low	Acceptable
16 years, female and older	<31	31−37	≥38
Pregnant, second trimester	<30	30−34	≥35
Pregnant, third trimester	<30	30−32	≥33
Hemoglobin, conc. MCHC[2] g/100 ml RBC[2]			
All ages	—	30−	≥30
Serum iron, mcg/100 ml			
0−5 months	—		—
6−23 months	<30		≥30
2−5 years	<40		≥40
6−12 years	<50		≥50
12 years, male	<60		≥60
12 years, female	<40		≥40
Transferrin saturation, percentage			
0−5 months	—		—
6−23 months	<15		≥15
2−12 years	<20		≥20
12 years, male	<20		≥20
12 years, female	<15		≥15
Red cell folacin, ng (nanogram)/ml			
All ages	<140	140−159	≥160−650
Serum folacin, ng/ml	3.0	3.0−5.9	≥6.0
Serum protein, gm/100 ml			
0−11 months		<5.0−	≥5.0
1−5 years		<5.5	≥5.5
6−17 years		<6.0	≥6.0
Adult	<6.0	6.0−6.4	≥6.5
Pregnant, second and third trimesters	<5.5	5.5−5.9	≥6.0
Serum albumin, gm/100 ml			
0−11 months		<2.5	≥2.5
1−5 years		<3.0	≥3.0
6−17 years		<3.5	≥3.5
Adult	<2.8	2.8−3.4	≥3.5
Pregnant, first trimester	<3.0	3.0−3.9	≥4.0
Pregnant, second and third trimesters	<3.0	3.0−3.4	≥3.5
Serum vitamin C, mg/100 ml			
0−11 months	—	—	—
1 year	<0.1	0.1−0.19	≥0.2
Plasma carotene, mcg/100 ml			
0−5 months		<10	≥10
6−11 months		<30	≥30
1−17 years		<40	≥40
Adult	<20[3]	20−39	≥40
Pregnant, second trimester		30−79	≥80
Pregnant, third trimester		40−79	≥80
Plasma vitamin A, mcg/100 ml			
0−5 months	<10	10−19	≥20
0.5−17 years	<20	20−29	≥30
Adult	<10	10−19	≥20

TABLE 10.10 *(Continued)*

| | CLASSIFICATION CATEGORY | | |
| | Less than Acceptable | | |
Determination	Deficient	Low	Acceptable
Urinary thiamin, mcg/gm creatinine			
1–3 years	<120	120–175	≥176
4–6 years	<85	85–120	≥121
7–9 years	<70	70–180	≥181
10–12 years	<60	60–180	≥181
13–15 years	<50	50–150	≥151
Adult	<27	27–65	≥66
Pregnant, second trimester	<23	23–54	≥55
Pregnant, third trimester	<21	21–49	≥50
Urinary riboflavin, mcg/gm creatinine			
1–3 years	<150	150–499	≥500
4–6 years	<100	100–299	≥300
7–9 years	<85	85–269	≥270
10–15 years	<70	70–199	≥200
Adult	<27	27–79	≥80
Pregnant, second trimester	<39	39–119	≥120
Pregnant, third trimester	<30	30–89	≥90
Urinary iodine, mcg/gm creatinine	<25	25–49	≥50

Source: Reprinted with permission from R. M. O'Neal, O. C. Johnson, and A. E. Schaefer, *Pediatrics Research*, 4:103, 1970 (**27**). Copyright © 1970 by Williams and Wilkins Co., Baltimore, Maryland.
[1]Excessively high levels may indicate abnormal clinical status or toxicity.
[2]MCHC is mean corpuscular hemoglobin concentration; RBC is red blood cells.
[3]May indicate unusual diet or malabsorption.

GUIDES FOR ADEQUATE FOOD INTAKES

Growing children, as well as adults, obtain most nutrients through their foods. All nutrients, with the possible exception of iron, can be obtained in adequate amounts through a varied diet by normal, healthy children. The USDA has developed guidelines for food intake that generally insure the intake of the essential nutrients. The most commonly used guide is the Four Food Groups (Figure 10.4). As was pointed out in Chapter 1, the USDA recently added a fifth group, Fats, Sweets, and Alcohol, to the basic food guide. Foods in this group supply large amounts of calories without making a significant nutritional contribution to the diet. The intake of such foods should be controlled carefully in any individual's diet and especially in that of the growing young person. For young people it is essential that nutrients required for normal growth not be replaced by empty calorie foods.

Children can obtain adequate amounts of the essential nutrients by consuming the recommended servings and by selecting intelligently from each food group to insure intakes of those nutrients found in relatively few foods.

Of course, some exceptions exist to this general statement. Children who are strict vegetarians or who for racial or cultural reasons do not consume the range of foods common in most households are unique and may require special attention. Dietary adjustments may be necessary for certain individuals to avoid excessive weight gain or to correct specific health problems. The guide is useful, however, as a general reference for most persons.

The USDA has developed food plans that give the amounts of various foods necessary to meet the nutritional needs of children and adults. Food plans have been developed for low-cost (Table 10.11), moderate-cost (Table 10.12), and liberal-cost (Table 10.13) foods. The estimates are based on food purchases for a week and consider usual losses such as discarded portions, plate waste, and spoilage. Adjustments for individuals are appropriate, but plans do give general food purchasing guidance for families or individuals.

To increase the effectiveness of any food guide, it is necessary for nutrition

TABLE 10.11   LOW-COST FOOD PLAN: AMOUNTS OF FOOD FOR A WEEK[1]

Family member	Milk, cheese, ice cream[2] (qt)	Meat, poultry, fish[3] (lb)	Eggs (no.)	Dry beans and peas, nuts[4] (lb)	Dark green and deep yellow vegetables (lb)	Citrus fruit, tomatoes (lb)	Potatoes (lb)
Child:							
7 months to 1 year	5.70	0.56	2.1	0.15	0.35	0.42	0.06
1–2 years	3.57	1.26	3.6	0.16	0.23	1.01	0.60
3–5 years	3.91	1.52	2.7	0.25	0.25	1.20	0.85
6–8 years	4.74	2.03	2.9	0.39	0.31	1.58	1.10
9–11 years	5.46	2.57	3.9	0.44	0.38	2.13	1.41
Male:							
12–14 years	5.74	2.98	4.0	0.56	0.40	1.99	1.50
15–19 years	5.49	3.74	4.0	0.34	0.39	2.20	1.87
20–54 years	2.74	4.56	4.0	0.33	0.48	2.32	1.87
55 years and over	2.61	3.63	4.0	0.21	0.61	2.38	1.72
Female:							
12–19 years	5.63	2.55	4.0	0.24	0.46	2.17	1.17
20–54 years	3.02	3.21	4.0	0.19	0.55	2.34	1.40
55 years and over	3.01	2.45	4.0	0.15	0.62	2.54	1.22
Pregnant	5.25	3.68	4.0	0.29	0.67	2.80	1.65
Nursing	5.25	4.16	4.0	0.26	0.66	2.99	1.67

Source: U.S. Department of Agriculture.

[1] Amounts are for food as purchased or brought into the kitchen from garden or farm. Amounts allow for a discard of about one-tenth of the edible food as plate waste, spoilage, and so on. Amounts of foods shown to two decimal places to allow for greater accuracy, especially in estimating rations for large groups of people and for long periods of time. For general use, amounts of food groups for a family may be rounded to the nearest tenth or quarter of a pound.

[2] Fluid milk and beverage made from dry or evaporated milk. Cheese and ice cream may replace some milk. Count as equivalent to a quart of fluid milk: natural or processed Cheddar-type cheese, 6 oz; cottage cheese, 2½ lb; ice cream, 1½ qt.

educators to understand the values and attitudes of growing children toward health, nutrition, and food and eating practices. There is a need for sound information on the nutritional status of youth as a whole, in fact. Studies of groups of growing children indicate tremendous variations in their nutritional status and support the view that a proportion of young people do have nutritional problems. Such children need to be identified and sought out for nutritional help. Functional nutrition education programs at the school age level require the cooperation of several professional groups, including teachers, school food service personnel, school nurses, guidance counselors, and others. Other ways to reach school age children in addition to the school setting must be identified. The mass media is often accused of having a detrimental effect on the eating patterns of children

TABLE 10.11 *(Continued)*

Other vegetables, fruit (lb)	Cereal (lb)	Flour (lb)	Bread (lb)	Other bakery products (lb)	Fats, oils (lb)	Sugar, sweets (lb)	Accessories[5] (lb)
3.43	0.71[6]	0.02	0.06	0.05	0.05	0.18	0.06
2.88	0.99[6]	0.27	0.76	0.33	0.12	0.36	0.68
2.95	0.90	0.30	0.91	0.57	0.38	0.71	1.02
3.67	1.11	0.45	1.27	0.84	0.52	0.90	1.43
4.81	1.24	0.62	1.65	1.20	0.61	1.15	1.89
3.90	1.15	0.67	1.88	1.25	0.77	1.15	2.61
4.50	0.90	0.75	2.10	1.55	1.05	1.04	3.09
4.81	0.93	0.71	2.10	1.47	0.91	0.81	2.11
4.92	1.02	0.62	1.73	1.23	0.77	0.90	1.16
4.57	0.75	0.63	1.44	1.05	0.53	0.88	2.44
4.17	0.71	0.55	1.31	0.94	0.59	0.72	2.13
4.57	0.97	0.58	1.24	0.86	0.38	0.64	1.11
4.99	0.95	0.66	1.52	1.06	0.55	0.78	2.56
5.33	0.78	0.61	1.55	1.16	0.76	0.91	2.70

[3]Bacon and salt pork should not exceed ⅓ lb for each 5 lb of this group.
[4]Weight in terms of dry beans and peas, shelled nuts, and peanut butter. Count 1 lb of canned dry beans—pork and beans, kidney beans, and so forth—as 0.33 lb.
[5]Includes coffee, tea, cocoa, punches, ades, soft drinks, leavenings, and seasonings. The use of iodized salt is recommended.
[6]Cereal fortified with iron is recommended.

TABLE 10.12   MODERATE-COST FOOD PLAN: AMOUNTS OF FOOD FOR A WEEK[1]

Family member	Milk, cheese, ice cream[2] (qt)	Meat, poultry, fish[3] (lb)	Eggs (no.)	Dry beans and peas, nuts[4] (lb)	Dark green and deep yellow vegetables (lb)	Citrus fruit, tomatoes (lb)	Potatoes (lb)
Child:							
7 months to 1 year	6.46	0.80	2.2	0.13	0.41	0.49	0.06
1–2 years	4.04	1.69	4.0	0.15	0.29	1.24	0.59
3–5 years	4.74	1.88	3.0	0.22	0.30	1.46	0.85
6–8 years	5.79	2.60	3.3	0.34	0.37	1.94	1.17
9–11 years	6.68	3.31	4.0	0.38	0.45	2.61	1.40
Male:							
12–14 years	7.02	3.77	4.0	0.48	0.48	2.44	1.52
15–19 years	6.65	4.65	4.0	0.29	0.47	2.73	2.00
20–54 years	3.38	5.73	4.0	0.29	0.59	2.92	1.94
55 years and over	2.97	4.64	4.0	0.19	0.70	2.91	1.69
Female:							
12–19 years	6.22	3.32	4.0	0.24	0.53	2.62	1.21
20–54 years	3.35	4.12	4.0	0.19	0.62	2.84	1.35
55 years and over	3.35	3.21	4.0	0.14	0.72	3.09	1.17
Pregnant	5.44	4.57	4.0	0.25	0.91	3.52	1.60
Nursing	5.31	5.01	4.0	0.26	0.91	3.76	1.73

Source: U.S. Department of Agriculture.

[1]Amounts are for food as purchased or brought into the kitchen from garden or farm. Amounts allow for a discard of about one-sixth of the edible food as plate waste, spoilage, and so on. Amounts of foods are shown to two decimal places to allow for greater accuracy, especially in estimating rations for large groups of people and for long periods of time. For general use, amounts of food groups for a family may be rounded to the nearest tenth or quarter of a pound.

[2]Fluid milk and beverage made from dry or evaporated milk. Cheese and ice cream may replace some milk. Count as equivalent to a quart of fluid milk: natural or processed Cheddar-type cheese, 6 oz; cottage cheese, 2½ lb; ice cream, 1½ qt.

(**28–30**). If such influence is as great as critics imply, the mass media could and should be used to positively influence food intake in this age group (**31**). A recent study demonstrated the effectiveness of the mass media approach in disseminating nutrition information to teenagers (**31**). The authors conclude that young people can be reached and knowledge improved through a short-term mass media promotion campaign if such a campaign has a special incentive for, and personal appeal to, the audience.

SPECIFIC CONCERNS RELATED TO NUTRITION DURING THE GROWING YEARS

Nutrition during childhood adolescence should result in the final maturation of biological growth and development. Although studies show that the majority of

TABLE 10.12 *(Continued)*

Other vegetables, fruit (lb)	Cereal (lb)	Flour (lb)	Bread (lb)	Other bakery products (lb)	Fats, oils (lb)	Sugar, sweets (lb)	Accessories[5] (lb)
3.98	0.64[6]	0.02	0.06	0.05	0.05	0.10	0.08
3.44	1.03[6]	0.26	0.81	0.33	0.12	0.28	0.79
3.51	0.74	0.27	0.82	0.73	0.41	0.81	1.42
4.39	0.84	0.39	1.14	1.11	0.56	1.03	1.97
5.76	1.03	0.51	1.47	1.51	0.66	1.31	2.63
4.66	0.94	0.56	1.69	1.54	0.85	1.34	3.65
5.45	0.80	0.67	1.98	1.82	1.05	1.15	4.41
5.93	0.76	0.65	1.97	1.65	0.95	0.96	2.95
5.88	0.89	0.53	1.58	1.45	0.87	1.05	1.50
5.38	0.68	0.56	1.34	1.22	0.56	0.97	3.36
4.94	0.54	0.49	1.28	1.08	0.65	0.81	2.89
5.50	0.81	0.52	1.20	0.98	0.45	0.73	1.39
6.13	0.73	0.83	1.77	1.28	0.46	0.85	3.50
6.52	0.74	0.81	1.84	1.42	0.69	1.00	3.79

[3]Bacon and salt pork should not exceed ⅓ lb for each 5 lb of this group.
[4]Weight in terms of dry beans and peas, shelled nuts, and peanut butter. Count 1 lb of canned dry beans—pork and beans, kidney beans, and so forth—as 0.33 lb.
[5]Includes coffee, tea, cocoa, punches, ades, soft drinks, leavenings, and seasonings. The use of iodized salt is recommended.
[6]Cereal fortified with iron is recommended.

young people have adequately nutritious diets, a significant minority consume low levels of calcium, iron, vitamin A, and ascorbic acid (**6, 15, 16**). The sporadic eating patterns of young people and the high nutritional needs associated with active growth accentuate the problem. Nutrition-related problems of concern to youth and/or those working closely with them include obesity, the effects of teenage pregnancy, nutrient supplements for the athlete, the use of fad diets, and the influence of oral contraceptives and drug abuse on nutrient status. Several of these topics were discussed in previous chapters. Here, the focus is on obesity in the adolescent and nutrition for the pregnant teenager and young athlete.

Obesity in the Rapidly Growing Young Person

Obesity is one of the major nutrition-related health problems in the United States. It is estimated that between 20 and 30 percent of the teenage population is

TABLE 10.13 LIBERAL-COST FOOD PLAN: AMOUNTS OF FOOD FOR A WEEK[1]

Family member	Milk, cheese, ice cream[2] (qt)	Meat, poultry, fish[3] (lb)	Eggs (no.)	Dry beans and peas, nuts[4] (lb)	Dark green and deep yellow vegetables (lb)	Citrus fruit, tomatoes (lb)	Potatoes (lb)
Child:							
7 months to 1 year	6.94	0.97	2.3	0.14	0.43	0.60	0.06
1−2 years	4.26	2.07	4.0	0.17	0.31	1.50	0.59
3−5 years	5.08	2.35	3.1	0.23	0.32	1.77	0.85
6−8 years	6.25	3.18	3.4	0.36	0.40	2.35	1.18
9−11 years	7.21	4.04	4.0	0.39	0.48	3.15	1.41
Male:							
12−14 years	7.57	4.57	4.0	0.50	0.51	2.94	1.52
15−19 years	7.18	5.59	4.0	0.31	0.50	3.29	2.01
20−54 years	3.64	6.83	4.0	0.32	0.62	3.51	1.95
55 years and over	3.24	5.54	4.0	0.19	0.76	3.52	1.68
Female:							
12−19 years	6.72	3.97	4.0	0.25	0.56	3.15	1.21
20−54 years	3.62	4.86	4.0	0.20	0.66	3.41	1.35
55 years and over	3.65	3.79	4.0	0.15	0.76	3.71	1.14
Pregnant	5.91	5.43	4.0	0.26	0.96	4.22	1.57
Nursing	5.76	5.97	4.0	0.28	0.97	4.51	1.72

Source: U.S. Department of Agriculture.

[1]Amounts are for food as purchased or brought into the kitchen from garden or farm. Amounts allow for a discard of about one-fourth of the edible food as plate waste, spoilage, and so on. Amounts of foods are shown to two decimal places to allow for greater accuracy, especially in estimating rations for large groups of people and for long periods of time. For general use, amounts of food groups for a family may be rounded to the nearest tenth or quarter of a pound.

[2]Fluid milk and beverage made from dry or evaporated milk. Cheese and ice cream may replace some milk. Count as equivalent to a quart of fluid milk: natural or processed Cheddar-type cheese, 6 oz; cottage cheese, 2½ lb; ice cream, 1½ qt.

significantly overweight, with 15−20 percent classified as genuine medical problems because of overweight (**32**). Nutritional surveys show that alarming numbers of adolescents do have serious overweight problems. The Ten-State Nutrition Survey indicated that obesity in white females sometimes begins as early as age 10 and often continues throughout the sixth decade (**16**). Obesity is also prevalent among upper-income adolescent males. These findings are especially disturbing since obesity that begins at an early age generally persists into adulthood, resulting in a severe condition which is extremely resistant to treatment.

The growth patterns of growing children have already been discussed. The greatest single physiological difference between adolescents and younger or older people is the rapidity and extent of their growth. Normal adolescent growth

TABLE 10.13   (Continued)

Other vegetables, fruit (lb)	Cereal (lb)	Flour (lb)	Bread (lb)	Other bakery products (lb)	Fats, oils (lb)	Sugar, sweets (lb)	Accessories[5] (lb)
4.71	0.64[6]	0.02	0.05	0.06	0.05	0.20	0.09
4.10	1.07[6]	0.28	0.82	0.35	0.13	0.27	0.95
4.18	0.76	0.27	0.79	0.78	0.45	0.85	1.74
5.21	0.85	0.39	1.08	1.23	0.60	1.08	2.41
6.83	1.04	0.51	1.39	1.67	0.71	1.38	3.21
5.52	0.95	0.56	1.60	1.71	0.92	1.40	4.47
6.45	0.84	0.69	1.92	2.05	1.07	1.20	5.36
6.99	0.79	0.66	1.91	1.86	0.95	1.00	3.54
6.97	0.89	0.54	1.49	1.57	0.94	1.09	1.82
6.34	0.71	0.59	1.31	1.35	0.54	0.98	4.09
5.81	0.56	0.51	1.24	1.22	0.66	0.84	3.47
6.42	0.74	0.54	1.17	1.12	0.48	0.77	1.66
7.17	0.70	0.87	1.70	1.45	0.46	0.87	4.20
7.66	0.75	0.84	1.76	1.58	0.68	1.02	4.52

[3]Bacon and salt pork should not exceed ⅓ lb for each 5 lb of this group.
[4]Weight in terms of dry beans and peas, shelled nuts, and peanut butter. Count 1 lb of canned dry beans—pork and beans, kidney beans, and so forth—as 0.33 lb.
[5]Includes coffee, tea, cocoa, punches, ades, soft drinks, leavenings, and seasonings. The use of iodized salt is recommended.
[6]Cereal fortified with iron is recommended.

is characterized by an increase in velocity of weight gain and linear growth. If the teenager overeats, the weight gain will be disproportionately greater than the increase in height, resulting in obesity.

Nutrition is very important during the demanding growth changes associated with adolescence, and the nutritional aspects of weight control in the adolescent are critical. Nutrient requirements during this stage are complex because the individual has not reached a state of stability in terms of growth. Any diet must meet the requirements of growth and development and at the same time result in a slowing of weight gain. The aim of any weight control program, therefore, should be the establishment of a nutritious life style rather than weight loss alone.

Food fads and periodic bouts of starvation seem to appeal to the adoles-

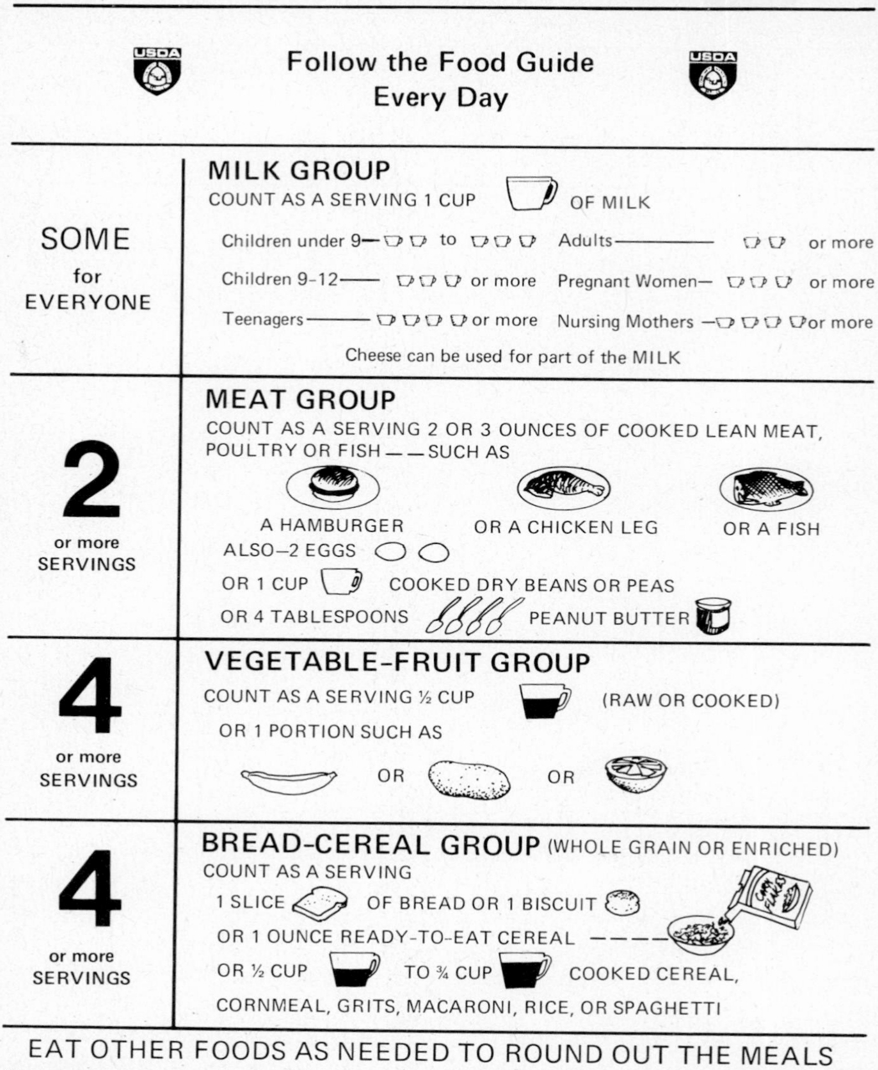

Follow the Food Guide
Every Day

SOME for **EVERYONE**	**MILK GROUP** COUNT AS A SERVING 1 CUP 🥛 OF MILK Children under 9— ▽▽ to ▽▽▽ Adults————— ▽▽ or more Children 9-12——— ▽▽▽ or more Pregnant Women— ▽▽▽ or more Teenagers———— ▽▽▽▽ or more Nursing Mothers —▽▽▽▽ or more Cheese can be used for part of the MILK
2 or more SERVINGS	**MEAT GROUP** COUNT AS A SERVING 2 OR 3 OUNCES OF COOKED LEAN MEAT, POULTRY OR FISH — —SUCH AS A HAMBURGER OR A CHICKEN LEG OR A FISH ALSO—2 EGGS ⬭ ⬭ OR 1 CUP 🥣 COOKED DRY BEANS OR PEAS OR 4 TABLESPOONS ⫯⫯⫯⫯ PEANUT BUTTER 🫙
4 or more SERVINGS	**VEGETABLE–FRUIT GROUP** COUNT AS A SERVING ½ CUP 🥣 (RAW OR COOKED) OR 1 PORTION SUCH AS 🍌 OR 🥔 OR 🍊
4 or more SERVINGS	**BREAD-CEREAL GROUP** (WHOLE GRAIN OR ENRICHED) COUNT AS A SERVING 1 SLICE 🍞 OF BREAD OR 1 BISCUIT 🥮 OR 1 OUNCE READY-TO-EAT CEREAL — — — — OR ½ CUP 🥣 TO ¾ CUP 🥣 COOKED CEREAL, CORNMEAL, GRITS, MACARONI, RICE, OR SPAGHETTI

EAT OTHER FOODS AS NEEDED TO ROUND OUT THE MEALS

Figure 10.4 *Daily food guide based on four food groups.* (*Source:* From U. S. Department of Agriculture.)

cent who is trying to lose weight. Such methods of weight loss need to be discouraged. The obese adolescent needs a diet which will supply adequate amounts of the nutrients required for normal growth and development and at the same time slow down or stop the rate of weight gain until a gain in height will accommodate the present weight. It is extremely important that calorie and nutrient intake not be cut in any way that will interfere with normal growth. Prolonged low calorie intake may retard linear growth in the rapidly growing

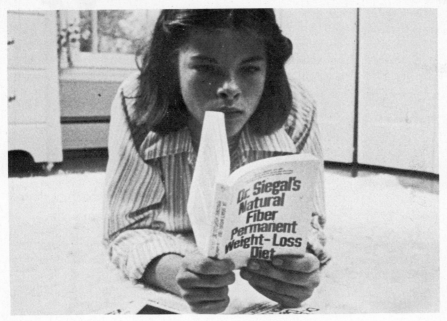

Adolescents are interested in nutrition as it relates to self-image.

adolescent and should be avoided, particularly by children who have not yet reached their peak in height velocity.

Basically, two weight control goals are appropriate for the obese adolescent. If the overweight teenager has not yet reached peak height growth, the most realistic and appropriate physiological goal is to try to stabilize weight so that the *individual* can gradually grow in height to accommodate weight. It is a significant achievement if the teenager does not lose any weight over a specified amount of time but adds 2 in. of height while maintaining present weight. The appropriate goal for the obese teenager who has attained peak height is a slow but relatively constant loss of weight. This loss should be at a rate of no more than 2 lb per week, aimed at achieving ideal body weight over a period of several months. It may take from several months to a year or more for the overweight teenager to achieve ideal body weight for height. Teenagers should understand that achievement of ideal body configuration will not necessarily be a steady process but that with perseverance the ultimate goal of successful weight control will be realized by changing one's eating habits.

Poor food habits resulting in poor selection of food and excessive eating is a major cause of adolescent obesity. Teenagers are inclined to eat only a limited number of foods. They often choose breads, pastas, sweet rolls, doughnuts, cookies, candies, and soft drinks and seldom eat fruits and vegetables. Many teens recognize that excess food intake leads to overweight but are so unaware of their actual food practices that they do not realize what or how much food they are actually consuming.

Nutrition counseling, therefore, can be a problem unless teenagers sincerely want to improve their nutritional habits. Health professionals must try to help adolescents understand nutrition as it applies to their individual physiological and psychological needs. The nutrition education of overweight young people in relation to their individual eating patterns is imperative if weight loss is to be maintained satisfactorily. Behavior modification techniques can be used to stress the importance of becoming aware of what individual eating patterns actually are. By studying patterns and trends noted in food records, young people can learn where behavior changes need to be made and how to begin those changes. A gradual growth toward normal weight for height can be achieved through good nutrition. It should be noted that many causative factors can be involved in the development of adolescent obesity, and health professionals should consider all causes when working with the overweight teen. Physical inactivity may play a major role in many teens' inability to control weight. Others may have problems that require the advice of a physician or psychologist before the teen can be helped with nutrition education.

Teenage Pregnancy

Teenage pregnancies are a national concern since there has been a dramatic increase of them over the last decade. The nutritional needs of pregnant teenagers warrant special consideration for several reasons. Teenagers may have little or no education concerning the nutritional needs and care of both mother and unborn child. In addition, in the pregnant teenager the nutritional stress of pregnancy is superimposed on the increased nutrient needs of growth and physical maturation.

The onset of menarche is considered a benchmark of maturity in women, since the most rapid period of growth precedes it with height increasing only an additional 2 in. or so after menarche. Girls are considered to be biologically mature at three years past menarche. The average age of menarche in the United States today is 13 years. Therefore, a young girl becoming pregnant before 16–17 may not yet have reached full biological maturity.

As discussed in Chapter 4, adolescent pregnancy can pose a serious threat to the life and health of a young woman and her child, so adequate nutrition during this period is of major importance. Girls 17 years of age or younger have greater nutritional requirements in relation to body size than do adult women because they are still actively growing. Table 10.14 shows the RDAs for the teenage girl in three age ranges and the additional requirements during pregnancy. In general, nutrient requirements are higher in younger age groups on a per weight basis.

The energy requirements suggested in Table 10.14 are based on growth requirements for both the actively growing teenager and the fetus. Teenage girls, often concerned with their weight, may restrict calorie intake without adequate supervision. Protein requirements, like those for energy, are related to maturation

TABLE 10.14 RDAs FOR FEMALES IN CHILDBEARING AGE GROUPS (REVISED 1980)

Age	11−14 years		15−18		19−22		Pregnant
Weight (kg) (lb)	46	101	55	120	55	120	
Height (cm) (in.)	157	62	163	64	163	64	

Nutrient Needs							
Energy (with range) (kcal)	2200 (1500−3000)		2100 (1200−3000)		2100 (1700−2500)		+300
Protein (g)	46		46		44		+30
Vitamin A[1] (mcg R.E.)	800		800		800		+200
Vitamin D[2] (mcg)	10		10		7.5		+5
Ascorbic Acid (mg)	50		60		60		+20
Folacin (mcg)	400		400		400		+400
Niacin (mg N.E.)[3]	15		14		14		+2
Riboflavin (mg)	1.3		1.3		1.3		+0.3
Thiamin (mg)	1.1		1.1		1.1		+0.4
Vitamin B_6 (mg)	1.8		2.0		2.0		+2.0
Vitamin B_{12} (mcg)	3.0		3.0		3.0		+1.0
Calcium (mg)	1200		1200		800		+400
Phosphorus (mg)	1200		1200		800		+400
Iron (mg)	18		18		18		—[4]

Source: Reprinted from Food and Nutrition Board, *Recommended Dietary Allowances,* 9th edition, National Academy of Sciences, Washington, 1980 (**5**).

[1] 1 R.E. = 1 mcg retinol or 6 mcg B carotene.
[2] As cholecalciferol. 10 mcg cholecalciferol = 400 IU vitamin D.
[3] 1 N.E. = 1 mg niacin or 60 mg dietary tryptophan.
[4] The increased requirement during pregnancy cannot be met by the iron content of habitual American diets or by the existing iron stores of many women. Therefore, the use of 30−60 mg of supplemental iron is recommended.

events in the growing female and in fetal growth. Adequate amounts of protein should not generally be a problem for the pregnant teenager unless she is unnecessarily restricting her food intake, is following a vegetarian life style, or unless her income is very limited. Vitamin A intake may present a problem in the pregnant adolescent if her intake of vegetables and fruits is low. If milk, fortified with vitamin D, is not included regularly in the diet the pregnant teenager may not receive enough of this fat-soluble vitamin. Vitamin C requirements increase during pregnancy. In addition to the increased physiological requirement associated with pregnancy, studies suggest that vitamin C requirements increase with various types of stress. The pregnant adolescent, at risk because of physiological immaturity, economic dependency, poor nutritional status, inadequate medical care, and lack of education, may experience stress to a greater degree than does the more adult pregnant female. Again, if the intake of fruits and vegetables is low, vitamin C intake by pregnant teens may be low. Requirements for folacin, niacin, riboflavin, thiamin, pyridoxine, and vitamin B_{12} all increase during pregnancy in relation to metabolic changes. The requirements for calcium and phosphorus increase because of their role as structural materials. The intake of these minerals can be a problem for the young woman not consuming milk and green leafy vegetables in adequate amounts. Iron is needed in increasing amounts during pregnancy, too; and it is especially important that the pregnant adolescent takes in enough iron to meet her own growth needs and those of the developing fetus. Although absorption of iron does increase during pregnancy, dietary intake alone is generally not sufficient to provide the levels of iron required by pregnant girls (**33**).

A limited number of studies have evaluated the nutritional status of pregnant teenagers. The results of such studies vary. Kaminetzky et al. (**34**) reported that intakes of protective foods and iron were below the recommended levels in the majority of 13–17-year-old girls studied. King et al. (**35**) have observed more frequently adequate nutrient intakes among pregnant teens. Calcium, iron, and vitamin A intake were the nutrients most likely to be inadequate, according to the study. A further study by Carruth (**36**) showed only folic acid and iron being consumed in amounts less than two-thirds of the RDA.

Table 10.15 shows the number of servings from each of the four food groups that should be eaten each day by the pregnant teenager. Such a menu pattern, however, may not fit the eating styles of today's teens. Sanjur (**6**) suggests that the Basic Food Groups as a measure of nutritional adequacy currently have limited use in assessing the changing food patterns and new food combinations of teenagers. Approximately 40 percent of the calories consumed by teens come from vendor-type or fast-food outlets (**36**). Thus the opportunity to eat adequate amounts of fruits, vegetables, and dairy products may well be limited. How well does the typical teenage diet of hamburgers, French fries, and soft drinks provide the nutrient needs of the pregnant teenager? Nutrient analyses show that such a meal is lacking in calcium, iron, vitamin A, vitamin C, thiamin, and riboflavin while providing excess calories in the form of fat and sugar.

A major factor contributing to inadequate nutrient intake in the pregnant teenager is the desire to be slim, coupled with the desire to continue to participate in normal teen social and peer groupings. Unfortunately, little thought may be given to the pregnancy or to the health of the unborn child. The young woman may drastically restrict food intake to control her weight. When she does eat, she may allow her food choices to be largely influenced by what her peers are eating. For these reasons, the pregnant teenager presents a major challenge to the nutrition educator. Motivating young girls to be concerned about their own well-being and

TABLE 10.15   SUGGESTED NUMBER OF SERVINGS
FROM EACH FOOD GROUP FOR PREGNANT TEENAGERS

Food group	No. of servings
Protein foods	2+
Milk and milk products	4+
Breads and cereals	5–6
Fruits and vegetables	4+ (vitamins C and A rich, plus others)

Source: U.S. Department of Agriculture.

that of the fetus can be difficult. As with any other age group, food habits will change slowly. In the short span of nine months, the pregnant teen may not modify her present eating habits enough to make a permanent impact on future eating habits (**36**). Health professionals working with pregnant teens should, therefore, suggest simple modifications to improve food intake based on information gained from a 24-hour dietary recall. The young girl herself should be involved in this meal planning. With the help of a nutritionist she should be able to choose foods that appeal to her, do not isolate her from her peers, and supply all required nutrients in adequate amounts. She should be reminded of the *importance* of her food selection to her own health and that of her child. The unborn child may not have much reality in many pregnant teenagers' thinking until late in pregnancy or even until birth. Thus a pregnant teenager's own growth and development may be a more tangible concept through which she can be persuaded to improve her nutrient intake. As has been stressed in previous sections of this text, a well-nourished pregravid state with adequate intake during pregnancy is most likely to produce a healthy baby and a healthy postpartum mother.

Nutrition for the Athlete

Amateur sports can be a highly competitive field. The strong desire to win and experience peer approval makes child athletes a prime target for nutrition information. Attention to proper nutrition is very important for the budding athlete, since deficiencies in caloric and nutrient intake can actually decrease performance (**37**). The energy requirements of a young athlete will depend on age, sex, body size, weight, type of sport, training level, and other factors. A nutritionally balanced diet designed to meet these energy requirements, therefore, is a major objective in feeding the athletic child.

Unfortunately, these athletes and their trainers, coaches, and parents are often highly susceptible to nutritional deception. A common misconception among young athletes and their coaches is that excess protein intake will result in the "building" of muscle tissue (**38**). Yet no scientific evidence exists to indicate that supplementing a basically sound diet can improve athletic performance (**39**). Although muscles are composed primarily of protein, muscle building is the process of strengthening existing muscle cells through physical exercise, not through excessive intakes of high protein foods or the use of protein supplements. In general, athletes do not require more protein than do nonathletes based on body size. Protein should supply from 10−15 percent of the caloric intake in a balanced diet. The normal young athlete generally has no problem in meeting this goal and, in fact, may consume much more protein than is necessary (**39**).

Another common misconception is that a high protein meal just prior to an athletic event will improve performance. The pregame meal, however, does not essentially supply for the upcoming event energy but may serve more of a psychological function. Any single meal prior to an event is not likely to improve performance to any great extent. The wrong choice of foods in a pregame meal could. however, detract from maximum performance. The pregame meal should be readily digestible and can include milk, fruit or juice, meat, bread and/or a starchy vegetable, and a plain dessert. Fat content should be kept to a minimum (**40**). Gas-forming foods should also be avoided (**40**). Excessive protein and bulk may increase urinary and bowel excretion. Two to three hours should elapse between the pregame meal and the athletic event to allow for proper digestion. The maintenance of blood glucose levels and prevention of dehydration are major objectives during the actual performance.

A nutritional practice associated with athletics that has achieved recent popularity, especially among marathon runners, is that of carbohydrate loading. This is the practice of manipulating the diet to increase glycogen stores in the muscles and thus delay eventual glycogen depletion and the accompanying fatigue during long distance runs. Muscles are exercised to exhaustion approximately one week in advance of the event to deplete glycogen stores. The athlete then follows a high-fat, high-protein, low-carbohydrate diet for three days to keep the glycogen content of the muscles low. About three days before competition, the athlete begins to eat large quantities of carbohydrate and normal amounts of fat and protein. The potential benefits associated with carbohydrate loading include increased efficiency, increased performance, decreased perception of fatigue, and delayed dehydration from a water storage associated with increased carbohydrate intake. Possible disadvantages include abnormal water retention, nutritional imbalance, possible breakdown of muscle fibers, and electrocardiogram abnormalities. It is suggested that carbohydrate loading not be attempted too frequently (**38**).

A dangerous nutritional practice that must be strongly discouraged is total starvation, semistarvation, or dehydration to control weight. Boxers and wrestlers routinely follow such practices to qualify for lower weight classes. In some cases coaches and trainers demand this weight loss. To accomplish this goal, the trainers impose water deprivation and/or caloric restriction on the young athlete. Coaches, parents, and the young athlete should recognize, however, that weight control by dehydration is only temporary. Moreover, they should recognize that the restriction of fluid intake can lead to serious, even fatal, consequences (**41**). A severe caloric restriction to lose weight can be highly detrimental to the growing child (**18**). The American Medical Association and the American College of Sports Medicine strongly condemn this practice (**42**).

Considerable amounts of body fluids are lost during strenuous exercise, especially under hot, humid conditions. Heat stroke and incapacitation are likely to occur if approximately 10 percent of the total body water is lost. A loss of 20 percent of a person's total body water is almost always fatal. The loss of 3 percent causes some physiological changes; a 5 percent loss brings symptoms of heat exhaustion, and hallucination may occur with a 7 percent loss (**43, 44**).

The replacement of water and electrolytes is limited by gastric emptying time. It is almost impossible to drink enough liquid to offset water loss during an athletic event, but partial replacement will prevent overheating. The athlete will need to ingest more water and possibly more salt than usual to replenish amounts lost during profuse sweating, especially during prolonged training or activity carried out in a hot, humid environment.

Athletes should be encouraged to drink water during practice or an event. Salt tablets, if taken without fluid replacement, may produce undesirable side effects such as nausea and dehydration (**45**), so salt should be supplied as much as possible in foods and beverages. A saline solution, prepared by dissolving one tablespoon of salt in one gallon of water can be used.

In general, nutritional regimes for the young athlete should focus on diets which provide enough calories for their very high activity levels. Foods should be provided that supply both energy and the other essential nutrients. Since no physiological reasons exist for many diets imposed by coaches who may have little or no knowledge about nutrition (**46, 47**), dietary practices such as the intake of excessive levels of protein, wheat germ, megavitamins, and others should be avoided. Supplements are not required in the majority of cases, although studies indicate that iron deficiency is common among athletic women, particularly during menstruation, and intakes should be increased accordingly (**48**).

SUMMARY

The period from early childhood to maturity is a critical time in the growth and development of the child and, as in other periods throughout life, is influenced by the nutritional environment. This chapter has reviewed the nutrient needs of the growing child and focused on the importance of adequate intakes of all essential nutrients, with special reference to those likely to cause problems in the growing youngster. The wide variations in food consumption patterns dictated by culture, race, income, and individual preferences were not considered in detail, but the student will recognize that such variations do exist.

Parents and health professionals are concerned with the nutrient intake of individuals or groups of growing children and with possible nutrient deficits. Records of food intake over predetermined periods of time can be analyzed for nutrient content and evaluated against nutrient intake guidelines to assess the adequacy of a diet. The nutritionist should exercise caution in drawing conclusions from this type of assessment. However, it does provide a useful guideline for indicating potential nutritional problems. In addition to nutrient intake, certain biochemical measures are useful in assessing the nutritional status of an individual.

Adequate amounts of most nutrients can be obtained through the consumption of a well-balanced diet containing a variety of foods. Several guidelines for food intake that generally insure adequate intake of the essential nutrients are available.

STUDY QUESTIONS AND TOPICS FOR INDIVIDUAL INVESTIGATION

1. Complete a 24-hour recall or a three-day food record for children of different cultural or economic backgrounds. Evaluate the children's food intakes using a food composition table and compare intakes of key nutrients to the RDA. How do these children compare with each other and to those in the Ten-State Nutrition Survey? What are "problem" nutrients? How would you suggest improving the diets of the children?
2. Examine the nutrient content, using available food composition data, of foods commonly consumed by young children as snacks. Do the same for teenagers. What problems might arise from high intakes of these foods?
3. Review the evidence in the nutrition literature used as the basis for establishing the RDA for a single nutrient for the growing child. For example, what is the basis for setting the RDA for vitamin B_6 at 2.0 mg for the 15–18-year-old male?
4. If you were a nutritionist working with families with growing children and the mother of a 15-year-old high school student tells you that the football coach is recommending an expensive protein supplement for her son, what advice will you give her? How can you help this parent be certain that her son is receiving adequate nutrients from his dietary intake?
5. Do you recognize overweight among young people as a possible nutritional problem on your campus? Approximately how many of your friends could lose a few pounds? What are their eating habits? Would these habits contribute to a weight problem? Does the student health center (or any other group on campus) offer overweight young people information and help with the problem? What kind of information is given out? Do you see a need for improvement? Explain your answer.

REFERENCES

1. Jelliffe, D. B. Nutrition in early childhood. *World Review of Nutrition and Dietetics,* 16:1, 1973.
2. Mitchell, H. H. *Comparative Nutrition of Man and Domestic Animals,* Vol. 1. Academic Press, New York, 1962.
3. Brasel, J. Factors that affect nutritional requirements in adolescents. In: *Nutritional Disorders of American Women,* ed. M. Winick. Wiley, New York, 1977.
4. Macy, I. G., and H. J. Kelly. *Chemical Anthropology: A New Approach to Growth in Children.* University of Chicago Press, Illinois, 1957.
5. Food and Nutrition Board, National Academy of Sciences. *Recommended Dietary Allowances,* 9th ed. Washington, D.C., 1980.

6. Sanjur, D. Teenagers and nutrition: contemporary issues. *Professional Nutritionist,* 11(3):1, 1979.
7. FAO/WHO Energy and Protein Requirements. World Health Organization Technical Report Series No. 522, 1973.
8. Holt, L. E., Jr., and R. McIntosh, eds. *Diseases of Infancy and Childhood,* 11th ed. Prentice-Hall, Englewood Cliffs, N.J., 1941.
9. Fomon, S. J. *Infant Nutrition.* Saunders, Philadelphia, 1967.
10. Mitchell, H. H., T. S. Hamilton, F. R. Steggerda, and H. W. Bean. The chemical composition of the adult human body and its bearing on the biochemistry of growth. *Journal of Biological Chemistry,* 158:625, 1945.
11. Abernathy, R. P., M. Speirs, R. W. Engel, and M. E. Moore. Effects of several levels of dietary protein and amino acids on nitrogen balance of preadolescent girls. *American Journal of Clinical Nutrition,* 19:407, 1966.
12. Nakagawa, I., T. Takahashi, and T. Suzuki. Amino acid requirements of children. *Journal of Nutrition,* 71:176, 1960.
13. Irwin, M. I., and D. M. Hegsted. A conspectus of research on amino acid requirements of man. *Journal of Nutrition,* 101:539, 1971.
14. Abernathy, R. P., and S. J. Ritchey. Protein requirements of preadolescent girls. *Journal of Home Economics,* 64:56, 1972.
15. U.S. Department of Health, Education, and Welfare. Ten-State Nutrition Survey, 1968–70. DHEW Publication No. (Health Services and Mental Health Administration) 72–8133, Atlanta, Ga., 1972.
16. First Health and Nutrition Examination Survey, Preliminary Findings, U.S. 1971–72. Dietary intake and biochemical findings. DHEW Publication No. (Health Resources Administration) 74–1219–1, Washington, D.C., 1974.
17. Guthrie, H. A. *Introductory Nutrition,* 4th ed. Mosby, St. Louis, 1979.
18. Hamilton, E. M., and E. Whitney. *Nutrition Concepts and Controversies.* West Publishing, St. Paul, Minn., 1979.
19. Irwin, M. I., and E. W. Kienholz. A conspectus of research on calcium requirements of man. *Journal of Nutrition,* 103:1019, 1973.
20. Hankins, W. W., V. G. Leonard, and E. Speck. The total body hemoglobin in children and its relation to calorie and iron requirements. *Metabolism,* 5:70, 1956.
21. Food and Nutrition Board, National Academy of Sciences. Iron Nutriture in Adolescence. DHEW Publication No. 77–5100, Washington, D.C., 1976.
22. Halsted, J., J. C. Smith, and M. I. Irwin. A conspectus of research in zinc requirements of man. *Journal of Nutrition,* 104:345, 1974.
23. Ritchey, S. J., M. K. Korslund, Laura Gilbert, Diana Fay, and Meredith Robinson. Zinc retention and losses of zinc in sweat by preadolescent girls. *American Journal of Clinical Nutrition,* 32:799, 1979.
24. Sandstead, H. H. Zinc nutrition in the United States. *American Journal of Clinical Nutrition,* 26:1251, 1973.
25. Watt, B., and A. Merrill. Composition of Foods—Raw, Processed, Prepared. Agriculture Handbook No. 8. U.S. Department of Agriculture, Washington, D.C., 1963.

26. Adams, C. Nutritive Value of American Foods in Common Units. Handbook No. 456. U.S. Department of Agriculture, Washington, D.C., 1975.
27. O'Neal, R. M., O. C. Johnson, and A. E. Schaefer. Guidelines for classification and interpretation of group blood and urine data collected as part of the national nutrition survey. *Pediatric Research,* 4:103, 1970.
28. Gussow, J. Counternutrition messages of TV ads aimed at children. *Journal of Nutrition Education,* 4:48, 1972.
29. Manoff, R. K. Potential uses of mass media in nutrition programs. *Journal of Nutrition Education,* 5:125, 1973.
30. Where the growth came in network TV in 1976. *Advertising Age, 48(7):34, 1977.*
31. Axelson, J., and D. Del Campo. Improving teenager's nutrition knowledge through the mass media. *Journal of Nutrition Education,* 10:30, 1978.
32. What to do about teenage overweight. What's New in Home Economics. September 1966, p. 104.
33. Wrigley, E. S. The pregnant adolescent. *Journal of the American Dietetic Association,* 66:588, 1975.
34. Kaminetzky, H. A., A. Langer, H. Baker, O. Frank, A. D. Thomson, E. D. Munves, A. Opper, F. C. Behrle, and B. Glista. The effect of nutrition in teenage gravidas on pregnancy and the status of the neonate. *American Journal of Obstetrics and Gynecology,* 115:639, 1973.
35. King, J. C., S. Cohenour, D. Calloway, and H. Jacobson. Assessment of nutritional status of teenage pregnant girls. *American Journal of Clinical Nutrition,* 25:916, 1972.
36. Carruth, B. R. Nutrition and teenage pregnancies. In: *Nutrition Update: Accent on Youth,* ed. B. Tanis. American Home Economics Association, Washington, D.C. June 1978.
37. Shils, M. E. Food and nutrition relating to work and environmental stress. In: *Modern Nutrition in Health and Disease,* 5th ed., eds. R. Goodhart and M. Shils. Lea & Febiger, Philadelphia, 1973.
38. Serfass, R. Nutrition for the athlete. *Contemporary Nutrition,* 2(5), May 1977.
39. Serfass, R. Dietary considerations for athletes. In: *Nutrition Update: Accent on Youth,* ed. B. Tanis. American Home Economics Association, Washington, D.C. June 1978.
40. Huse, D. M., and R. A. Nelson. Basic, balanced diet meets requirements of athletes. *Physical Fitness and Sports Medicine,* 5:53, 1977.
41. Consolazio, C. F. Physical activity and performance of the adolescent. In: *Nutrient Requirements in Adolescence,* eds. J. I. McKigney and H. N. Munro. MIT Press, Cambridge, Mass., 1976.
42. American College of Sports Medicine. Position stand on weight losses in wrestlers. *Medicine and Science in Sports,* 8:11, 1976.
43. Adolph, E. F. *Physiology of Man in the Desert.* Wiley, New York, 1947.
44. Johnson, R. E. Feeding problems in man as related to environment. Quartermaster Food and Container Institute for the Armed Forces, Chicago, 1946.

45. Ryan, A. Round table—balancing heat stress, fluids, and electrolytes. *Physical Fitness and Sports Medicine,* 3:43, 1975.
46. American Association of Health and Physical Education. Nutrition for Athletes. The Alliance. Washington, D.C., 1971.
47. Williams, J. G. P. Diet and the athlete. *Practitioner,* 201:324, 1968.
48. Buskirk, E. R., and E. Hames. Nutrient requirements for women in sport. Women and Sport: A National Research Conference. Penn State HPR Series No. 2, 1972.

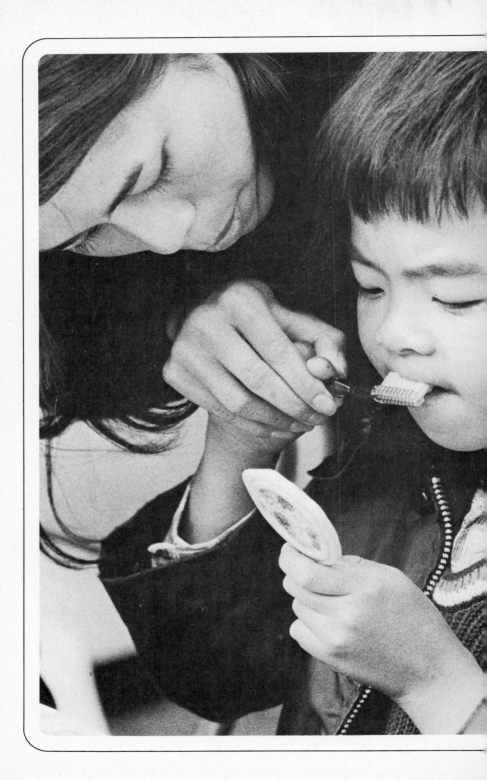

CHAPTER 11

NUTRITION AND DENTAL HEALTH

$\mathbf{T}$ he mouth is often referred to as the "mirror of health" because many signs of nutritional deficiencies and problems as well as evidence of numerous other disease conditions, appear in or near the mouth (**1**). The maintenance of sound oral health is, itself, essential to general good health throughout the life cycle. Problems with the teeth and gums confront many persons from very early in life until death, so most public health professionals recognize dental caries and related difficulties as major health problems. Thus an understanding of the development of the teeth, prevention of dental caries and other oral diseases, and the role of nutrition in these conditions is an important aspect of any book on maternal and child nutrition.

Nutrition plays an important role in the formation, development, and maintenance of teeth and supporting oral tissues. The growth phases of these tissues are similar to those of all other body tissues (see Chapter 5). The development of the teeth and associated structures is related to the availability of nutrients, and, as with other parts of the body, a lack of nutrients will retard and/or block sound development of the teeth.

DEVELOPMENT OF TEETH

Tooth development begins very early in life. The dental lamina, or the ridge along the jaw, begins to appear as early as the thirty-fourth day of embryonic life (**2**), and the tooth buds of the ten primary teeth are formed by the sixth week of gestation. As the epithelial cells increase the tooth buds move into the underlying tissue. This movement stimulates the connective tissue to produce the dental papillae, the organs responsible for the subsequent formation of the dentin and pulp portions of the tooth. The epithelial cells produce the enamel (the caplike cover) and the bell-shaped enamel organ. The developing tooth is shown in Figure 11.1.

The *ameloblasts* are cells responsible for laying down the enamel matrix and are derived from the inner layer of cells. The dental papillae are largely encased in the bell. The *odontoblasts*, connective tissue cells forming the outer surface of the dental pulp, differentiate from the peripheral cells of the papillae. The membrane separating the ameloblasts from the odontoblasts eventually becomes the junction between the dentin and enamel parts of the calcified crown of the tooth. The dental pulp is derived from the connective tissue within the dental papillae. The outer layers of the enamel epithelium serve as a mechanism for the movement of nutrients when calcification begins. This process of calcification is initiated during the fourth to sixth month of pregnancy and begins at the junction of dentin and enamel. All 20 primary teeth are involved, even though they may not erupt or appear in the mouth for several years.

After the dentin and enamel form, the roots begin to develop. It is also during this period, about the fifth month of pregnancy, that the tooth germs of the permanent teeth begin to appear. The central incisors appear first and the permanent tooth germs continue to appear through the tenth month of life after birth when the second bicuspid is apparent. Tooth germs of the permanent molars come still later.

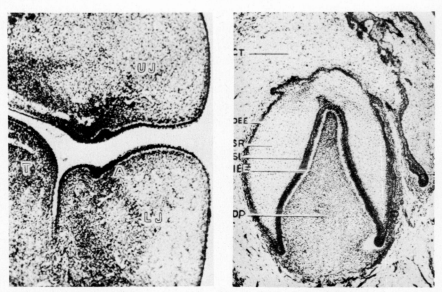

Figure 11.1 *Section through the developing tooth during the advanced "bell" stage. The fetus is about four months of age. CT, connective tissue; OEE, outer enamel epithelium; SR, stellate reticulum; SI, stratum intermedium; IEE, inner enamel epithelium; DP, dental pulp. (Source:* Reproduced with permission from *Growth and Development of Children,* 7th edition, by G. H. Lowrey. Copyright © 1978 by Year Book Medical Publishers, Inc., Chicago.)

A matrix of protein forms during the early stages of tooth development. Calcification begins around this matrix of protein prior to birth and continues until the child is approximately 16 years old. Key nutrients in this calcification process are calcium, phosphorus, vitamin D, and vitamin C. The parts of a healthy tooth are shown in Figure 11.2

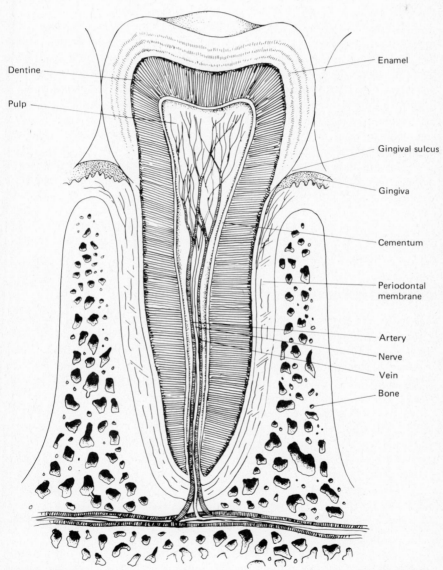

Figure 11.2 *The major components of a healthy tooth and supporting tissues. (Source:* Reproduced with permission from D. P. DePaola and M. C. Alfano in *Nutrition Today* magazine, May/June 1977. Copyright © 1977 by Nutrition Today, Annapolis, Maryland.)

Malnutrition during critical periods of growth will alter the development of the teeth. Conversely, good nutrition during the period of gestation is important to the development of sound teeth, since deficiencies of protein, calcium, vitamin D, and perhaps other nutrients during pregnancy may result in poor tooth development (**3**). Malnutrition or poor nutrition during gestation may indeed cause irreversible damage to the developing tooth. Later, the teeth and bones of the head and face may not develop properly in those growing children who suffer from malnutrition.

During the child's growth, the crowns of the permanent teeth develop, the roots of the primary teeth are resorbed, and the permanent teeth erupt. Through this process the primary teeth are replaced by the permanent ones (**2**). The life cycle of dental development may be divided into six periods: (1) growth, (2) calcification and maturation, (3) eruption of the primary teeth, (4) resorption of the roots of the primary teeth, (5) eruption of the permanent teeth, and (6) attrition or loss of permanent teeth. The time range involved in the cycle of tooth development can be varied. The average times for the development of primary and permanent teeth are presented in Table 11.1.

The eruption of the tooth is the process that takes the tooth from its developmental crypt and places it in the appropriate site with other teeth. The degree of physical growth of the individual may influence the eruption of both the primary and permanent teeth (**5**). For example, the teeth of premature infants erupt later than those of full-term babies. Times for primary tooth development are presented in Table 11.2. The normal sequence of the eruption of the permanent teeth is presented in Table 11.3.

COMPOSITION OF TEETH

The tooth is composed of four major tissues (Figure 11.2): enamel, dentin, cementum, and pulp. The enamel is approximately 96 percent mineral matter, 3 percent water, and 1 percent organic material (**7**), making it the most highly mineralized structure of the body. Enamel is comparatively inert, has neither cells nor cytoplasm, and neither synthesis of new material nor repair of present material occurs after the initial formation.

Dentin is composed of about 70 percent mineral matter, 10 percent water, and approximately 20 percent organic material. Most of the organic matter is collagen, a structural type protein associated with connective tissue. Dentin has the same basic composition as bone. Dentin has cells and is, to a limited extent, metabolically active.

The outer surface of the root is covered by a layer of cementum, a substance not as hard as enamel. Cementum has cells and is an active tissue. At the center of the root is the pulp containing blood, lymph vessels, and nerves. The pulp provides nutrients to the tooth through its vascular components.

The mineral structure of teeth is a complex crystal lattice of hydroxyapatite with calcium and phosphorus as the major components. Other minerals, however, are found in teeth. These elements may replace, in part, the calcium and

TABLE 11.1 AVERAGE TIMES OF THE DEVELOPMENT OF TEETH IN THE HUMAN

PRIMARY DENTITION

Tooth	Calcification Begins		Crown Completed		Eruption		Exfoliation	
	Maxilla (weeks *in utero*)	Mandible (weeks *in utero*)	Mandible (month)	Maxilla (month)	Maxilla (month)	Mandible (month)	Maxilla (year)	Mandible (year)
Central incisor	14	14½	1½	2½	9⅓	7½	6–7	6–7
Lateral incisor	16	16½	2½	3	11	13¼	7–8	7–8
Cuspid	17	17	9	9	19½	19⅔	10–12	9–12
First molar	5	15½	6	5½	15⅔	16	9–11	9–11
Second molar	19	18	11	10	28	26½	10–12	10–12

PERMANENT DENTITION

Tooth	Calcification Begins		Crown Completed		Eruption		Root Completed	
	Maxilla	Mandible	Maxilla (year)	Mandible (year)	Maxilla (year)	Mandible (year)	Maxilla (year)	Mandible (year)
Central incisor	3–4 months	3–4 months	4½	3½	7–7½	6–6½	10–11	8½–10
Lateral incisor	10–12 months	3–4 months	5½	4–4½	8–8½	7¼–7¾	10–12	9½–10½
Cuspid	4–5 months	4–5 months	5½–6½	5½–6	11–11⅔	9¾–10¼	12½–15	12–13½
First premolar	1½–1¾ year	1¾–2 years	6½–7½	6½–7	10–10⅓	10–10¾	12½–14½	12½–14
Second premolar	2–2¼ years	2¼–2½ years	7–8½	7–8	10¾–11¼	10¾–11½	14–15½	14½–15
First molar	32 weeks *in utero*	32 weeks *in utero*	4–4½	3½–4	6–6⅓	6–6¼	9½–11½	10–11½
Second molar	2½–3 years	2½–3 years	7½–8	7–8	12¼–12¾	11¾–12	15–16½	15½–16½
Third molar	7–9 years	8–10 years	12–16	12–16	20½	20–20½	18–25	18–25

Source: From Lowrey (**2**). Reproduced with permission from Lowrey, G. H.: *Growth and Development of Children,* 7th edition. Copyright © 1978 by Year Book Medical Publishers, Inc., Chicago.

TABLE 11.2   ERUPTION AGES IN MONTHS FOR PRIMARY TEETH

		PERCENTILES					
	Early			Average		Late	
	Minimum	10	30	50	70	90	100
Mandibular central incisor	4	5	6	7.8	9	11	17
Maxillary central incisor	5	6	8	9.6	11	12	15
Maxillary lateral incisor	6	7	10	11.5	13	15	21
Mandibular lateral incisor	6	7	11	12.4	14	18	27
Maxillary first molar	8	10	13	15.1	16	20	28
Mandibular first molar	8	10	14	15.7	17	20	29
Mandibular cuspid	8	11	16	18.2	19	24	29
Maxillary cuspid	8	11	17	18.3	20	24	29
Mandibular second molar	8	13	24	26.0	28	31	34
Maxillary second molar	8	13	24	26.2	28	31	34

Source: From Horowitz and Hixon (**6**). Reprinted with permission from *The Nature of Orthodontic Diagnosis* by S. L. Horowitz and E. H. Hixon. Copyright © 1965 by S. L. Horowitz. C. V. Mosby Company, St. Louis, Missouri, 1965.

TABLE 11.3   NORMAL SEQUENCE OF ERUPTION OF THE PERMANENT TEETH

Mandible	Maxilla
1. First molar	2. First molar
3. Central incisor	5. Central incisor
4. Lateral incisor	6. Lateral incisor
7. Cuspid	8. First bicuspid
9. First bicuspid	10. Second bicuspid
11. Second bicuspid	12. Cuspid
13. Second molar	14. Second molar

Source: From Lowrey (**2**). Reproduced with permission from *Growth and Development of Children,* 7th ed., by G. H. Lowrey. Copyright © 1978 by Year Book Medical Publishers, Inc., Chicago.
NOTE: The numbers indicate the usual sequence of eruption.

phosphorus or may be added during mineralization and with the addition of subsequent layers during eruption (**8**).

Numerous reports have appeared on the mineral composition of teeth. One of the more comprehensive analyses in recent years is reported in Table 11.4 and represents analyses of 175 sound permanent teeth from a variety of individuals (**9, 10**).

SALIVA

Saliva bathes the teeth and tissues of the mouth with a continual flow, but the amount may vary from 0.5 to 1.5 ml per minute under usual conditions. Stimulation may cause the flow of saliva to increase up to 5 ml per minute. Saliva is derived

TABLE 11.4 MINERAL COMPOSITION OF ENAMEL AND DENTIN PORTIONS OF PERMANENT TEETH

Mineral	Enamel	Dentin
Macro (percentage of dry weight)		
Calcium	37.1	26.9
Phosphorus	18.1	13.2
Magnesium	0.77	1.45
Sodium	0.72	0.58
Potassium	0.03	0.02
Chlorine	0.78	0.06
Micro (ppm in dry weight)		
Fluorine	104.6	175.6
Iodine	5.6	3.7
Managanese	7.0	5.6
Copper	23.4	13.9
Iron	39.5	42.8
Zinc	185.7	174.7
Selenium	0.5	0.3
Cobalt	34.3	31.8
Aluminum	89.9	64.9
Strontium	285.6	180.1
Lead	45.2	43.3

Source: From Derise, Ritchey, and Furr; and Derise and Ritchey (**9, 10**). Reprinted with permission from N. L. Derise, S. J. Ritchey and A. K. Furr, *Journal of Dental Research 53,* 847, 1974 and *53,* 853, 1974. Copyright © 1974 by the North American Division of the International Association for Dental Research, American Dental Association, Champaign, Illinois.

from several glands and is primarily water, along with sodium, potassium, chloride, carbonate, sulfate, trace elements, and calcium carbonate. Protein, amino acids, mucin, several enzymes, and small amounts of other compounds are also present (**4, 11, 12, 13**). The components of saliva provide an environment that maintains the integrity of the teeth, since dental caries occur very rapidly when saliva is not present (**14**).

ORAL DISEASES

Two major oral diseases affect humans: periodontal disease and dental caries (**15, 16**). Estimates of the incidence of these two problems suggest that approximately 75 percent of the world's people are affected by inflammatory periodontal disease, a chronic inflammation of the periodontal tissues (Figure 11.3). Dental caries affect approximately 90 percent of the population (**4**). Caries is the destruction of the enamel followed by inflammation of the dentin and the tooth pulp (Figure 11.3).

Both dental caries and periodontal disease are influenced by three different

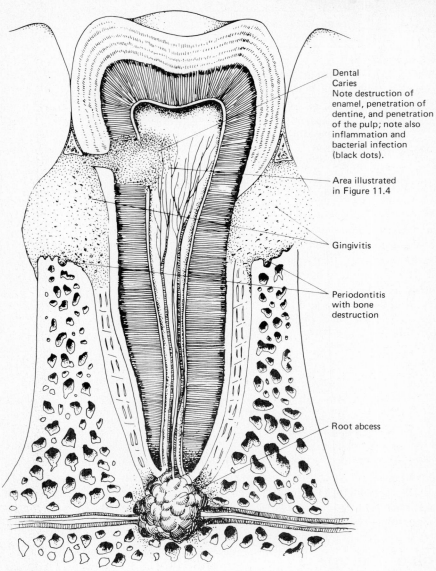

Dental
Caries
Note destruction of
enamel, penetration of
dentine, and penetration
of the pulp; note also
inflammation and
bacterial infection
(black dots).

Area illustrated
in Figure 11.4

Gingivitis

Periodontitis
with bone
destruction

Root abcess

Figure 11.3 *The effects of periodontal disease and caries in a typical tooth.* (*Source:* Reproduced with permission from D. P. DePaola and M. C. Alfano in *Nutrition Today* magazine, May/June 1977. Copyright © 1977 by Nutrition Today, Annapolis, Maryland.)

major factors or types of environmental forces. Each of these is discussed in the following sections (**17**).

Host Factors

This group of influences includes the tooth itself and its development and morphology, the enamel and its potential resistance, the size of the tooth, and the composition and flow of saliva in the mouth. Most people's teeth are susceptible to decay. A few, however, seem to have resistant teeth, but these are rare cases.

Microbial Factor

This factor is often referred to as the "dental plaque." Masses of bacteria come in contact with the oral tissues and the teeth. Dental plaque, or the colony of bacteria on the tooth surface, is the precursor of both caries and periodontal disease (Figure 11.4). Indeed, bacterial plaque is probably the primary cause of periodontal disease. This plaque can become located in the gingival crevice, the space between the surface of the tooth and the gingiva. It can be removed mechanically from the surface of sound teeth by brushing or by the use of dental floss.

Diet or Food

A person's choice of food plays a key role in his or her dental health. Diet is, in fact, probably the major environmental or etiological factor responsible for the very high incidence of dental caries in this country (**18**). The nutrient composition of foods influences the teeth at two stages:

1. *Prior to Eruption*. Nutrients may affect the time of eruption and the composition of the teeth.
2. *After Eruption*. Nutrients may play two different roles, both important in dental health: they may change the formation of dental plaque on the surface of the enamel, or they may alter the rate of flow and the composition of saliva that bathes the teeth (**17**).

The primary effect of food appears to be its role in the development and activity of the plaque microflora. The pattern of food intake, however, is probably as important as the type and amount of food. Dietary habits have changed in the past few years to the extent that the United States is now a country of nibblers rather than meal eaters. This food consumption pattern is a primary cause of dental caries and other oral diseases (**14, 17**). The following discussion provides information about the known, as well as certain postulated, roles of diet in the development of dental caries and periodontal disease.

Periodontal Disease. The ideal growth and development of an infant to maturity includes the development of a healthy mouth and sound teeth. Should these tissues become diseased and/or destroyed, the long-term health of the individual is impaired. Periodontal disease results in the destruction of the gingiva, the tissue that covers the neck of the tooth and the supporting base (**4**).

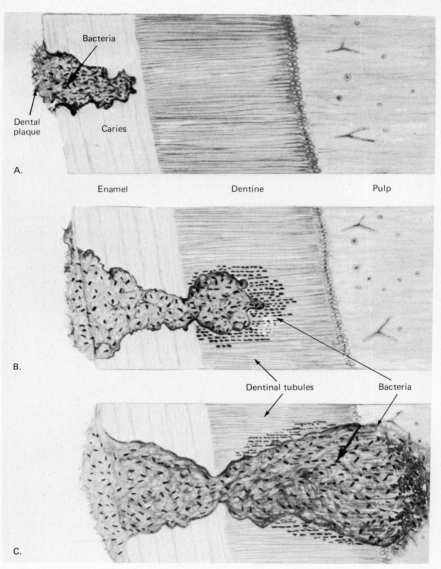

Figure 11.4 *Pathology of a decaying tooth. (A) Dental plaque is a colony of mixed bacteria invaded in an intercellular matrix that adheres to the enamel. The primary mechanism of tooth decay is demineralization by organic acids produced by bacteria of the dental plaque. (B) Once the lesion penetrates the hard enamel layer, it enlarges at a more rapid rate in the relatively softer denture. The bacteria invade the dental tubules and advance toward the pulp chamber. (C) The lesion has penetrated the pulp chamber. (Source:* Reproduced with permission from D. P. DePaola and M. C. Alfano in *Nutrition Today* magazine, May/June 1977. Copyright © 1977 by Nutrition Today, Annapolis, Maryland.)

The periodontal ligament (or the connective tissue by which the tooth is attached to the bone) and the bone that supports the tooth in the jaws (or the alveolar bone) are also affected. Causes of periodontal disease are not clearly known. Bacteria, however, are not the sole cause. Anything that irritates the gums, weakens their resistance to infection or places unusual stress on the supporting structures of the teeth promotes the development of periodontal disease. One such cause is poor oral hygiene that permits collection of food at the gum margins. In the case of periodontal disease, the diet is also important at the systemic level. The effect of nutrition is more pronounced in affecting the general health of the periodontum than is food within the mouth that directly affects the oral tissues. Prevention of periodontal disease is important and includes a well-balanced diet, regular tooth cleansing, and dental care.

Dental Caries. Two major nutritional factors are implicated in the prevention and/or development of dental caries: (1) the role of carbohydrate in the diet and (2) the role of fluoride in lowering the incidence of caries. Other nutrients, including strontium and other trace elements, have been suggested as playing a role in the prevention of caries (**19**), but the evidence for the involvement of these nutrients is not as clear as that for carbohydrate and fluoride.

Role of Carbohydrate. Among the theories advanced concerning the cause of dental caries is one suggesting that bacteria in the mouth ferment carbohydrate and produce organic acids that, in turn, demineralize the tooth enamel. This theory is the one most widely accepted by health professionals. As a result, considerable evidence has been collected to demonstrate the specific role of carbohydrate in the formation of dental caries.

The potential role of sugars or sweets in tooth decay was recognized by Aristotle who wondered about the relationship between soft, sweet figs and damage to the teeth of those who ate them (**14**). Epidemiological evidence suggests that the introduction and increased use of refined foods leads to increased problems with dental caries. Both the Eskimos and the African Masai tribesmen began to have more caries and related problems when refined foods were introduced into their cultures.

The per capita consumption of sugar has increased in the United States since about 1900 (Figure 11.5). This increased consumption of sugars or simple carbohydrates is a contributing factor to the increased incidence of caries (**4**). It is known that restricting sugar can lead to a reduction in the number of caries (**20, 21, 22**). Data from several clinical studies support this concept (Figure 11.6).

Carbohydrates do not all have the same effect in the production of caries (**2**). Studies with both animals and human subjects demonstrate that sucrose is a leading cause of caries, producing an excessive amount of dental plaque. Sucrose produces approximately five times the amount of plaque that glucose does. Other carbohydrates in addition to sucrose can support the production of caries. A comparison of several carbohydrates is made in Figure 11.7 which shows the relative caries-producing properties of these sugars. Caries can result

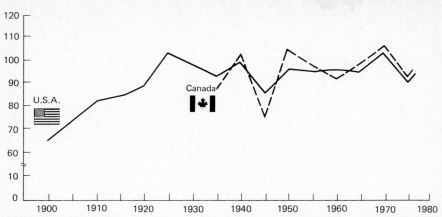

Figure 11.5 *Per capita consumption of sugar in the U. S. and Canada from 1900 to 1976.* (*Source:* Reproduced with permission from D. P. DePaola and M. C. Alfano in *Nutrition Today* magazine, May/June 1977. Copyright © 1977 by Nutrition Today, Annapolis, Maryland.)

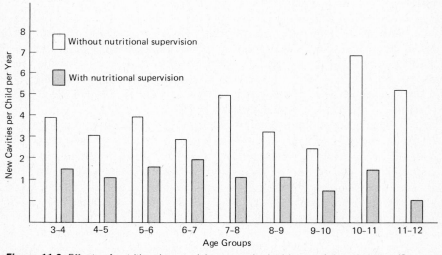

Figure 11.6 *Effects of nutritional supervision upon the incidence of dental caries.* (*Source:* Reproduced with permission from Percy R. Rowe, Ruth L. White and Mark D. Elliott, *Journal of the American Dental Association* 29:39, 1942 **[22]**. Copyright © 1942 by the American Dental Association, Chicago.)

from the consumption of both crude and refined carbohydrates. The form of the sugar actually may be more important than other properties (**24**). If the sugar tends to become stuck to the teeth and gums it likely will be more cariogenic, or caries producing, than a carbohydrate that is easily rinsed away by drink or by the normal flow of saliva. For example, caramel candy, sticky dried fruits, and soft bread may stick to the surface of the tooth. Apples, oranges, cucumbers, and carrots do not stick to the tooth surface and may actually have a natural cleansing effect on teeth as they move between and around teeth during chewing. The physical form of the carbohydrate determines the length of time it will be present in the mouth. This, in turn, affects the length of time the bacteria in the mouth can act on the carbohydrate to produce acids that dissolve the enamel of the tooth.

The pattern and frequency of carbohydrate intake are also important considerations in the development of dental caries (**4**). Actual contact between the teeth and sugars is necessary for caries to form. For example, in experiments with animals, the feeding of sugars by tube to avoid contact with the teeth prevented the development of caries (**14**). Reducing the amount of time carbohydrates come in contact with the teeth or reducing the time in which the sugar remains in the mouth is important in reducing caries development in both children and adults. The avoidance of sticky foods, particularly as between-meal snacks, is essential, since most damage to the teeth is done 15–20 minutes after sweet foods are eaten. Dental caries increase when children do not immediately brush their teeth after eating. Snacking, particularly on sugar in a form that sticks to the teeth and gums, is much more damaging than the intake of sucrose at regular meals (**26**). A recent evaluation of snack type foods indicates that the form of the food was an important characteristic in the appearance of conditions favorable to the development of dental problems (**27**). The influence of snacking on the development of caries has been demonstrated many times (Figure 11.8). An example of a study demonstrating the disappearance of glucose when consumed in different forms or patterns of feeding is provided in Table 11.5.

Role of Fluoride.   Although a relationship between fluorine and dental health was demonstrated in the 1930s the role of fluorine continues to be controversial (**28**). Bitter arguments have divided communities during delibera-

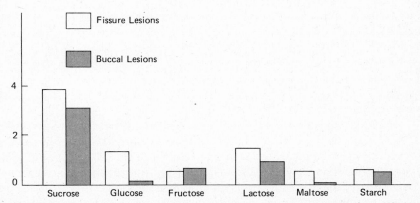

Figure 11.7 *Relative caries producing potential of different carbohydrates.* (*Source:* Reproduced with permission from E. J. Wakeman, J. K. Smith, M. Zeppelin, W. B. Sarles, and P. H. Phillips, *Journal of Dental Research* 27:489, 1948 [**23**]. Copyright © by the American Dental Association, North American Division of the International Association for Dental Research, Champaign, Illinois.)

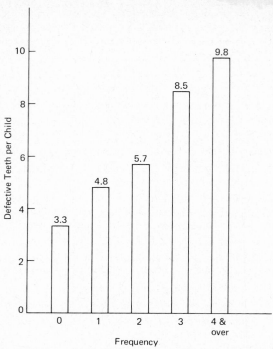

Figure 11.8 *Effect of frequency of snacking on defective teeth in preschool children.* (*Source:* Reproduced with permission from R. L. Weiss and A. H. Trihart in *American Journal of Public Health* 50: 1097, 1960. Copyright © 1960 by the American Public Health Association, Washington, D.C.)

tions about the usefulness of adding fluorine to the public water supply. Clear evidence exists that fluorine can have both positive and negative effects on the dental health of a given population, thus the controversies are based on legitimate concerns. Public health officials, however, recognize that the concentration of fluorine in water is critical. The maximum health benefits, with a minimum risk of problems, are found when there is about 1 ppm of fluoride in the water, and when public water supplies are fluoridated the concentration is usually at this level. At that concentration, a person consuming 1000–1500 ml of water daily would ingest from 1.0–1.5 ppm of fluorine.

Fluoridation of the public water supply at concentrations between 0.8 and 1.2 ppm leads to improved dental health of the population (**31, 32**). The results of a large study relating dental caries and fluoride concentration of the public water supply are shown in Figure 11.9. Studies also demonstrate that when fluorine is removed from the water supply the incidence of dental caries increases, especially in growing children. The benefits of fluoride supplements in the form of liquid sodium fluoride have been demonstrated in children from birth to about 12 years of age (**33**), with residual benefits manifested through fewer carious teeth four or five years later in the same children (**34**).

TABLE 11.5   GLUCOSE CONCENTRATION (MG 100 ML) AT
INTERVALS FOLLOWING INGESTION OF 500 MG OF GLUCOSE

How used	Time in minutes				
	0	2	9	16	30
Eaten (cake)	18	1425	68	20	14
Sucked (wafer)	18	3304	1860	1125	229
Rinsed (solution)	21	832	105	25	17
Chewed (gum base)	23	725	204	144	27

Source: From Vocker (**26**). Reprinted by permission from J. F.
Vocker, *Journal of the American Dental Association 51,* 285, 1955
(**26**). Copyright © 1955 by the American Dental Association, Chicago.

Studies such as those, coupled with other evidence from epidemiological
studies, have led to the recommendation that infants and young children receive
supplements of fluoride (**35**). During the first 6 months of life, infants should
receive fluoride at the level of 0.25 mg daily either in the form of a supplement or in
formula (see Chapter 7). After 6 months, fluoride should be present in commercial
dry cereals or should be provided as a supplement.

The mechanism by which fluoride functions to reduce caries is not precisely
known at the present time (**28**), but the most commonly postulated mechanisms
are these:

1. Fluorine is incorporated into the structure of the tooth, as well as into
   bone, and causes the formation of a stronger, more resistant tooth.
2. Fluorine is taken up by the tooth enamel when applied directly and
   results in a more resistant tooth.

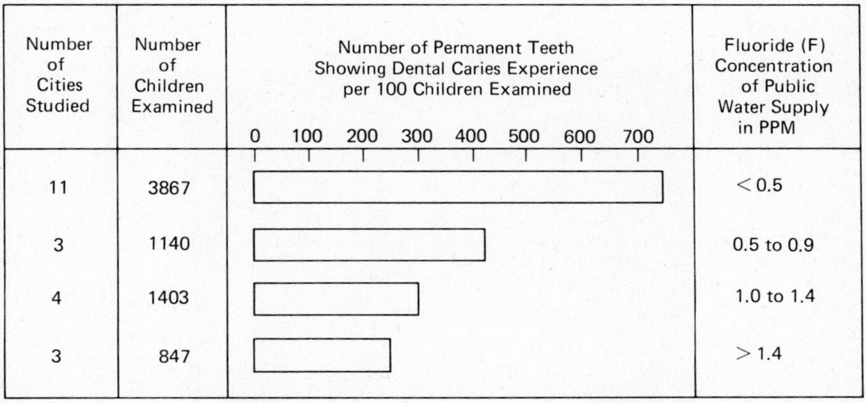

Number of Cities Studied	Number of Children Examined	Number of Permanent Teeth Showing Dental Caries Experience per 100 Children Examined	Fluoride (F) Concentration of Public Water Supply in PPM
11	3867		< 0.5
3	1140		0.5 to 0.9
4	1403		1.0 to 1.4
3	847		> 1.4

Figure 11.9 *Number of dental caries in 12 to 14-year-old children living in different cities
and states with varying concentrations of fluorine in the water supply. (Source:* Reproduced
with permission from H. T. Dean, F. A. Arnold, Jr., and E. Elvore, *Public Health Reports* 57:
1155, 1942 **[36]**. Copyright © Public Health Reports, Rockville, Maryland.)

3. Fluorine may reduce the activity of bacteria in the mouth and lessen the production of acids from carbohydrates.

Fluoride may actually function in more than one of these ways or through a mechanism not yet postulated or explored. Nevertheless, the effect of fluorine on lowering the incidence of dental caries has resulted in the recognition of fluorine as an essential nutrient by the FNB, National Academy of Sciences (**37**). It recommends fluoridation of public water supplies when natural fluorine levels are low.

The teeth become mottled at fluorine concentrations above 2−3 ppm (**38**). The syndrome, initially described in the early 1900s, is most often referred to as "mottled tooth enamel," "mottled teeth," or "dental fluorosis." The problem is not significant in the mild form, but loss of enamel and pitting of the teeth occur in the more severe form (**28**). The condition is characterized further by chalky white patches, scattered irregularly over the surface of the teeth. If severe, there will be excessive wear of the tooth and chewing may be affected. Damage to the enamel is permanent. An example of a mottled tooth is shown in Figure 11.10.

The critical nature of the fluoride concentration as related to fluorosis or mottled teeth is shown in Figure 11.11. The following summarizes the relationship between dental health and concentration of fluorine:

Fluorine Concentration (ppm)	Probable Condition of Population
1.0	Higher incidence of dental caries
0.8−1.2	Lowered incidence of caries
2−3	Very mild mottling
4	Mild mottling
5−6	Moderate mottling
Up to 14	Moderate to severe mottling
7−8	Chance of effects on growth and development

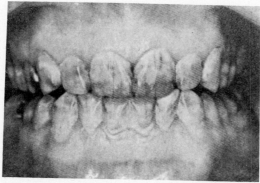

Figure 11.10 *Mottled tooth enamel resulting from high concentrations of fluorine or fluorosis.* (*Source:* Reproduced with permission from *Nutrition in Preventive Dentistry: Science and Practice,* by A. E. Nizel. Copyright © 1972 by W. B. Saunders Co., Philadelphia.)

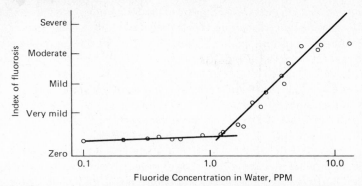

Figure 11.11 *Relationship between dental fluorosis and fluoride concentration.* (*Source:* Reproduced with permission from H. C. Hodge, *Journal of the American Dental Association* 40:436, 1950 **[39]**. Copyright © 1950 by the American Dental Association, Chicago.)

NURSING BOTTLE SYNDROME

"Nursing bottle syndrome" is one of the most crippling conditions involving the teeth and mouth of young children (**40**). The condition results in the decay of all the upper teeth and sometimes the decay of the lower back teeth. The lower front teeth are rarely involved. The condition is caused by the direct contact of the teeth with sugar, honey, and other sweeteners added to water, milk or fruit juice and consumed from a nursing bottle.

In nursing bottle syndrome, the bottle with a sweetened solution is used to pacify the child, often beyond the normal age of nursing or using a bottle for feeding. The major problem occurs when the child falls asleep while sucking the bottle. As long as there is an active sucking motion an increased flow of saliva washes the sugar and other ingredients from the mouth. But when sleep comes and sucking ceases, the saliva flow decreases and the sugar solution accumulates around the teeth. Then, as in the older child or adult, bacterial action produces acids that affect the tooth enamel. The lower front teeth seem not to be affected because the tongue protects them from the pooling of sugar.

The result of nursing bottle syndrome and other damaging activities is that young children have a high incidence of dental caries. By 2 years of age, from 5 to 10 percent of all children have caries; by age 3 or 4, from 40 to 55 percent are affected, and by age 5, about 75 percent have damaged teeth. The incidence of caries in the young child is shown here:

Age (years)	Average Number of Decayed and Filled Teeth
2	0.3
3	1.0
4	2.5
5	4.6
3–4 (nursing bottle syndrome)	> 10.0

Nursing bottle syndrome and other maladies that cause decay and loss of teeth may have serious consequences for the child. Certain of these may have long-term effects causing impairment throughout life. The following are commonly found in nursing bottle syndrome:

1. Pain and discomfort that causes the child to be irritable.
2. A lisp in the speech.
3. Malformation and malocclusion of the permanent teeth.
4. Usual chewing function may become impaired.

Nursing bottle syndrome can be prevented. If at all possible, the bottle should not be used as a pacifier. The child should not be permitted to take a bottle containing a sugar solution to bed and then fall asleep. In those instances when the bottle is used as a pacifier, the solution in it should be plain water or milk. Sugars and sweetened solutions should be avoided.

PREVENTION OF DENTAL DISEASE

The control and prevention of oral disease and dental caries involves numerous essential components (**14**). The following factors are suggested as important in the maintenance of sound oral health:

1. Improvement in the structural quality of the teeth during development through the consumption of an adequate diet to meet general nutritional needs.
2. Treatment of the surfaces of the teeth with fluoride applications during the period of development to increase tooth resistance to acids.
3. Mechanical removal and chemical inhibition of plaque bacteria.
4. Consumption of foods that have less potential for creating an environment conducive to caries formation.
5. Alteration of eating habits to reduce factors that cause caries by reducing the consumption of sweets, particularly between-meal snacks.
6. Consumption of fluoridated water if at all possible.

Dental caries as a general problem can be prevented in the young child. The teeth of the child should be cleaned with a brush or gauze pad after each feeding to remove sticky particles of food and bacterial plaque from the surface of the teeth. The incidence of caries can be lowered by using water with a fluoride concentration of approximately 1 ppm. Lozenges with added fluoride may be useful, particularly if the public water supply is not fluoridated or has a low concentration (less than 0.8 ppm). For children under 3 years of age the lozenge should contain about 0.5 mg of fluoride. For children above 3 years of age, the lozenge may contain 1.0 mg of fluoride. As a means of establishing good dental health habits and repairing minor problems of the teeth, the child should begin regular dental examinations early in life. This practice should be established no later than 2 years of age.

The recognition is increasing that nutrition is an important component in the development of healthy teeth. Dental students are now given information about nutrition and are being taught techniques for applying nutrition knowledge in their relationships with patients (**41, 42**).

SUMMARY

Genetic inheritance can be a determinant of whether teeth are sound or not. In addition, nutrition plays a role in future tooth development, even before birth. Tooth development begins very early in life at approximately the thirty-fourth day of embryonic life. Therefore, a well-balanced diet consumed by the mother is of extreme importance to the normal tooth development of the child. Key nutrients involved in the calcification process are calcium, phosphorus, vitamin D, and vitamin C. Malnutrition during critical periods of growth will alter the development of the teeth.

Nutritional factors govern the health of the teeth following eruption whether present in the mouth or by operating through interior systemic pathways to affect the general health of oral tissue. Some major influences in the oral environment that affect the incidence of dental caries are the oral microorganisms, the carbohydrates the microorganisms must have to multiply and produce tooth-destroying substances, and the amount and composition of the saliva controlled by systemic influences not well understood and beyond individual control. One can reduce tooth decay by altering the diet to include less sticky, tooth-adhering carbohydrates; by reducing the time the teeth are exposed to carbohydrates, especially sucrose; and by a suitable program of tooth cleansing and regular care by a dentist. Proper use of fluorides will also help to decrease the incidence of dental caries. Fluoride intake at levels of about 1 mg per day seem to lower the incidence of dental caries in the growing child.

The decay-producing capabilities of certain foods can be influenced by people's eating habits. For example, the potential for extreme dental decay in the very young child is established when a habit of frequent night bottle feeding is continued beyond a reasonable age. Educational programs directed toward new parents can be particularly effective in preventing tooth decay in the young child. Good nutrition and proper dental care throughout life will promote a healthy oral condition and normal growth and development. The development of sound teeth begins early in life, and the prevention of caries and periodontal disease is a continuous, lifelong process.

STUDY QUESTIONS AND
TOPICS FOR INDIVIDUAL INVESTIGATION

1. Examine the role of food habits in the etiology and in the prevention of dental caries. How might children be educated or trained to lower the incidence of caries? Develop a 30-minute nutrition education program on "Nutrition and Its Value to Dental Health" for use with a kindergarten class. Focus on the causes of dental caries, the importance of oral hygiene, and the nutrients essential for dental health. You might use food models, posters, colorful pictures of foods, puppets, songs, cartoon characters, and so on, to present your main ideas. Include some means of assessing the children's present food habits. Have a tasting party. Introduce the children to tasty, colorful, appealing snack foods conducive to sound dental health. You might include celery stuffed with cheese, cheese dips and vegetable sticks, radishes, wedges of lettuce, carrot and celery sticks, cucumber rings, apples, bananas, grapes, peaches, tangerines, pears, cheese and meat cubes, and crisp crackers. For a beverage serve milk, tomato juice, or unsweetened fruit juices in attractive glasses.

2. Nursing bottle syndrome can be prevented through a timely educational program to new parents. What information would you include in a pamphlet for distribution to parents concerning the relationship of good nutritional habits and sound dental health? You might write to the American Dental Association, 211 East Chicago Avenue, Chicago, Illinois 60611, for a copy of the pamphlet *Nursing Bottle Mouth* or to the American Society of Dentistry for Children, at the same address, for a copy of *A Warning to Parents* to get some ideas on what you may need to include in such a program and to see what is already available in this area.

3. The popularity of incorporating nutritional assessment and counseling in dental care has increased tremendously in the past few years. Why not conduct a survey of dental offices in your locality? A lack of valid nutrition information in some areas has been due to the absence of competent, well-trained nutritionists and dietitians whom the dental health team can contact for advice. Determine the extent to which nutrition counseling is offered through dental offices in your area, techniques used in dental and nutrition counseling, availability of nutritional resources for use by dentists, and so forth.

4. Do you have a sweet tooth? Sugar may be found in some foods that are thought to be sugarless or exist in amounts greater than you expected. Try to find information on the sugar content of your favorite snack foods. Read package labels. Is sugar a major ingredient? Look at the recipes for some common snacking foods, for example, chocolate chip cookies, fudge, fruit pie. How much sugar is there in the whole recipe? How much in one piece or in the amount consumed for an afternoon snack? Where can you make changes in your snacking habits to avoid foods conducive to caries formation?

5. Outline the eruption process and the sequence in which the teeth appear. Why might this process be different for individual children?
6. Relate the role of food to the development of dental plaque.
7. Develop a position defending the fluoridation of public water supplies in a community in which a referendum is scheduled on the issue.

REFERENCES

1. National Institutes of Dental Health. *Nutrition and Dental Health,* Bethesda, Md., 1970.
2. Lowrey, G. H. *Growth and Development of Children,* 7th ed. Year Book Medical Publishers, Inc., Chicago, 1978.
3. Navia, J. M. Nutrition, diet and oral health. Food and Nutrition News, National Livestock and Meat Board 50:3, 1979.
4. De Paola, D. P., and M. C. Alfano. Diet and oral health. *Nutrition Today,* 12:6, 1977.
5. Garn, S. M., A. B. Lewis, and R. S. Kerensky. Genetic, nutritional and maturational correlates of dental development. *Journal of Dental Research,* 44:228, 1965.
6. Horowitz, S. L., and E. H. Hixon. *The Nature of Orthodontic Diagnosis.* Mosby, St. Louis, 1965.
7. Sognnaes, R. F. Dental aspects of the structure and metabolism of mineralized tissues. In *Mineral Metabolism,* Vol. 1B, eds. C. L. Comar and F. Bronner. Academic Press, New York, 1960.
8. Tuttle, W. W., and B. A. Schotteliens. *Textbook of Physiology.* Mosby, St. Louis, 1969.
9. Derise, N. L., S. J. Ritchey, and A. K. Furr. Mineral composition of normal human enamel and dentin and the relation of composition to dental caries. I. Macrominerals and comparison of methods of analyses. *Journal of Dental Research,* 53:847, 1974.
10. Derise, N. L., and S. J. Ritchey. Mineral composition of normal human enamel and dentin and the relation of composition to dental caries: II. Microminerals. *Journal of Dental Research,* 53:853, 1974.
11. Krasse, B. The effect of nutrition on saliva and oral flora. *Sympos. Smed. Nutr. Found,* 3:21, 1965.
12. Darves, C. Effects of diet on salivary secretion and composition. *Journal of Dental Research,* 49:1263, 1970.
13. Caldwell, R. C. The organic components of human salivary secretion. In: *Dental Caries Research,* ed. R. S. Harris. Academic Press, New York, 1968.
14. Nizel, A. E. *Nutrition in Preventive Dentistry: Science and Practice.* Saunders, Philadelphia, 1972.
15. Anonymous. Nutrition and oral health. *Dairy Council Digest,* 49:3, 1978.

16. Navia, J. M. Dental Health: Nutrition's Special Role. *Professional Nutritionist*, Foremost Foods, 1977.

17. Savara, B. S. Nutrition and oral health: prediction of dental caries. *Nutrition News*, National Dairy Council 31, No. 1, 1968.

18. Nizel, A. E. Nutrition and oral problems. *World Review of Nutrition and Dietetics*, 16:227, 1973.

19. Anonymous. Strontium, other trace elements and dental caries. *Nutrition Reviews*, 36:334, 1978.

20. Jay. P. The role of sugar in the etiology of caries. *Journal of the American Dental Association*, 27:293, 1940.

21. Beeks, H. Carbohydrate restriction in the prevention of dental caries using the L. A. count as one index. *Journal of the California Dental Association*, 26:53, 1950.

22. Howe, R. P., R. L. White, and M. D. Elliott. The influence of nutritional supervision on dental caries. *Journal of the American Dental Association*, 29:38, 1942.

23. Wakemann, E. J., J. K. Smith, M. Zepplin, W. B. Sarles, and P. H. Phillips. Microorganisms associated with dental caries in the cotton rat. *Journal of Dental Research*, 27:489, 1948.

24. Konig, K. G., and H. R. Muhlemann. The cariogenicity of refined and unrefined sugars in animal experiments. *Archives of Oral Biology*, 12:1297, 1967.

25. Weiss, R. L., and A. H. Trihart. Between meal eating habits and dental caries experience in preschool children. *American Journal of Public Health*, 50:1097, 1960.

26. Vocker, J. F. Relation of oral biochemistry of sugars to the development of caries. *Journal of the American Dental Association*, 51:285, 1955.

27. Martin, J. B., and C. W. Berry. Cariogenicity of selected processed machine-vended and health food snacks. *Journal of the American Dietetic Association*, 75:159, 1979.

28. Underwood, E. J. *Trace Elements in Human and Animal Nutrition*, 3rd ed. Academic Press, New York, 1971.

29. Cholak, J. Fluorides: A critical review. I. The occurrence of fluoride in air, food and water. *Journal of Occupational Medicine*, 1:501, 1959.

30. Hodge, H. C., and F. A. Smith. *Fluorine Chemistry*, Vol. 4, ed. J. H. Simons. Academic Press, New York, 1965.

31. Clifford, P. A. Report on fluorine. *Journal of the Association of Official Agricultural Chemists*, 28:277, 1945.

32. McClure, F. J. Water fluoridation. The search and the victory. National Institute of Dental Research. Superintendent of Documents, Washington, D.C., 1970.

33. Aasenden, R., and T. C. Peebles. Effects of fluoride supplementation from birth on human deciduous and permanent teeth. *Archives of Oral Biology*, 19:321, 1974.

34. Aasenden, R., and T. C. Peebles. Effects of fluoride supplementation from birth on dental caries and fluorosis in teenaged children. *Archives Oral Biology,* 23:111, 1978.
35. Fomon, S. J., L. J. Filer, T. A. Anderson, and E. E. Ziegler. Recommendations for feeding normal infants. *Pediatrics,* 63:52, 1979.
36. Dean, H. T., F. A. Arnold, Jr., and E. Elvove. Domestic waters and dental caries. V. Additional studies of the relation of fluoride domestic waters to dental experience in 4425 white children age 12−14 years, of 13 cities in four states. *Public Health Report,* 57:115, 1942.
37. Food and Nutrition Board. *Recommended Dietary Allowances,* 8th ed. National Academy of Sciences, Washington, D.C., 1974.
38. American Academy of Pediatrics, Committee on Nutrition. Fluoride as a nutrient. *Pediatrics,* 49:456, 1972.
39. Hodge, H. C. The concentration of fluorides in drinking water to give the point of minimum caries with maximum safety. *Journal of the American Dental Association,* 40:436, 1953.
40. Nizel, A. E. Nutrition News, National Dairy Council, Vol. 38, Chicago, 1975.
41. DePaola, D. P., C. L. Modrow, and J. K. Wittemann. An integrated nutrition education program for dental students. *Journal of Nutrition Education,* 10:160, 1978.
42. Wittemann, J. K., D. P. DePaolo, C. L. Modrow, and J. K. Odom. A strategy for evaluating nutrition counseling skills of dental students. *Journal of Nutrition Education,* 10:164, 1978.

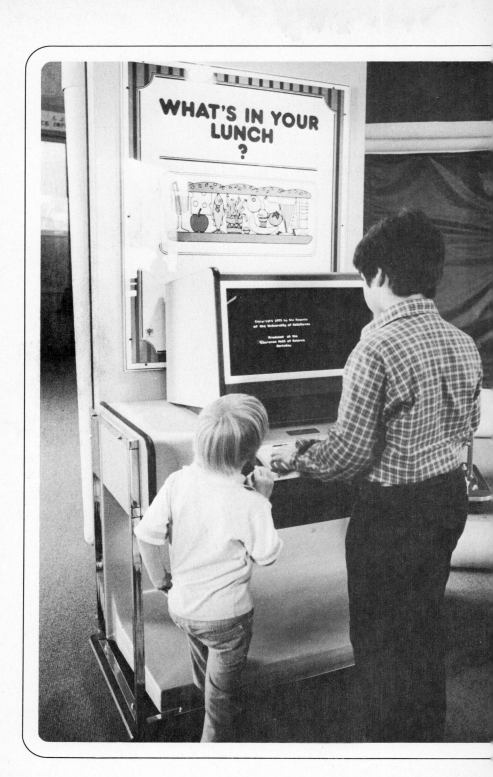

CHAPTER 12

NUTRITION PROGRAMS FOR MOTHER AND CHILD

A 4-year-old is taken to a day care center every morning by his working mother. Along with 20 other boys and girls from homes where both parents work, he is served a nutritious lunch at noon. A fifth grader in another part of the country chooses between three different entrees served by her school at lunchtime. A mother, with her 3-month old daughter, attends a clinic in still another part of the country and is provided with food vouchers to buy nutritious foods for her daughter and herself. What do these people have in common? They exemplify millions of people all over the United States who are participating in programs designed to improve the nutritional status of children and their families.

FOOD PROGRAMS OF THE USDA

Increased sensitivity on the part of the public to the existence of hunger and malnutrition in this country has brought forth new legislation, increased funding and resources, and more general recognition of the plight of millions of people who lack adequate diets (**1**). Over the years many different family assistance programs have existed at the federal, state, and local levels. Prior to the White House Conference on Food, Nutrition, and Health, essentially two existing effective programs provided food assistance to those in need. These included programs administered under the 1935 Commodities Section of Public Law 74-320 (as modified by the Agricultural Act of 1949), and the National School Lunch Act of 1946. Since 1969 the number of children and families receiving help through USDA food assistance programs has increased dramatically. Current federal programs providing food assistance include the School Lunch; School

Breakfast; Special School Milk; Special Nonschool Food Service; Special Supplemental Food Program for Women, Infants, and Children; and Food Stamp programs. The general purpose of such programs is to increase the well-being of children nationwide through better nutrition and to create educational opportunities for the development of sound nutrition habits. Each year child nutrition programs assist schools and other child care institutions across the country to establish, strengthen, and expand food service programs in reaching millions of children.

The Food and Nutrition Service is the agency of USDA that administers food assistance programs. The agency's national headquarters are in Washington, D.C. A series of seven regional offices administer the programs across the country. Figure 12.1 shows the area of each regional office, and office addresses are listed in Table 12.1. Each regional office operates the family and child feeding programs through the appropriate state agency (agricultural, educational, welfare, or health) in its region.

School Lunch Program

The National School Lunch Program, the largest and most comprehensive feeding program in the world, had its beginnings in the 1930s when the federal government distributed surplus foods to schools for use in free lunches (3). In 1943, the USDA began providing cash reimbursements to partially cover the cost of foods purchased locally by any school system. Finally in 1946 the National School Lunch Act was passed establishing a program of cash assistance to schools (4). The stated goal of the National School Lunch Program is to offer lunches of nutritional benefit to students. Through such a program, students should gain a better understanding of nutrition and acquire good food habits for

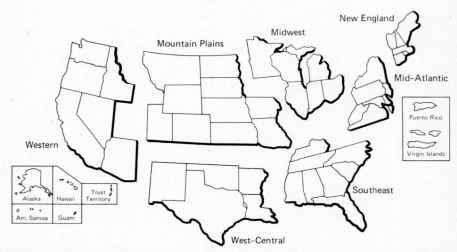

Figure 12.1 *Food and Nutrition Service Regions of the U. S. Department of Agriculture.* (*Source:* From U. S. Department of Agriculture [**2**])

TABLE 12.1 FOOD AND NUTRITION SERVICE REGIONAL OFFICES OF THE USDA

New England Regional Office:
Food and Nutrition Service
U.S. Department of Agriculture
33 North Avenue
Burlington, Mass. 01803
Connecticut, Maine, Massachusetts,
New Hampshire, Rhode Island,
Vermont

Mid-Atlantic Regional Office:
Food and Nutrition Service
U.S. Department of Agriculture
One Vahlsing Center
·Robbinsville, N.J. 08691
Delaware, Maryland, New Jersey,
New York, Pennsylvania, Virginia,
West Virginia, Puerto Rico,
Virgin Islands

Southeast Regional Office:
Food and Nutrition Service
U.S. Department of Agriculture
1100 Spring Street, NW
Atlanta, Ga. 30309
Alabama, Florida, Georgia,
Kentucky, Mississippi, North
Carolina, South Carolina,
Tennessee

Midwest Regional Office:
Food and Nutrition Service
U.S. Department of Agriculture
536 South Clark Street
Chicago, Ill. 60605
Illinois, Indiana, Michigan,
Minnesota, Ohio, Wisconsin

Mountain Plains Regional Office:
Food and Nutrition Service
U.S. Department of Agriculture
2420 W. 26th Avenue, Suite 415-D
Denver, Colo. 80211
Colorado, Iowa, Kansas, Missouri,
Montana, Nebraska, North Dakota,
South Dakota, Utah, Wyoming

Southwest Regional Office:
Food and Nutrition Service
U.S. Department of Agriculture
1100 Commerce Street
Dallas, Tex. 75202
Arkansas, Louisiana, New Mexico,
Oklahoma, Texas

Western Regional Office:
Food and Nutrition Service
U.S. Department of Agriculture
550 Kearny Street
San Francisco, Calif. 94108
Alaska, American Samoa, Arizona,
California, Guam, Hawaii,
Idaho, Nevada, Oregon, Trust
Territories, Washington

Source: From U.S. Department of Agriculture (**2**).

life. Since 1946, the program has grown from 6.5 million children to more than 25 million. The number of schools with operating programs doubled to 90,000 during this time, and 90 percent of American school children now have access to low-cost nutritious school lunches (**5**). Over 40 percent of the lunches are provided free or at a reduced price. The number of participating needy children (those receiving free or reduced price meals) has tripled to 11 million since 1946. However proposed changes in federal support during 1981 may result in dramatic changes.

Schools and child care institutions providing school lunch must conduct the program on a nonprofit basis for all children regardless of race, color, or national origin; furnish free or reduced price meals to any child unable to afford a full price meal without discrimination against or identification of these children; and provide meals that meet an established nutrition criterion (**3**).

The National School Lunch Program regulations require that each fiscal year the secretary of agriculture establish the family size and income criteria to be used in determining eligibility for free or reduced price lunches. In some instances, children from families with incomes greater than the amount specified for free or reduced price meals may be eligible for assistance. Factors considered include unusually high medical bills, home costs, special educational expenses because of abnormal mental or physical conditions of a child or disaster and casualty losses.

The Type A lunch established by USDA supplies approximately one-third of the RDAs set forth by the National Research Council for 10–12-year-old children. Until recently, it included a serving of meat or a meat alternate, fruit and/or vegetables, bread or a suitable equivalent, milk, and butter or fortified margarine (Table 12.2). The Type A lunch pattern is revised periodically to accommodate new information about food consumption, eating patterns, food preferences, and the nutritional needs of children. Local schools are thus provided maximum flexibility to satisfy children's food tastes. Cultural and economic backgrounds of children must be considered when planning for food service, since children tend to prefer familiar foods. For example, pizza, lasagne, or tacos are nutritionally sound if they are served as part of a well-balanced lunch.

Commodity foods, purchased by the federal government on the open market in relation to the supply situation, have long been used in the School Lunch Program (**6**). When too much of one crop appears on the market at once, prices may drop, causing cash returns to farmers to be extremely low. To prevent this, the government buys some of these foods and puts them to use in the School Lunch Program. The individual school's only costs for such commodity items are handling and shipping expenses within the state.

Recently, highly processed or engineered foods have made their appearance in the School Lunch Program (**7, 8**). Engineered foods can offer good nutrition at reduced cost, greater convenience in preparation, improved storage properties, and improved acceptability (**9**). School food service personnel need to be aware of changes in children's dietary habits concerning convenience foods,

---

TABLE 12.2   FOODS INCLUDED IN TYPE A PATTERN LUNCH

- ½ pint of fluid milk
- 2 oz of cooked lean meat, poultry, or fish; or 2 oz of cheese; or one egg; or ½ cup of cooked dry beans or peas; or 4 tablespoons of peanut butter; or an equivalent quantity of any combination of these
- ¾ cup of two or more vegetables or fruits or both
- 1 slice of whole grain or enriched bread or an acceptable bread alternate
- 2 teaspoons butter or fortified margarine

Source: U.S. Department of Agriculture.

as well as nutritional qualities of processed foods so that they can provide these foods in nutritionally balanced lunches.

Several recent changes have been initiated in the School Lunch Program to help schools more adequately meet the nutritional needs of children (**4, 10**). Many schools in the United States do not have kitchen facilities to operate a School Lunch Program, and the concept of "satellite kitchens" was developed to serve such areas. A central kitchen is used to prepare lunches that are then shipped to individual schools, heated, and kept in special ovens or delivered hot to schools immediately before the lunch hour. The satellite kitchen concept enables more children to share in the benefits of nutritious hot lunches.

Recently, the Food and Nutrition Service of USDA conducted a pilot project to develop a computer bank of the numerous recipes used in the School Lunch Program, costed and measured in terms of nutritive value. Such a computer bank would allow local schools to select least-cost menus meeting certain nutritional and palatability standards. This approach to menu planning should eventually result in an overall reduction in food costs and at the same time give greater assurance of meeting children's nutritional requirements (**11, 12**).

Universal concern about world food supplies and conservation of resources has increased awareness of the problem of food waste associated with the School Lunch Program (**13, 14**). In 1975, USDA conducted a review of the Type A pattern. This review and recent legislation resulted in some proposed changes in the Type A pattern (**15, 16**). Table 12.3 shows differences in the current and proposed requirements. Some of these changes have already been enacted. The adjustment of serving sizes compatible with the stage of growth and development of children at different age levels should diminish plate waste without endangering the nutritional quality of school lunches. Also, senior high school students, offered the complete Type A lunch, need only choose three of the five required items. The requirements for butter or fortified margarine with each meal essentially has been eliminated. Additional changes in the lunch pattern are being considered, including defining minimum portions of food to meet the nutritional requirements of five age groups. Reduced amounts of food would be served to younger children under this proposal. Lunch could also be served at two sittings that together would meet lunch pattern requirements in order to accommodate those youngsters with extremely small appetites. Growing children with increased appetites and nutrient needs would be offered the choice of more food. Bread alternates would be expanded to include enriched or whole grain rice and macaroni, noodles, and other pasta products. Students would be offered the choice of unflavored fluid low-fat, skim, or buttermilk, in addition to unflavored or flavored whole milk. This provision is aimed at keeping dietary fat at a moderate level for students who need to control fat intake. Schools would be required to involve students in their school lunch programs through activities such as menu planning, program promotion, and related activities. If enacted, the proposed changes should have the following effect on the School Lunch Program (Table 12.4). These and other proposed changes will be tested and revised in accordance with public reaction. The USDA is also continually searching for alterna-

TABLE 12.3 NATIONAL SCHOOL LUNCH PROGRAMS

CURRENT REQUIREMENTS AND RECOMMENDATIONS

	Elementary School		Secondary School
	6–10	10–12	12–18
Meat and/or alternate	2 oz	2 oz	3 oz
Vegetable and/or fruit	¾ cup	¾ cup	1 to 1½ cups
Bread	1 slice	1 slice	1–3 slices
Fluid milk	½ pint	½ pint	½ pint
Butter or fortified margarine			

PROPOSED REQUIREMENTS

	Elementary School		Secondary School
	Age 6–9	9–12	12 and over
Meat and/or alternate	1½ oz	2 oz	3 oz
Vegetable and/or fruit (at least 2 kinds)	½ cup	¾ cup	¾ cup
Bread and/or alternate	8 servings per week	8 servings per week	10 servings per week
Fluid milk	¾ cup	½ pint	½ pint

Source: U.S. Department of Agriculture, Food and Nutrition 7:11, 1977 (**15**).

TABLE 12.4 NATIONAL SCHOOL LUNCH
PROGRAM EFFECT OF CHANGES IN PROPOSED PATTERN

Current type A pattern	Changes	Results
1. One required lunch pattern with recommendations for various age groups	Lunch patterns required for various age groups.	Makes portion sizes more suitable for each age group
2. Based on RDA and dietary consumption data that are outdated	Reflects changes in dietary consumption habits and more recent RDA (1974)	Establishes minimum serving sizes designed to meet the nutritional goal
3. Bread requirement specified on daily basis	Bread/bread alternate requirement specified on a weekly basis. Now can include rice and pasta	Increases menu flexibility; reflects food preferences and cultural habits
4. All students required to accept minimum portion sizes	Children 12 years and older may take smaller portion sizes	Minimizes plate waste; increases child's independence in food selection

Source: U.S. Department of Agriculture, Food and Nutrition 7:11, 1977 (**15**).

394

tives to the Type A lunch pattern. The feasibility of a "nutrient standard" approach to menu planning has been considered. Such an approach allows for the planning of menus to meet a predetermined nutrient level rather than a food pattern made up of specific types and amounts of foods.

It is difficult to measure the direct cause-and-effect relationship between hunger and behavior or performance in school. Nutritionists, however, believe that the School Lunch Program, as it has evolved to the present and will continue to change in the future, is a positive influence on the behavior and learning capacity of the nation's children.

School Breakfast Program

Eating breakfast at school may be a new idea for some children, but for others it is something they have been doing for years. In 1966 an amendment to the Child Nutrition Act authorized federal cash assistance for a school breakfast program on a pilot basis (**3, 4**). The program originally was conceived to accommodate those children from homes where working mothers left the home before the children had breakfast, low-income homes where a nutritionally adequate breakfast was not always a financial possibility, and areas where children were forced to travel long distances to school. The school breakfast program was not meant to be in competition with or replace a breakfast served at home. School districts were judged eligible for the program on the basis of economy and time and distance of bus travel to school. The pilot program was patterned after the School Lunch Program to meet specified nutrition standards and provide free or reduced-price breakfasts to particularly needy children. Orange juice, cereal, French toast, scrambled eggs and toast, and milk are among the foods served in the breakfast program (Table 12.5).

Teachers note that the school breakfast program results in less dragging and drowsiness in the late morning hours in those children who participate (**17, 18**). A nutrition awareness campaign associated with school breakfast has encouraged some children, not previously accustomed to doing so, to start eating breakfast at home. The Child Nutrition Legislation of October 1975 authorized the School Breakfast Program as a permanent federal program. It was to be made available to all schools throughout the United States if the individual schools chose to participate in the program.

TABLE 12.5 FOODS INCLUDED IN SCHOOL BREAKFAST

- Fruit or juice daily
- Milk daily
- Bread or cereal daily
- Protein-rich foods as often as possible

Source: U.S. Department of Agriculture.

Special Milk Program

In the 1940s a federally subsidized school milk program existed, known as the Penny Milk Program (**3**). This program supplied ½ pint of whole milk daily to supplement the meals of children receiving inadequate diets at home. In 1954 Congress established a Special School Milk Program enabling the USDA to reimburse schools for milk served in addition to that available with the Type A lunch (**4**). The Special Milk Program was incorporated into the Child Nutrition Act in 1966 (**4**). For some time the program was discontinued in those schools with school lunch and/or breakfast programs and was, therefore, available only where no other food service program was in operation. In low-income areas, especially, some children may bring a bag-lunch from home rather than participate in the School Lunch Program. For such children, milk offers an excellent nutritional supplement to their carried lunch. To meet this need, the Special Milk Program is now available in schools with other food service programs.

Special Nonschool Food Service Program

In 1968 an amendment to the National School Lunch Act provided for the Special Food Service Program for Children (**4**). This legislation made federal cash and food assistance available for both preschool and school-age children in nonschool, nonresidential situations. These included public and nonprofit private institutions and group activities such as day care centers, summer day camps, and other recreational programs. The Child Care Food Program began in 1968 in areas of economic need and with high concentrations of working mothers. In 1975 legislation extended eligibility to all public or nonprofit licensed day care centers (**19**). The 1975 legislation also opened participation to family and group day care homes.

The main purpose of the program is to enable states and local communities to improve the nutritional status of preschool and school-age children by providing nutritious meals, including breakfast and/or lunch and/or dinner and/or in-between-meal supplements (Table 12.6). The program is administered through

TABLE 12.6 FOODS INCLUDED IN SPECIAL NONSCHOOL FOOD SERVICE PROGRAM	
Breakfast	● Milk
	● Fruit or juice
	● Bread or cereal
Lunch or supper	● Milk
	● Meat or other protein-rich food
	● Two or more vegetables or fruit
	● Bread
	● Butter or margarine
Supplemental food between meals	● Milk
	● Fruit or vegetable juice
	● Bread or cereal

Source: U.S. Department of Agriculture.

USDA which donates food and financial aid up to 75 percent of the cost to buy and/or rent necessary food service equipment. Meals served through this program must meet minimum nutritional requirements established by the USDA.

The Summer Food Service Program for Children (**19**) spans the gap in the school nutrition programs by providing meals during extended school vacation periods. Sponsors serve nutritious meals at recreation sites, schools, camps, and other convenient locations.

Children age 18 and younger and living in areas of economic need are eligible for the program. The Summer Food Service Program for Children operates during the summer or any vacation period longer than three weeks in districts with continuous school year calendars.

Any public, or private nonprofit, nonresidential institution may sponsor the program in areas where at least one-third of the children are eligible for free or reduced-price school meals. Camps may also sponsor summer food services and be reimbursed for meals served to economically needy children. Examples of sponsoring agencies include units of county and municipal school systems, recreation departments, social service organizations, and churches.

All meals are served without charge to eligible children. The USDA reimburses sponsors for the operating cost of the food service up to a specified maximum rate for each meal provided. In addition, sponsors are reimbursed for planning, operating, and supervising expenses.

FOOD PROGRAMS FOR MOTHERS AND CHILDREN

The USDA has two programs to meet the special needs of low-income mothers and children (**2**). One is the Special Supplemental Food Program for Women, Infants, and Children, commonly known as WIC. The other is the Commodity Supplemental Food Program (CSFP).

As a result of the Ten-State Nutrition Survey and Senate hearings, the need for a supplemental food program became evident to meet the needs of pregnant and nursing women, infants, and young children. Supplemental nutrition to these groups is recognized as having potential lifelong beneficial effects on the health and development of the nation's young people. In 1972 an amendment to the Child Nutrition Act resulted in a special supplemental food program (WIC) designed to curb malnutrition in low-income, nutritionally at-risk mothers, infants, and children (**21**). A pilot program was initiated in 1974 to help low-income women provide nourishing foods both for themselves and their children during the critical early years.

The WIC program is administered at the state and local levels by state departments of health with funds granted by the USDA at the federal level (**22**). The program operates through health clinics serving low-income areas, providing special foods to pregnant and lactating women, infants, and children up to 5 years of age. Individuals who are determined to be at risk nutritionally by nutritionists and health professionals and who cannot afford to purchase an adequate diet are eligible. The foods supplied are generally high in protein, calcium, iron, and vitamins A and D. They include iron-enriched formula and cereal, whole fluid milk, and vitamin C-rich fruit juices for infants (Table 12.7); whole fluid milk, evaporated or skim milk, low fat or nonfat dry milk, cheese, iron-fortified cereals, fruit and vegetable juices rich in vitamin C, products rich in vitamin A and D, and eggs for mothers and children 1–5 years of age (Table 12.8). Participants receive different combinations of these foods, depending on their particular needs. Supplemental foods are distributed at health clinics, or food vouchers that are redeemable at authorized food stores may be issued.

Nutrition education must accompany the distribution of foods if the WIC program is to be effective in improving the nutritional status of participants. Legislation was passed in 1975 that mandated that nutrition education must be an integral part of every WIC program to insure that the program would positively affect food habits. State agency offices are responsible for planning, directing, and coordinating the nutrition education component of the program under the supervision of a nutritionist or dietitian. Nutrition education material presented must be compatible with the recipient's level of understanding, and take into account socioeconomic, educational, cultural, and other environmental factors. Lectures, films, newspaper articles, radio, TV, leaflets, posters, and one-to-one instruction methods are all used to present information on the importance of proper diet and eating habits relevant in terms of language, lifestyles, and food practices of participants.

The WIC program is anticipated to have a positive effect on the infant mortality rate in some areas of the country and on the level of knowledge about proper food and nutrition practices and health care. The nutritional status of participants can be expected to improve, since the program provides essentially 100 percent of the RDAs for infants and up to 35 percent or more of key nutrients to mothers pre- and postnatally. Although the special supplemental foods are of inestimable value, the program provides additional benefits that may be equally

---

TABLE 12.7   FOOD LIST—INFANTS

Monthly Allowance

1. Infant formula (31 13-oz cans)
   These brands are allowed
   Enfamil with Iron
   Similac with Iron
   SMA with Iron
2. Dry infant cereal (3 8-oz boxes) any brand
3. Infant fruit juice (15 4-oz cans or 92 fluid oz of single strength juice), any brand
   Whole fluid milk—beginning at age 6 months, may be substituted for formula at rate of 1 qt of whole milk per 13 fluid oz of concentrated formula
   Evaporated milk—at 6 months may be substituted for whole milk at rate of 13-oz can per quart of whole milk or can of formula

---

Source: U.S. Department of Agriculture.
NOTE: The food is planned to meet individual needs. The foregoing is the maximum monthly allowance. A nursing mother may receive the cereal and juice for her baby with only part or no formula. Likewise, cereal and juice can be started at the age recommended by the physician.

TABLE 12.8   FOOD LIST—WOMEN AND CHILDREN

Monthly Allowance

1. Milk (28 qt per month)—whole, skim, low-fat milk or buttermilk; **or**
   Instant nonfat dry milk (5-qt box)—may substitute at rate of 1 lb per 5 qt milk; **or**
   Evaporated milk (13-oz can)—substitute at rate of one can per quart of whole milk; **or**
   Cheese (1 lb) natural Cheddar, Monterey Jack, Colby—may substitute for whole milk at
   rate of 1 lb per 3 qt
2. Eggs (1 dozen)—large, any brand, 2½ dozen per month
3. Fruit juice (46-oz can)—these juices are allowed:
   Orange juice, any brand
   Grapefruit juice, any brand
   Orange-grapefruit, any brand
   Tomato juice, Campbell's Homestyle, or Del Monte
   Frozen juices (12 6-oz cans monthly)—these are allowed:
   Orange or grapefruit, any brand
   Pineapple, Dole Concentrate
4. Cereal (36-oz dry cereal monthly)
Bucwheats	Kellogg's Concentrate
Total	Fortified Oat Flakes
Corn Total	Cream of Wheat
Product 19	Post 40% Bran Flakes

   Must have 28 mg iron per 100 gm of cereal

Source: U.S. Department of Agriculture.

as important. The WIC program is not simply another food assistance program. Rather, the program's efforts are coupled with those of the local health department. This valuable aspect means that WIC serves as an incentive in encouraging women to visit health centers for important prenatal care. Diseases or problems that might otherwise have gone unnoticed are being detected, and positive changes in patient attitudes and health habits noted.

The Commodity Supplemental Food Program distributes USDA-donated foods to low-income women and children certified by local health agencies. Those eligible include infants, children up to age 6, and pregnant or breastfeeding women vulnerable to malnutrition. To take part in the CSFP, women and children must be determined to be in nutritional need. In addition, they must qualify for benefits under an existing federal, state, or local food, health, or welfare program for low-income people.

Participating women and children get prescribed food items that they pick up at a distribution facility. Foods available through the Commodity Supplemental Food Program include infant formula or evaporated milk and corn syrup blend; instant, nonfat dry milk; instant mashed potatoes; enriched quick-cooking farina; egg mix; peanut butter; canned boned chicken or turkey or canned beef with natural juices; canned fruit and vegetable juices; canned vegetables; and canned fruits.

The CSFP now serves approximately 100,000 people monthly in 11 states and the District of Columbia. Nutrition education is a vital part of the program.

COMMODITY DISTRIBUTION PROGRAM

Since the mid-1930s the Commodity Distribution Program providing food assistance to low-income families has varied in size and scope. A commodity distribution program consists essentially of the distribution of supplemental enriched and/or fortified foods to low-income families. In 1960 a revival of the food stamp approach meant a general decrease in participation in commodity distribution programs. Food stamps, first used in 1939–1943, increased food purchasing power by giving money normally spent for food in exchange for food stamps of higher monetary value. In 1961 the Food Stamp Program was initiated on a pilot basis, and the Food Stamp Act was passed in 1964. Localities theoretically can select which of the two programs they will use to provide food assistance. Most areas of the country have transferred from commodity distribution to the Food Stamp Program. In the early 1970s over two-thirds of the counties in the United States were using the Food Stamp Program (Figure 12.2).

FOOD STAMP PROGRAM

The Food Stamp Program that is known today had its beginnings in the food assistance programs of the depression. To help both farmers and consumers during that time, the federal government distributed surplus foods to hungry people all across the country. In the late 1930s a Food Stamp Plan similar to the

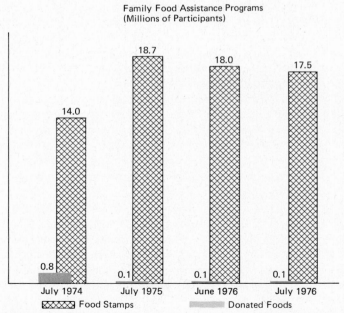

Family Food Assistance Programs
(Millions of Participants)

18.7   18.0   17.5   14.0   0.8   0.1   0.1   0.1

July 1974   July 1975   June 1976   July 1976

Food Stamps   Donated Foods

Figure 12.2 Family food assistance programs. (*Source:* U. S. Department of Agriculture [**23**])

one in use now evolved. Under this plan, families exchanged money for stamps of equal value to purchase regular food items. In addition they received stamps to buy certain surplus foods at retail stores. This program terminated in 1943 when World War II reduced food surpluses and created new jobs. In the mid-1950s certain areas of the country reestablished a system for distributing surplus foods to needy individuals. As a result interest in a food stamp program increased. In 1961 President John F. Kennedy directed the USDA to establish a new food stamp program on a pilot basis, and by 1964 the program was in operation in 43 project areas. The Food Stamp Act of 1964 established the Food Stamp Program as a permanent program.

The Food Stamp Program enables low-income families to buy more food of greater nutritional value than their income level would normally permit. Based on family size, net monthly income, and other factors, participants obtain free food stamps or pay a small amount of money for food stamps. These stamps can then be used in certain food stores to purchase more food than the family would have received if the food had been paid for directly. A household voluntarily fills out a form listing all its resources, income, and expenses. These forms are then evaluated to determine if the household is eligible to receive or purchase food stamps. Households with a net monthly income of approximately $20 or less per member may receive food stamp coupons without paying any money. Others may "purchase" food stamps. The purchase price varies with the net income of the household, increasing as income increases. In no case does it amount to more than 30 percent of the household's net income or take-home pay. Food stamps can be used at approved food stores to purchase food for home consumption only. In essence they supply a family with greater purchasing power than it effectively has and, it is hoped, improve the nutritional status of family members by supplying nutritious foods in greater variety and larger amounts than would otherwise be possible.

In September 1977, the Food Stamp Act of 1977 (**24**) passed, making major reforms in the Food Stamp Program, simplifying program administration and making it easier for eligible people to participate. Under the new program, the USDA must also develop education materials to help people with low reading levels understand the relationship between diet and health and how to buy and prepare nutritious, economical meals.

NUTRITION EDUCATION IN GOVERNMENT FEEDING PROGRAMS

Simply making additional money available is not assurance that people will learn to use it wisely (**8**). Evidence that income is a major factor in determining nutritional status is strong, but increased income, years of schooling, or amount of money spent on food alone do not guarantee an adequate diet. Massive numbers of Americans are eating improperly. This is not because they cannot afford a better diet but because they are ignorant of what is needed to keep themselves healthy. Some are simply unwilling to apply the information they do have. A problem exists because a major emphasis in many nutrition programs is placed on supplying nutrition facts rather than concentrating on ways in which individuals can use these facts to develop and maintain good eating habits (**25**). Effective nutrition education components are long overdue in many of the present food assistance programs (**26**). The nutrition education of parents and the establishment of good food habits in children is essential (**27, 28**). Supplemental food programs offer excellent opportunities for providing this education. When positive, long-term changes in the feeding patterns of recipients are being considered, nutrition education is as important as the supplemental food itself. It must be carried out at all levels by government, industry, mass media, and within the family unit (**29**).

Nutrition education must be a high priority in all child nutrition programs (**30**). Although the original act of Congress that created school feeding programs has as a major aim the teaching of nutrition and the formation of good eating habits, in practice, nutrition education is lacking in most school lunchrooms. The school food service programs have excellent potential for becoming important educational tools if used for that purpose (**31, 32**). In many areas, however, such programs are merely feeding operations. Until children participating in these programs have a sound knowledge of and a positive attitude about the importance of nutrition to health, significant improvements in the development of good food habits cannot be expected.

Too often schoolchildren are told what to eat without being properly motivated to do so. As nutrition educators we need to create a desire in children to change their food habits (if necessary) and develop habits conducive to good health. The concepts of nutrition will become part of one's thinking only when the education given guides the learner to see relationships between nutrition facts and his or her own experience. People knowledgeable in nutrition need to speak in simple, warm, and human terms to students to further the kind of major breakthrough needed. The learner's motivation is the key to his or her willingness to learn. Students' needs, wants, drives, and concerns must be the central focus in their education (**33**). Maslow's framework for analyzing human motivation provides useful guidance for the nutrition educator (**34**). Maslow suggests that man's needs arrange themselves on a hierarchy and that one need must be reasonably satisfied before the need at the next level emerges. Needs are arranged as follows: physiological needs (hunger and thirst); safety needs (security); love needs (affection, acceptance); esteem needs (self-respect, recognition by others); and self-actualization (self-fulfillment). Strategies to arouse motivation are too seldom applied to the real life setting of the school cafeteria. Although no one bag of motivational tricks can be used to induce people to behave in desirable ways, several schools throughout the country are trying innovative techniques to encourage student interest in good nutrition and thereby increase participation in the school lunch program (**35–37**).

Some schools are motivating students by involving them in the actual planning of menus and the preparation, service and cleanup of school meals. Others are organizing student "taste panels" in which groups of students taste unusual foods or try out new recipes. The students then discuss these foods with their classmates who are encouraged to try new foods on the lunch line. Schools in some states set up their cafeteria lines to resemble short-order restaurants. The fast-food lunch, based on the Type A pattern, is proving to be extremely popular. Still other schools offer a choice of several entrees to students. Some devise build-your-own sandwich lines. One school system adopted a smorgasbord approach. Student servers in colorful smocks hand out silver and plates to fellow students who then help themselves to a variety of foods all meeting Type A requirements. These can be Mexican food, soul food, chicken and rice seasoned in the Puerto Rican style, and even chow mein and noodles straight from Chinatown traditions. Serving style can vary in other ways. Family style service is well accepted in some elementary schools. Popular with some students is the practice of serving a complete box-packed Type A lunch that can be eaten out of doors.

Many possibilities exist for using school feeding programs as a laboratory to teach nutrition (**32**). Individual schools throughout the country are continually seeking and developing effective ways to involve school food service personnel beyond the food preparation and serving stages (**38–43**). Those who plan school menus, purchase, prepare, and then serve food to children and instructors who teach nutrition principles are working together to bring about positive change in some areas (**44**). Theories of good nutrition learned in the classroom can then be directly related to the learning and development of constructive food habits in the school cafeteria (**45**).

Recently, the federal government intensified its efforts to develop nutrition education along with supplemental feeding programs (**16**). Both the USDA and the Department of Health, Education, and Welfare (now Health and Human Services) provide grant money for the development of nutrition education curriculum for elementary and secondary schools. In 1977 legislation to revise and expand child nutrition programs established specific guidelines for nutrition education programs. A firm commitment to nutrition education emphasizes support for the concept of preventative health care in child nutrition programs.

RELIABLE SOURCES OF NUTRITION INFORMATION

A question nutritionists are frequently asked is "Where can I go to find reliable information about nutrition?" The general public is confused by the vast number of paperback books, newspapers, and magazine articles, all promoting various, often conflicting, views of what good nutrition really is. Books with catchy titles and promises of the panacea for the ills of humankind have a great deal of popular appeal and frequently become best-sellers. As the number of resources dealing with nutrition and health care increases, both professionals and lay people need help in evaluating and determining which of these sources are dependable and which are not. Nutritionists need to assume a role of leadership in acquainting the public with sound nutrition information and with sources of where this information can be obtained.

Many channels are available to provide reliable nutrition information to the large numbers of people who do consume inadequate diets. Federal and state government agencies and various professional organizations continually battle against false and misleading information. The government does not have the authority to suppress the publication of books or other sources of misleading information. It, therefore, becomes essential for the general public to be better educated and aware of what reliable information is and where it can be obtained.

Health departments in some states have compiled lists of available nutrition books. They state which books they would recommend as accurate in an effort to increase public knowledge and protect people from misleading claims and harmful diets or food fads. Much nutrition information also can be found in bookstores operated by Government Printing Offices in many cities. These carry numerous books and pamphlets developed by government agencies and can supply current lists of most government publications. Other reliable sources of nutrition information include professional nutritionists who teach and carry out research programs; a variety of government agencies operating at the local, state, and federal levels; and numerous private and professional organizations that offer nutrition information as a public service. In the following pages the nutrition-related activities of some of these organizations are discussed. A more complete list of companies or organizations that provide free and/or inexpensive reliable education materials in the area of foods, nutrition, and health is presented in Table 12.9.

Government Agencies

USDA. The Consumer and Food Economics Institute is responsible for a national program of basic and applied research designed to improve the diets of families. The Institute has prepared many research-based guidance materials for use in nutrition education programs. Materials provided include food plans to help families with preschool and school-age children select affordable, nutritious, and satisfying meals. The Institute also cooperates with the Food and Nutrition Service, USDA, to develop special materials for use in child feeding programs and publishes *Nutrition Program News,* providing nutrition education information for all population groups, including children and youth.

The Agricultural Research Service, USDA, conducts a research program to provide a sound basis for dietary recommendations for the average person.

The Food and Nutrition Service is a government agency developed in 1969 to administer the various federal food programs in cooperation with state agencies. The food programs administered by the Food and Nutrition Service include family-oriented programs such as the Commodity Distribution and Food Stamp Program and the various child nutrition programs.

Rising food costs, an increased awareness about nutrition, the availability of new food products, and changing lifestyles all intensify the need for more knowledge about human nutrition throughout the country. The Smith Lever Act of 1914 authorized the USDA through the Cooperative Extension Service of land-grant colleges to give instruction and practical demonstrations in agriculture,

TABLE 12.9 RELIABLE SOURCES OF NUTRITION INFORMATION

A. U.S. Government
  1. U.S. Department of Agriculture
      Agriculture Research Service
      - Consumer and Food Economics Institute
        Federal Center Building
        Hyattsville, Md. 20782
      - Human Nutrition Research Laboratories
        Agricultural Research Center
        Beltsville, Md. 20705
      - Extension Service
        USDA
        Room 5038, South Building
        Washington, D.C. 20250
      - Food and Nutrition Service
        USDA
        Washington, D.C. 20250
  2. U.S. Department of Health and Human Services
      Washington, D.C. 20204
  3. U.S. Government Printing Office
      Superintendent of Documents
      Washington, D.C. 20204

B. Professional Organizations
  - American Academy of Pediatrics
    P.O. Box 1034
    Evanston, Ill. 60204
  - American Dental Association
    211 East Chicago Avenue
    Chicago, Ill. 60611
  - American Dietetic Association
    620 North Michigan Avenue
    Chicago, Ill. 60611
  - American Home Economics Association
    2010 Massachusetts Avenue, NW
    Washington, D.C. 20036
  - American Medical Association
    Section of Nutrition Information
    535 North Dearborn Street
    Chicago, Ill. 60610
  - The American National Red Cross
    Food and Nutrition Consultant
    National Headquarters
    Washington, D.C. 20006
  - Food and Agriculture Organizations of the United Nations
    North American Regional Office
    1325 C Street, SW
    Washington, D.C. 20025
  - Food and Nutrition Board
    National Academy of Sciences
    2101 Constitution Avenue, NW
    Washington, D.C. 20418

(Continued)

TABLE 12.9 *(Continued)*

- The Food and Nutrition Information and Educational Materials Center
  National Agriculture Library
  10301 Baltimore Boulevard, Room 304
  Beltsville, Md. 20705
- National Dairy Council
  111 North Canal Street
  Chicago, Ill. 60606
- The National Foundation-March of Dimes
  1275 Mamaroneck Ave.,
  White Plains, N.Y. 10605
- Nutrition Today
  101 Ridgely Avenue
  P.O. Box 465
  Annapolis, Md. 21404
- Society for Nutrition Education
  2140 Shattuck Avenue, Suite 1110
  Berkeley, Calif. 94704

C. Trade Organizations

- Campbell Soup Company
  Food Service Products Division
  375 Memorial Avenue
  Camden, N.J. 08101
- Del Monte Kitchens
  Del Monte Corporation
  215 Fremont Street
  San Francisco, Calif. 94119
- General Mills
  P.O. Box 113
  Minneapolis, Minn. 55440
- Gerber Products Company
  445 State Street
  Fremont, Mich. 49412
- H. J. Heinz
  Consumer Relations
  Post Office Box 57
  Pittsburgh, Pa. 15230
- Hunt Wesson Foods
  Educational Services
  1645 West Valencia Drive
  Fullerton, Calif. 92634
- Kellogg Company
  Department of Home Economics Services
  Battle Creek, Mich. 49016
- Mead Johnson Nutritionals
  2404 Pennsylvania Avenue
  Evansville, Ind. 47721

Source: Compiled by the authors.

home economics, and related areas to those not attending land-grant colleges. The Cooperative Extension Service helps families and individuals identify and solve their home and community problems through the use of research of USDA and the state land-grant colleges. The Extension Service, through a network of federal, state, and county offices, has staff carrying out education programs in almost all counties of the United States. Programs are directed to people of all ages and socioeconomic levels and are conducted through trained volunteer leaders, Extension technicians, and Extension agents using mass media and group teaching techniques. All state Extension programs include nutrition education. The Extension Service is concerned with the development of skills and application of knowledge by individuals and families to help them enjoy improved health through better nutrition.

In the mid-sixties, an increasing consciousness of adverse conditions that affected large numbers of people in this country resulted in the identification of inadequate nutrition as a major area of concern. In 1968 the Extension Service developed the Expanded Food and Nutrition Education Program (EFNEP) in an attempt to improve the dietary intake of low-income families by teaching good nutrition practices on a one-to-one basis in the home or in small groups (**8**). Counties selected to participate in the EFNEP program are chosen according to guidelines established by the USDA and the Federal Extension Service. Factors involved in selection include the percentage of low-income families in the area, the willingness of the locality to support the program, and local support for Extension. Paraprofessional aides from low-income areas are being trained under the supervision of professional home economists to teach low-income homemakers on an individual and group basis. These aides work to improve the nutritional quality of diets by helping homemakers plan, purchase, and prepare nutritionally balanced meals. One-to-one contact methods are used to teach homemakers nutrition by telling, showing, working with them, and repeating each process until they become confident enough to use the nutrition information on their own. More than 240,000 families in over 1500 city and county sites have been reached since EFNEP began in 1968. EFNEP has shown that educational programs tailored to the interests, needs, competencies, and economic and educational levels of the homemaker can be effective in producing positive changes in eating habits.

Extension 4-H programs reach young people with nutrition information. Nationally developed project manuals geared for particular age groups improve young people's knowledge of the importance of nutrition. Camping programs sponsored by 4-H were expanded in 1970 in some states to include nutrition day camps. Learning nutrition was made fun through the use of nutrition games, songs, puppet shows, and drama. Teenagers working as "junior leaders" with younger 4-H'ers learned more about nutrition themselves.

U.S. Departments of Health and Human Services and Education.   In 1980, the U.S. Department of Health, Education, and Welfare was split into two departments: the Department of Health and Human Services and the Department of Education. Prior to this split, several agencies within the Department of Health,

Education, and Welfare were responsible for nutrition-related activities. The responsibilities described here are now carried out through one of the two new departments.

A principal goal of the Department of Education is to develop nutrition education opportunities specifically to meet the needs of children within the school system. In the elementary grades children from families with a background of limited meal patterns are exposed to a wide variety of foods, their origins, how to prepare them, and how they are ultimately related to good health. Junior and senior high school students receive a more concentrated study of food and nutrition incorporated into subjects such as science, biology, health, and physical education. The Future Homemakers of America, a national organization of students in home economics courses, sponsors projects to improve teenage eating habits. The young people in this organization expand their understanding of food and nutrition through such activities as assisting with elementary children at lunchtime and operating fruit and juice bars at athletic games.

The Bureau of Head Start and Child Services Programs, Office of Child Development, operates Project Head Start. This is a comprehensive child development program designed to meet the total needs, including nutrition, of preschool children (**46, 47**). The Project Head Start Nutrition Packet contains seven nutrition publications designed to serve as guidelines and provide information to support the Head Start Food and Nutrition Program. Over 450,000 children between the ages of 3 and 6 from low-income families are enrolled in year-round half- or full-day programs or in summer programs under the direction of Head Start. The Office of Child Development also operates Parent-Child Centers where children under 3 years of age and their parents are included in nutrition education programs.

The Public Health Service works to eliminate inequities in the access to or receipt of care by certain disadvantaged people. Programs have been developed under the auspices of the Public Health Service to provide food and nutrition education to specific groups such as migrant workers and their families.

The Indian Health Service, within the Public Health Service, provides food and nutrition education programs designed to help infants and preschool children where nutrition-related illness and underachievement in growth and development are prevalent. Special emphasis is also given to nutrition programs for teenagers and females in the childbearing years.

The Maternal and Child Health Service, also a branch of the Public Health Service, deals with health care projects for expectant mothers and infants. Through this agency, nutrition services and nutrition education are made available to increasing numbers of low-income mothers and children. Families are provided with information about the nutritional needs and food habits of infants and children. Special efforts are also made to reach children with nutrition education as early as possible.

Professional and Other Organizations

The American Home Economics Association is one of the largest professional organizations with associations in each of the 50 states, the District of Columbia, and Puerto Rico. The purpose of the Association is to improve the quality and standards of individual and family life through education, research, cooperative programs, and public information. Members of the association support numerous nutrition-related activities.

The American Dietetic Association is a professional society for dietitians. Members of this group accept a professional responsibility to develop and encourage better nutritional care. Through publications, programs, and other contacts, the American Dietetic Association helps individuals and families choose foods for adequate nutrition in health or disease throughout the life cycle.

The American Medical Association has developed several nutrition education programs geared to health professionals. Desired audiences are then reached through the health professionals. Pamphlets on nutrition addressed to children and teenagers are distributed through physicians' offices.

The American National Red Cross is another organization active in prompting the principles of good nutrition. Various health and nutrition education materials developed by the Red Cross are used in elementary and secondary schools across the nation. Nutrition education is incorporated into Red Cross programs on mother-infant care and home nursing. The Red Cross has also played a role in certain of the USDA supplemental food programs where it has helped with certification of participants, transportation of food to homes, and nutrition education.

The National Foundation-March of Dimes is responsible for developing a massive attack on maternal malnutrition, especially among low-income women and adolescents. The Foundation has cosponsored several training institutes for health professionals working with local WIC units as part of its effort to improve nutrition during pregnancy. The scientific basis for nutritional guidance during pregnancy and techniques for counseling pregnant women on nutrition are taught at these institutes. The March of Dimes has developed many nutrition educational materials for use by individuals and agencies on request.

The foundation of the Dairy Council program is nutrition research and the adaptation of scientifically acceptable nutrition information obtained from such research to promote good eating habits, including the use of dairy foods. The National Dairy Council develops many nutrition education materials for use with different age groups. This information includes newer approaches to nutrition education based on certain behavioral objectives. The Big Ideas program, for use with school children from kindergarten through senior high, combines the basic concepts of nutrition with innovative and sound educational techniques. Each year the National Dairy Council also brings together researchers with newspaper and magazine food editors to update them on current nutrition problems.

The food industry can play a major role in educating the consumer about foods and the nutrients they contain. The food industry recently has been active in promoting a nutrition awareness campaign. Many nutrition education instruments are developed by the food industry for use by schools, government agencies, and private groups. Highly skilled communication experts associated with individual companies have produced several extremely high-quality teaching aids.

The Industry Council for Nutrition Education is a group of manufacturers, distributors, and members of advisory boards of different industries who have joined together in an effort to make nutrition awareness a focal point of all child feeding programs. They are accomplishing their goal by pooling resources to develop, publish, and distribute free nutrition education materials for use in elementary schools.

SUMMARY

The nutritional status of the American public and what can be done to improve it is a complicated issue. Children are a key group in the process of educating the nation to adopt better nutritional practices. However, there are children and youth of every age, hungry and malnourished, often because families are too poor to buy nutritional food or lack knowledge of sound nutrition practices. Food assistance programs have been developed to alleviate this hunger and nutrition gap. In 1970, 98 percent of the U. S. population lived in localities with family and child feeding programs. Federal food assistance programs reach children through child nutrition programs in school and other child care institutions and through family food programs that reach children in their homes. One of the greatest unmet needs in attaining top nutritional and health status for all children is nutrition education for all consumers. This education should give special attention to teaching children the relationship between nutrition and health.

Changes in the nutritional attitudes, knowledge, behavior, and status of children can be affected positively through carefully planned nutrition education programs. Good comprehensive nutrition education programs continue to be expensive and time consuming simply because the development and maintenance of good eating habits is a long-term process. Motivation is equally as important as nutrition education and presents a problem even more difficult to solve. There are no easy answers to the problem of motivating individuals to eat wisely. Nutrition education programs, as a component of all federal food assistance programs, will be essential in the future if health professionals are to realize success in helping a majority of the people of the United States achieve good nutritional health.

STUDY QUESTIONS AND
TOPICS FOR INDIVIDUAL INVESTIGATION

1. Several reliable sources of nutrition information have been mentioned in this chapter. Try to find out which sources are most active in your community. Do you make appropriate use of such sources? What factors exist in your community that might undermine reliable nutrition education efforts by making misleading information available to the public. Conduct a survey of college students to determine which sources they would most readily turn to for nutrition information.

2. In the United States today what do you perceive to be one of the greatest nutrition problems that could be alleviated (to some extent, at least) with a viable, innovative educational program? Who should carry out such a program? Narrow your problem down to a specific one rather than describing a broad general nutrition education program.

3. You have been asked to speak to a group of representatives from your state who are interested in looking at the health and nutritional needs of the people in the state and getting a better understanding of how they may be met. What will you discuss with the group in an effort to influence the establishment of laws or policies that will improve the nutritional health of people in your state? Include in your discussion any problems you see in existing nutrition programs and what you visualize as needed programs—if any.

4. In many areas the School Breakfast Program has not been widely accepted. Many schools offering breakfast have low participation. Conduct a study of the program in your vicinity. Try to answer the following questions:

    (a) Why do school districts elect (or elect not) to participate?
    (b) What are the benefits and problems experienced by participating schools?
    (c) Why do students not take advantage of the Breakfast Program when offered?
    (d) Is any information available on the number of children who do not get breakfast either at school or at home?
    (e) How can programs be developed to encourage student participation?
    (f) Is there any other relevant information dealing with the extent of need in your area?

5. "Okay, I guess I like green beans; I don't love them, but I like them." This was the response of one little boy whose teacher used the School Lunch Program as a nutrition education opportunity for stressing the importance of trying new foods. In addition to trying new foods on the lunch line, children participated in taste-testing parties where unfamiliar foods were introduced. Choose one of the following situations, and using a school feeding program as the setting, develop an innovative approach for teaching nutrition.

(*a*) A large population of children attending an elementary school are Spanish. The children do not seem to like the traditional foods served in the School Breakfast Program. What ideas can you come up with to meet the dietary needs and cultural preferences of these youngsters?

(*b*) Teenagers will not eat the school lunch simply because it is nutritious and cheap. Develop some appealing menus and innovative ideas to sell teens on school lunch and good nutrition.

(*c*) First graders are not familiar with many of the foods served in the school cafeteria or why they are good for them. Think of ways that nutrition education in the classroom and the school lunch program can be used together to teach first graders the basics of nutrition.

6. WIC offers an excellent opportunity for providing nutrition information to pregnant women and mothers of young children. Develop a 15-minute videocassette program that women could listen to when attending a WIC clinic or devise a colorful, informative leaflet for distribution at such clinics. Include information on one or more of the following topics:

(*a*) Nutrient needs of the pregnant woman
(*b*) Nutrient needs during lactation
(*c*) Nutrient needs of infants
(*d*) Nutrient needs of young children

7. The following journals provide useful information on nutrition education programs and techniques. You may want to subscribe to these individually or as a class. At least try to obtain copies of these journals either from the library or perhaps from faculty members. Become familiar with some of the happenings and research being conducted in the area of nutrition education.

(*a*) *Journal of Nutrition Education*
Society for Nutrition Education
2140 Shattuck Avenue, Suite 110
Berkeley, Calif. 94704

(*b*) *Nutrition Today*
Nutrition Today, Incorporated
703 Giddings Avenue
P.O. Box 1829
Annapolis, Md. 21401

(*c*) *Food and Nutrition*
Food and Nutrition Service
U.S. Department of Agriculture
Washington, D.C. 20250

REFERENCES

1. Butz, E. The success of the federal food assistance programs. *Nutrition Today,* 7:12, 1972.
2. U.S. Department of Agriculture. Food Programs of the U.S. Department of Agriculture Program Aid No. 1161. March 1977.
3. National Dairy Council. Child nutrition programs. *Dairy Council Digest,* 45:1, 1974.
4. Pearson, J. Child nutrition programs of the Food and Nutrition Service, USDA. *Nutrition Program News,* May–June:1, 1973.
5. U.S. Department of Agriculture. Lunch at school. *Food and Nutrition,* 9(3),:6 1979.
6. Lyng, R. The commodities controversy: Food for your lunch. *School Food Service Journal,* 26:30, 1972.
7. Yeutter, C. How can we strengthen school food service? *Food and Nutrition,* 3:2, 1973.
8. Senti, F., L. Page, and M. Hill. Nutrition awareness in the USDA. *Journal of the American Dietetics Association,* 61:17, 1972.
9. Lachance, P. Nutritional aspects of engineered foods and delivery systems in school food service. *Proceedings, Nutrition Education Seminar,* July:125, 1971.
10. Rosenfield, D. Feeding children through USDA programs. *Food Technology,* 27:36, 1973.
11. U.S. Department of Agriculture. National School Lunch Program—25 Years of Progress. Food and Nutrition Service PA–980. 1971.
12. Feldman, L. School food service: putting computers to work. *Food and Nutrition,* 6(6):2, 1976.
13. Jenkins, D. Plate waste—views on a complex tissue. *Food and Nutrition,* 6:10, 1976.
14. Head, M., and R. Weeks. Conventional vs. formulated foods in school lunches. II. Cost of food served, eaten, and wasted. *Journal of the American Dietetic Association,* 71:629, 1977.
15. U.S. Department of Agriculture. Lunch patterns proposed. *Food and Nutrition,* 7(5):11, 1977.
16. Jenkins, D. New legislation for child nutrition programs. *Food and Nutrition,* 6(1):2, 1976.
17. Koonce, T. Does breakfast help? *School Food Service Journal,* 16:54, 1972.
18. U.S. Department of Agriculture. Breakfast for energy. *Food and Nutrition,* 9(3):8, 1979.
19. U.S. Department of Agriculture. Child use and food. *Food and Nutrition,* 9(3):10, 1979.
20. U.S. Department of Agriculture. Serving mothers and children. *Food and Nutrition,* 9a(3):4, 1979.
21. Watts, M., T. Gregory, and C. Jensen. WIC: the special supplemental food program for women, infants, and children. *Food and Nutrition,* 7(1):2, 1977.

22. U.S. Department of Agriculture. Federal Agency Statement. Nutrition Education and the Special Supplemental Food Program for Women, Infants, and Children (WIC). Food and Nutrition Service, Extension Service, Bureau of Community Health Service, Indian Health Service, June 1977.

23. U.S. Department of Agriculture. Food and Nutrition. Newsletter of the Food and Nutrition Service, No. 48, October 1976, p. 4.

24. U.S. Department of Agriculture. The new Food Stamp legislation. *Food and Nutrition,* 7(5):2, 1977.

25. Lachance, P. National nutrition programs—perspective and policy. *Journal of the American Dietetics Association,* 71:487, 1977.

26. Schorr, A. Income maintenance. In *U.S. Nutrition Policies in the Seventies,* ed. J. Mayer. Freeman, San Francisco, 1973.

27. Smith, H., and C. Justice. Effects of nutrition programs on third grade students. *Journal of Nutrition Education,* 11(2):92, 1979.

28. U.S. Department of Agriculture. Teaching kids about food: parents get involved. *Food and Nutrition,* 9(2):10, 1979.

29. Ulrich, H., and G. Briggs. Improving education concerning nutrition—the general public. In: *U.S. Nutrition Policies in the Seventies,* ed. J. Mayer. Freeman, San Francisco, 1973.

30. American Dietetic Association. A.D.A. president testifies on child nutrition education act of 1973. *Journal of the American Dietetic Association,* 63:280, 1973.

31. Callahan, D. You can't teach a hungry child. *School Lunch Journal,* 25:26, 1971.

32. Stewart, M. Nutrition and learning—implications for schools. *Nutrition Program News,* March–April:1, 1971.

33. Gifft, H., H. Washbon, and G. Harrison. *Nutrition, Behavior, and Change.* Prentice-Hall, Englewood Cliffs, N.J., 1972.

34. Maslow, A. A theory of human motivation. *Psychological Review,* 50:37, 1943. 1943.

35. U.S. Department of Agriculture. How can we get kids to eat. *Food and Nutrition,* 6(5):12, 1976.

36. Thomas, K., and M. Watts. Child nutrition bicentennial project. *Food and Nutrition,* 5(5):6, 1975.

37. U.S. Department of Agriculture. Attracting school lunch customers. *Food and Nutrition,* 9(2):12, 1979.

38. Montoy, B. Two ways to make school lunch fun. *Food and Nutrition,* 3(5):8, 1973.

39. Sears, K. Nutrition education is as easy as 1, 2 . . . 9. *School Food Service Journal,* July–August:57, 1976.

40. Brand, E. Type A—the ethnic way. *Food and Nutrition,* 3(5):14, 1973.

41. U.S. Department of Agriculture. A look at high schools: What makes lunch sell? *Food and Nutrition,* 3(5):5, 1973.

42. Watts, M., and L. Klein. Lunch and learning. *Food and Nutrition,* 6(6):4, 1976.

43. Rhodes, R., and C. D'Arrezo. How two lunch programs save money. *Food and Nutrition,* 6(1):6, 1976.
44. Dickey, R., and J. Duran. Keeping nutrition in mind. *School Food Service Journal,* July—August:103, 1976.
45. Fisk, D. A successful program for changing children's eating habits. *Journal of Nutrition Education,* 14(3):6, 1979.
46. U.S. Department of Health, Education, and Welfare. Project Head Start. Nutrition Instructor's Guide. U.S. Department of Health, Education and Welfare, Washington, D.C. 20201, 1969.
47. U.S. Department of Health, Education, and Welfare. Project Head Start. Nutrition, Better Eating for a Head Start. U.S. Department of Health, Education and Welfare, Washington, D.C. 20201, 1969.

GLOSSARY

acetate a salt or ester of acetic acid

acidosis a condition in which the body's alkali reserve is below normal due to faulty metabolism

accretion growth in size by addition or accumulation of material

adenoids growths of lymphoid tissue in the upper part of the throat, behind the nose

ad libitum feeding regime that permits intake of food as desired by the individual

advisable nutrient intake intakes of a nutrient to take care of estimated requirements

allergy physiological reaction resulting from the interaction of an antigen with an antibody

alveolar duct a duct originating from and related to the air pockets in the lungs

alveolus a small hollow air cell in the lung

ameloblasts cells responsible for laying down the enamel matrix

amine a derivative of ammonia in which hydrogen atoms have been replaced by radicals containing hydrogen and carbon atoms

amniotic fluid a watery fluid surrounding the embryo and enclosed by the amnion membrane

amphetamine a colorless, volatile liquid used in its phosphate or sulfate forms as a drug to overcome mental depression, fatigue, and so on, and to lessen the appetite in dieting

amylopectin starch containing both 1,4 and 1,6 linkages; is branched chain

anabolism the process of building up living tissue; constructive metabolism

anion a negatively charged atom

anorexia lack or loss of appetite for food

antibiotic chemical substance having the capacity to inhibit the growth of or to destroy bacteria and other microorganisms

anticoagulant a drug or substance that delays or prevents the clotting of blood

antihistamine a drug used to minimize the action of histamine in such allergic conditions as hay fever and hives

atonic lacking bodily tone or muscle tone

atrophy a wasting away of body tissues or organs or the failure of an organ to grow or develop because of insufficient nutrition

barbiturate any salt or ester of barbituric acid used as a sedative or to induce sleep

basal metabolism amount of energy required to maintain the essential processes of life

bile substance secreted by the liver and

found in the gall bladder. It is discharged into the duodenum and aids in digestion, especially of fats

bilirubin a yellowish-red substance found in bile

bronchiole any of the small subdivisions of the bronchi

bronchus either of the two main branches of the trachea or windpipe

carboxyhemoglobin a compound of carbon monoxide and hemoglobin formed in the blood in carbon monoxide poisoning

casein a major protein in milk

catabolism the breaking down of living tissue into waste products of a simpler chemical composition

catalyze to speed up or, sometimes, slow down the rate of a chemical reaction by the addition of some substance that itself undergoes no permanent chemical change

cation a positively charged atom

cementum outer covering of the roots of the tooth

cerebellum the section of the brain behind and below the cerebrum. It functions as the coordinating center for muscular movement

cerebrosides class of compounds found in the brain

cerebrum the upper, main part of the brain. It is the largest part and is believed to control conscious and voluntary processes

cheilosis fissures of the lips and angles of the mouth

chondroplasia the formation of cartilage

chylomicrons particles of emulsified fat found in the blood

cm abbreviation for centimeter, a unit of measure equal to one hundredth of a meter

collagen a fibrous protein found in connective tissue, bone, and cartilage

colostrum secretion from the mammary glands during the first few days after birth

conception the origination of a new individual by union of a spermatozoon and ovum

congenital existing at birth as a result of development during one's prenatal environment

conjunctiva delicate membranes lining the eyelids and covering the eyeball

cranium the skull, specifically the bones encasing the brain

creatinine a nitrogen compound found in blood, muscle, and urine, where measurement of its excretion is used to evaluate kidney function

deciduous teeth first teeth formed that are temporary and will be replaced by permanent teeth

dendritic process a long branching protoplasmic process, such as the branches conducting impulses toward the body of a nerve cell

dental lamina ridge along the jaw in which the teeth erupt

dentin major substance of the teeth

deoxyribonucleic acid an essential component of all living matter and a basic material in the chromosomes of the cell nucleus. It contains the genetic code and transmits the hereditary pattern

dermatitis inflammation of the skin; can result from a variety of conditions

desensitization process of removing allergic reaction from the body

diploid having twice the number of chromosomes normally occurring in a mature germ cell. Most somatic cells are diploid

diuretic a drug or other substance that increases the secretion and flow of urine

diverticular the formation of a blind pouch in the intestinal tract

duodenum the first section of the small intestine, between the stomach and the jejunum

edema an abnormal accumulation of fluid in intercellular spaces of the body

electroencephalographic descriptive of the changes in electric potential produced by the brain

enamel the caplike cover of the tooth; is the most highly mineralized structure of the body

enzyme a proteinlike substance that acts as an organic catalyst in initiating or speeding up specific chemical reactions

epiphyseal relating to the portion of a bone that in early life is distinct from the shaft

estimated requirements least amount

of a nutrient needed to promote optimal health

familial conditions that tend to occur in families; may be genetic in origin, but the basic mechanism is often unknown

FAO/WHO Food and Agriculture Organization of the World Health Organization

fibrinogen a protein of the blood plasma that is converted to fibrin by the action of the enzyme thrombin in the clotting of blood

gestational pertaining to the period of carrying young in the uterus from conception to birth

glial pertaining to the supporting structure of the brain and spinal cord

globulin any of a group of proteins, fully soluble only in salt solutions, found in both animal and vegetable tissue

glomerulus a small convoluted mass of capillaries, especially a cluster of vascular tufts in the kidney

gluconeogenesis the production of carbohydrates, especially glycogen, from substances other than glucose

hallucinogen a drug or other substance that produces hallucinations

hemolysis the destruction of red corpuscles with liberation of hemoglobin into the surrounding fluid

hemopoietic relating to the formation of blood or blood corpuscles

hepatic refers to the liver

homeostatic descriptive of the tendency to maintain normal, internal stability in an organism by coordinated responses of the organ systems that automatically compensate for environmental changes

hydrocephaly a condition characterized by an abnormal increase in the amount of fluid in the cranium, especially in young children, causing enlargement of the head and destruction of the brain

hydrogenation the addition of hydrogen to another substance; usually refers to the addition of hydrogen to fats

hyperbilirubinemia an excess of "bilirubin" (a red pigment produced by degradation of hemoglobin in the spleen and liver) in the blood

hypercalcemia an excess of calcium in the blood

hypercholesterolemia above normal levels of cholesterol in the blood plasma or serum

hyperirritability excessive irritability or reaction; often results from a nutrient deficiency that affects the central nervous system

hyperlipoproteinemias high levels of lipoprotein and lipids in the blood

hyperopic descriptive of the condition of being farsighted

hypertension abnormally high blood pressure or a disease of which this is the chief sign

hypocalcemia low concentrations of calcium in the blood. Concentration is usually related to plasma or serum

hypoglycemia low levels of blood sugar

hypophosphatemic condition of low concentrations of phosphorus

hypothalamus the part of the brain that forms the floor of the third ventricle and regulates many basic body functions such as temperature

immunological protective mechanism derived through the immunoglobulins or antibodies

interstitial fluid fluid found between the cellular components of an organ

intrauterine within the uterus

involution the decrease in size and/or function of an organ that occurs with age

jaundice a condition in which the eyeballs, skin, and urine become abnormally yellow as a result of bile pigments in the blood

kernicterus a severe form of infant jaundice involving the brain and spinal cord

ketoacidosis acidosis resulting from the excessive formation of ketone bodies

ketogenic causing the formation of ketones in the body as a result of the incomplete oxidation of organic compounds such as fatty acids or carbohydrates

ketone an organic chemical compound containing the divalent carbonyl group, CO, in combination with two hydrocarbon radicals

ketonuria excretion of ketone bodies in the urine

ketosis excessive formation of ketones in the body; ketone bodies in the urine represents ketone production in excess of the body tissues' capacity to metabolize these compounds

kilocalorie (kcal) amount of heat necessary to raise 1 kilogram (kg) of water from 15 to 16° C; equivalent to 4184 joules (J)

kilojoule (kJ) energy used when 1 kg is moved 1 meter (m) by 1 newton (n); equivalent to 4.2 kcals

kwashiorkor severe deficiency of protein

larynx the structure of muscle and cartilage at the upper end of the human trachea containing the vocal cords

leukocyte small, colorless cells in the blood, lymph, and tissues important in the body's defenses against infection

lobulated divided and subdivided into small lobes

lumen a passage within any tubular organ, for example, intestine

macrocephaly a condition in which the head is abnormally large

marasmus severe deficiency of energy; often is a combination of nutrient deficiencies resulting from the lack of food

masticatory of, or for mastication; specifically, adapted for chewing

maturation the act or process of maturing, especially of becoming full grown or fully developed

mcg abbreviation for microgram, one millionth of a gram (g)

menarche the first menstrual period of a female in puberty

metabolic balance studies controlled studies in which nutrient intakes and excretions are carefully measured

mg abbreviation for milligram, one thousandth of a gram

micelle a structural unit composed of a group of molecules

miscarriage the expulsion of a fetus from the womb before it is sufficiently developed to survive

microcephaly a condition in which the head is abnormally small

morbidity the rate of disease or proportion of diseased persons in a given locality

mortality the proportion of deaths to the population of a region; death rate

mottled tooth enamel teeth with chalky white patches, pitted areas, and loss of enamel

myelin the white, fatty substance forming a sheath around certain nerve fibers

myelinization the production of myelin around the axon of a nerve cell

mucosa a mucus-secreting membrane lining body cavities such as the alimentary canal and respiratory tract

narcotic a drug, such as opium or any of its derivatives (morphine, heroin, codeine), used to relieve pain and induce sleep. Narcotics are often addictive

nasogastric the provision of nutrients via tubes inserted through the nasal passages

neonatal occurring during the first month of life; refers to the newborn

nephron a single urinary tubule in the vertebrate kidney

niacin equivalent (N.E.) 1 mg of niacin or 60 mg of dietary tryptophan

occiput the back part of the skull or head

odontoblasts cells that form the outer surface of the dental pulp during embryonic development of the teeth

organogenesis the origin and development of organs

ossification the process of changing or developing into bone

osteogenesis the development of bones

osteoporosis abnormal porosity of bone resulting from decalcification; the canals of the bone are enlarged

ovary either of the pair of female reproductive glands producing eggs

oviduct duct or tube through which ova (eggs) pass from an ovary to the uterus or to the outside

perinatal occurring during the period closely surrounding the time of birth

periodontal disease inflammation of the periodontal tissues

peristaltic pertaining to the rhythmic wavelike motion of the walls of the alimentary canal

pernicious anemia a form of anemia characterized by a gradual reduction in the number of the red blood cells and by gastrointestinal and nervous disturbances

pharynx the muscular and membranous cavity of the alimentary canal leading from the mouth and nasal passages to the larynx and esophagus

phocomelia the congenital absence or abnormal shortening of arms or legs, often with only short flipperlike limbs projecting from the body

phospholipid a phosphoric acid containing lipid. One of a class of compounds found in all animal cells, being abundant in the brain and spinal cord

physiological characteristic of or promoting normal, or healthy, functioning

phytate materials found in plants that may form chelates with the inorganic elements and render them not available to the individual

pituitary gland small, oval endocrine gland attached by a stalk to the base of the brain and consisting of an anterior and a posterior lobe. It secretes hormones influencing body growth and metabolism

plasma the fluid part of blood, as distinguished from the cells; used for transfusions

platelet a round or oval nonnucleated disk, smaller than a red blood cell and containing no hemoglobin, found in the blood of mammals, and associated with the clotting process

preconceptional prior to conception

primipara a woman who is pregnant for the first time or who has borne just one child

progestational related to hormones that, in female mammals, precede, prepare for, or are active in ovulation and pregnancy

protein efficiency ratio (PER) a measure of protein quality. Usually based on tests with laboratory animals and defined as the amount of weight gained, divided by the amount of protein consumed. Casein is the usual standard to which other proteins are compared

protein isolate proteins isolated from foods or other materials; used frequently in developing infant formulas based on proteins from soy

proteinuria the presence of protein in the urine

proteolytic descriptive of the breaking down of proteins, as by gastric juices, to form simpler substances

pureed foods that have been homogenized or cut into very fine particles

quadratic descriptive of an equation in which the second power, or square, is the highest to which a quantity is raised

radius the shorter and thicker of the two bones of the forearm on the same side as the thumb

Recommended Dietary Allowances (RDA) intakes of nutrients recommended for the maintenance of good nutrition of practically all healthy people in the United States

renal refers to the kidney

respiratory quotient the ratio between the volume of carbon dioxide eliminated and the volume of oxygen consumed by an organism during a given period of time

retinol equivalent (R.E.) 1 microgram (mcg) of retinol or 6 mcg B-carotene

saturated refers to fats in which the carbon atoms are holding the maximum number of hydrogens

sebaceous descriptive of the skin glands that secrete "sebum," a semiliquid, oily secretion

sigmoid having a double curve, like the letter *S*

solute materials in solution; may refer to concentration of materials in body fluids, urine, blood plasma, and so on

specific dynamic action the amount of energy expended or lost as the result of ingesting food

steatorrhea excess fat in the fecal material

subscapular site on back of body situated beneath the scapula, either of two flat triangular bones in the back of the shoulder

sulfonamide any of the sulfa drugs

surfactant a surface-active agent, specifically a substance active on the surface of the lung

synovial the viscous fluid found within the joints

thermogenesis the production of heat, especially by physiological action in an animal

thrombophlebitis the formation of a clot in a vein, resulting from irritation of the vein's inner lining

thrombosis coagulation of the blood in the heart or a blood vessel, forming a clot

tocopherol equivalent (T.E.) 1 mg D-α-tocopherol

trachea the tube extending from the larynx to its division into the two bronchi

transferrin a plasma protein that functions as an iron carrier

triceps the large muscle at the back of the upper arm that extends the forearm when contracted

unsaturated refers to fats in which the carbon atoms can combine with additional hydrogens

uterus hollow muscular organ in females in which the ovum is deposited and the embryo and fetus are developed

xanthomas yellow neoplastic growths on the skin; composed of large numbers of fat cells

INDEX

Absorption sites, 91
Adipose tissue
  brown adipose tissue, 94
  cell size, early life, 276
  cell size in obese children, 169
  formation in fetus, 94
Adult female
  nutritional requirements, 2
  nutritional status, 2
Alcohol, during pregnancy, 124
Alimentary tract
  changes in pregnancy, 56
Allergies, 300
  desensitizing, 301
  milk, 244, 300
  wheat, 300
Ameloblasts, 366
Amino acids
  branched chain metabolism, 309
  content of milk, 220
  estimated requirements, 217
  growth, 333
  inborn errors of metabolism, 301–310
  infant requirements, 217
  needs of low birth-weight infants, 282
  needs of preadolescent children, 336
  placental transport, 54
Amniotic sac, 48
Anemia
  folic acid, 111
  iron deficiency in children, 338
  megaloblastic, 111
  pernicious, 112
  pregnancy, 110
  vitamin B_{12}, 112
Anorexia nervosa, 200
Antibiotics, during pregnancy, 121
Anticoagulants, during pregnancy, 123
Apgar score, 108
Arm circumference
  limits in obesity, 170
Ascorbic acid. See Vitamin C
Athlete, 357
  carbohydrate loading, 358
  fluids, 358
  weight control, 358

Bacterial plaque, 373
Basal metabolism, 330
  age effects on, 331
  rates, 331
Biological rhythms, 277
Biotin, 21
Birth weight
  effects of drugs on, 123
  malnutrition and, 105
  maternal age and, 119
Blood
  blood pressure in infants, 149
  changes during pregnancy, 55
  development, 148
  normal values of, 149, 150
Body composition
  infants and children, 220

Brain
 effects of malnutrition on, 108
 fetal development, 86
Breast feeding, 65
 advantages, 233
 allergy protection, 234
 colostrum, 228
 contaminants, 236
 disadvantages, 235
 nutrient content of breast milk, 229
 patterns, 227
 weight gains in infants, 235
Breast milk, 227
 composition, 229
 immunological properties, 232
 nutrient composition, 227–228

Calcium, 22
 accretion during growth, 338
 infant intakes, 224
 needs during growth, 337
 needs during lactation, 67
 needs during pregnancy, 60
Carbohydrates, 9–12
 changes in consumption of, 187
 consumption patterns, 11
 disaccharides, 10
 fetal metabolism, 90
 glycogen, 10
 infant formulas, 240
 monosaccharides, 10
Cardiovascular
 changes during pregnancy, 56
 disease in children, 314
 plasma volume, 55
 prevention of disease, 274
Celiac sprue, 296
Cellular growth, 78
Central nervous system
 development, 146
 spinal cord, 146–148
Children
 growth patterns in, 326
 hypertension in, 277–278
 illnesses of, 293–294
 obesity, 275–276
 underweight, 272–273
Chlorine, 24
Chondroplasia, 145
Chromium, 27–28
Cigarettes, 124
Circulatory system
 development, 148
 infant heart rates, 149
Cobalt, 27
Colostrum
 composition, 228–229
 secretion at birth, 65
Commodity Distribution Program, 400
Commodity Supplemental Food

Program, 399
Copper, 26
 concentration in milk, 226
 infant intakes, 226
Corpus luteum, 51
Cultural influences, 183–184
Cystic fibrosis, 296

Dental caries, 371–373
 diet effects, 373
 nursing bottle syndrome, 381–382
 prevention, 382
 role of carbohydrate, 375–377
 role of fluoride, 377–380
Dental plaque, 373
Dentin, 366
 composition, 368
Deoxyribonucleic acid (DNA), 78
 organ content of fetus, 79
Diabetes Mellitus, 301–302
Diet history, 340
Diets
 food fads, 195–196
 supplements, 197
 vegetarian, 196
 weight control, 198–204
 Zen macrobiotic, 196
Differentiation, 47, 77
Digestive system, 152
Drugs
 effects during pregnancy, 120–124
 effects on lactation, 70
 oral contraceptives, 125–127

Electrolytes
 placental transport, 53
Embryo, 49
Enamel, 366
 mottled teeth, 380
Energy
 activity, 8
 adolescent needs, 327
 adult needs, 6
 basal needs, 330
 breast milk, 218
 carbohydrates, 9
 fast foods, 201
 fats (lipids), 12
 growth needs, 327, 333–334
 guides, infants and children, 294
 infant formulas, 238
 infant needs, 219
 kilocalorie (kcal), 330
 kilojoule (kJ), 330
 needs during lactation, 66
 needs during pregnancy, 59
 needs of children and adolescents, 334
 needs of low birth weights, 281
 specific dynamic action, 330
 stages of growth, 326

Enzyme systems, 143
Estrogen, 51
Expanded Food and Nutrition Education
    Program (EFNEP), 407
Extracellular fluid, 153

Familial hyperbetalipoproteinemia, 312
    abnormal patterns, 312
    dietary treatment, 313
Fast foods, 192
    caloric content, 202
Fasting, 200
Fat. *See* Lipids
Fat depots, 170
Feeding skills, 180
Feedings, 254
    baby foods, 259
    schedules, 258
    solid foods, 257
    techniques, 255
Female reproductive system, 46
    cervix, 46
    fallopian tubes, 46
    ovaries, 46
    placenta, 51
Fetus, 49
    Apgar scoring, 107
    birth weight of, 104
    malnutrition in, 104
    mortality of, 106
    nutrient accumulation in, 89
Fluids
    body fluid compartments, 153
    requirements for infants and children, 295
Fluoridation, 378
Fluorine, 29
    concentration in water, 380
    dental caries and, 377
    functions of, 379
    infant intakes of, 226
Fluorosis, 380
Folacin (Folic Acid), 20
    anemia during pregnancy, 111
    infant intakes of, 223
    pregnancy requirements of, 60
Food
    advertising, 189
    appearance, 180
    baby foods, 259
    composition of infant foods, 261, 270
    daily food guide, 30
    dietary counseling, 36
    fast food service, 192
    home-prepared baby foods, 268
    lactation, food guide, 68
    natural foods, 195
    needs during pregnancy, 61
    nutritive value, baby foods, 262
    organic foods, 195
    planning for adult female, 30

    pregnant teenagers, food guide, 356
    solid foods, guide, 258
    solid foods introduction, 257
Food and Nutrition Service, 390, 404
    regional offices, 391
Food composition, 340
Food consumption recall, 340
Food habits
    acceptability of foods, 183
    appearance of food, 180
    behavior modification, 201
    consumption changes, 187
    cultural influences on, 183
    development of, 178
    dietary fads, 195
    dietary supplements, 197
    effects of advertising on, 189
    factors affecting, 183
    fasting, 199
    feeding skills, 180
    influence of fast food service on, 192
    influence of television on, 191
    introduction of new foods, 181
    natural foods, 195
    nutrition education, 204
    processing changes, 187
    regional influences, 184
    religious influences, 184
    snacking, 193
    social factors influencing, 182
    weight control, 198
    working mothers, 191
    vegetarian, 196
    vending machines, 194
Food intake, weighed, 340
    related health problems, 272
Food plans, 346
Food programs, 389
    commodity distribution, 400
    commodity supplemental foods,
      399
    food stamps, 400
    non-school programs, 396
    nutrition education component, 401
    school breakfast, 395
    school lunch, 390
    special milk program, 396
    for women, infants and children, 397
Food record, 340
Food Stamp Program, 400
Formulas
    cow's milk, 242
    energy sources, 240
    infant, 237
    nutrient content of, 239
    regulations, 242
    special formulas, 297
    types of, 242
    weight gain in infants, 235
Four Food Groups, 352

Galactose
  malabsorption, 296
Galactosemia, 303
Gases
  placental transport, 52
Gastrointestinal tract
  fetal development, 87
Glucose, 10
  malabsorption, 296
  placental transport, 54
  tolerance tests, 302–304
Glycogen storage disease, 305
Gout, 310
Growth
  body parts, 82
  bone, 145
  cellular, 78
  cessation of, 167, 168
  of children, 326
  definition of, 139
  growth charts, 155–164
  of infants, 81
  measurement of, 155
  nutritional needs for, 327
  in obese children, 167
  organ growth, 143
  patterns, 139
  rate of, 140
  recommended daily allowances, 328
  standards, 154
  types of, 142

Hallucinogens, 123
Handicaps, 314
  development of feeding skills, 316
  feeding disabilities, 315
HANES study, 3
Head circumference, 156
  average values, 165
Head Start, 408
Heart
  composition of fetal heart, 86
  development, 85
Hemoglobin
  development, 148
  levels in pregnancy, 111
Homocystinuria, 308
Hormones
  actions, 97
  hierarchy of, 97
  use during pregnancy, 122
Hyperbilirubinemia, 317
Hyperlipoproteins, 311
  "broad beta" disease, 313
  hyperbetalipoproteinemia, 312
  hyperchylomicronesia, 314
  hyperpre-B-lipoproteinemia, 314
  lipoprotein patterns, 312
Hyperplasia, 143
Hypertension, 277

  in children, 277
  sodium intakes and, 277
Hypertrophy, 143

Immunoglobulins, 51
Inborn metabolic errors, 301
Infant
  early feedings, 281
  feeding schedules, 255
  formulas, 237
  nutritional requirements, 213
  parenteral feeding, 280
  recommended allowances, 215
  sucking and swallowing, 253
  weight gain, 220
  weight loss, 213
Insulin deficiency, 303
Iodine, 26
  infant intakes, 226
  pregnancy requirements, 61
Iron, 25
  anemia during pregnancy, 110
  anemia in infants, 273
  anemia in low birth-weight infants, 283
  anemia in women, 25
  content of infant foods, 266
  deficiency in children, 339
  fortification of infant foods, 274
  infant intakes, 225
  needs during growth, 337
  pregnancy requirements, 60

Kidney
  change during pregnancy, 56
  development in fetus, 84

Label, baby food, 264
Lactation
  drugs, 70
  fluid intake, 64
  food guides, 68
  nutrient supplements, 69
  nutritional needs, 66
Lactose, 10
  intolerance, 244
Larynx, 152
Lean body mass, 106
  changes during growth, 167
Linoleic acid
  infant, 218
Lipids
  in breast milk, 218
  cellular uptake, 92
  consumption changes of, 187
  fatty acids in milk, 219
  fetal metabolism, 91
  in infant formulas, 238
  placental transport of, 54
  plasma concentrations, 311

Liver
  development in fetus, 84
  placental transport, 54
  synthesis in fetus, 93
  triglycerides, 12
Low birth-weight infants
  feeding requirements, 282
  survival times, 279
Lymphatic system
  development, 152

Magnesium, 24
  infant intakes, 225
  pregnancy requirements, 60
Malnutrition
  birth weight, 105
  brain development, 108
  cell growth, 109
  effects on placenta, 106
  fetal malnutrition, 104
  mortality, 106
Maltose, 10
Mammary system, 64
Manganese, 26
Maple Syrup Urine Disease (MSUD), 309
Maturation, 80
Menarche, 46, 354
Milk
  allergy, 300, 344
  feeding after weaning, 243
  intake by children, 244
  lactose intolerance, 244
Minerals. See also separate entries for each
    mineral
  absorption of, 95
  adult female requirements of, 22
  content in baby foods, 271
  in infant formulas, 241
  needs during growth, 337
  needs during lactation, 337
  needs during pregnancy, 60
  placental transport, 54
  trace elements in baby foods, 267
Mottled tooth enamel, 380
Mouth, 366
Muscle
  cell number, 144
  growth, 143

Narcotics, during pregnancy, 123
Niacin, 19
  infant intakes of, 223
  pregnancy requirements of, 60
Nursing bottle syndrome, 381
Nutrients
  accumulation by fetus, 89
Nutrition education, 204
  government programs, 401
  Maslow's hierarchy, 402
  students' involvement in, 402

Nutrition information, 403
  Agriculture, 404
  American Dietetic Association, 409
  American Home Economics Association,
    408
  American Medical Association, 409
  American National Red Cross, 409
  Dairy Council, 409
  Health and Human Services, 407
  Industry Council for Nutrition Education,
    409
  March of Dimes, 409
Nutritional status
  of the adult female, 2
  blood data, guidelines, 343
  nutrient intake guides, 341
  urine data, guidelines, 343

Obesity
  arm circumference, 170
  behavior modification, 201
  biological rhythms, 277
  cell size and number, 277
  in children, 167
  fat depots, 170
  fatfold, 169
  feedings of infants, 276
  in teenagers, 349
  triceps skinfold, 169, 170
  weight control goals in children, 357
  weight reduction, 200
Odontoblasts, 366
Oral contraceptives
  complications arising from use of, 125
Organ weights, 154
Organogenesis, 80
Ossification, 145
  primary centers, 147
  secondary centers, 147
  skull growth, 166
Overnutrition, 274

Pantothenic acid, 21
Parenteral feeding, infants, 280
Periodontal disease, 373
Phenylketonuria, 305
  phenylalanine restricted diets, 307
Phosphorus, 23
  infant intake, 224
  needs during growth, 337
  pregnancy requirements, 60
Placenta, 48
  circulation, 89
  endocrine function of, 51
  immunological functions of, 51
  transport of nutrients across, 51
Potassium, 24
  pregnancy requirements, 60
Pregnancy
  anemias, 110

Pregnancy (*Continued*)
  drugs, 120
  hormonal aspects, 51
  implantation, 48
  patterns of weight gain, 115
  physiological changes during, 47
  recommended allowances during, 59
  respiratory system in, 56
  teenage pregnancy, 118
  toxemias, 112
  weight gains, 57, 114
Premature infants, 278–284
Progesterone, 51
Protein, 14
  amino acids and, 15
  content of early foods, 261
  deposition in fetus, 94
  growth, 333
  guidelines, infants and children, 294
  in infant formulas, 239
  infant intakes, 265
  lactation needs, 67
  placental transport of, 54
  pregnancy requirements of, 59
  recommended allowances, infants, 216
Purine metabolism, 310
Pyridoxine. See Vitamin B_6

Recommended dietary allowances
  for the adult female, 5
  during child-bearing years, 355
  for children, 328
  for infants, 215
Recumbent length, 155
Regional food patterns, 185
Respiratory system, 83
  changes in pregnancy of, 56
  development of, 152
  growth and development of, 83
  respiration rate, 153
Riboflavin, 19
  infant intakes, 223
  pregnancy requirements, 60

Saliva, 370
Salivary glands, 152
Salt
  in infant foods, 266
School breakfast, 395
  foods included, 395
School Lunch Program, 390
  current requirements, 394
  education component, 402
  historical bases of, 390
  income criteria, 392
  recent changes in, 393
  type A lunch, 392
Selenium, 27
Sensory system development, 148

Sitting height, 165
Skeleton development, 145
Skin development, 145
Smith-Lever Act, 404
Sodium, 23
  content in baby foods, 267
  needs during pregnancy, 60
Soy-based formulas, 242
Special formulas, 297
Special milk program, 396
Special non-school food service
  foods included, 396
  program, 396
  summer program, 397
Specific dynamic action, 330
Spinal cord, 146
Standing height, 155
Stomach, 152
Sucking instinct, 253
Sucrase deficiency, 296
  complications of pregnancy, 119
Sucrose, 110
Surfactant, 83
  lung development, 83
Swallowing, 90

Teenage pregnancy, 118, 354
  nutritional needs, 354–357
Teeth, 365
  calcification of, 367
  components, 367
  composition, 368
  development, 365
  disease effects on, 372
  eruption ages of, 370
  pathology of decay of, 374
Thiamine, 19
  infant intakes, 222
  needs during pregnancy, 60
Tidal air, 153
Toxemias
  during pregnancy, 112
  edema, 114
  proteinuria, 114
  weight gain, 113
Tranquilizers, 123
Triceps skinfolds, 170
  limits in obesity, 170
Tyrosinemia, 306

Underweight, 272
  low birth weight, 278
Urinary system, 84
  average secretion of urine, 153
  development, 84
Urine
  formation, 84
  secretion, 153
  status guides, 343

Vital capacity, 153
Vitamin A, 16
    intake by infants, 221
    pregnancy requirements of, 60
Vitamin B$_6$, 20
    intake by infants, 223
    pregnancy requirements of, 60
Vitamin B$_{12}$, 20
    anemia during pregnancy, 112
    infant intakes, 223
    pregnancy requirements of, 60
Vitamin C, 21
    infant intakes, 223
Vitamin D, 16
    infant intakes, 223
    pregnancy requirements of, 60
Vitamin E, 17
    infant intakes, 222
    pregnancy requirements of, 60
Vitamin K, 18
    hemorrhagic disease, 283
    intake by infants, 222
Vitamins
    absorption, 95
    adult female requirements, 16
    infant formulas, 240
    infants, advisable intakes, 221
    needs during lactation, 67

needs during pregnancy, 60
placental transport, 54

Water, 28
    content in infant foods, 265
    daily balance of, 29
    fetal concentration of, 93
    infant intakes of, 222
    needs during lactation, 69
    placental transport of, 52
    retention during pregnancy, 57
Weaning, 243
Weight
    changes in pregnancy, 57
    control of, 198
    gain by infants, 220
    gains during breast-feeding, 235
WIC. See Women, Infants and Children
Width-length index, 166
Women, Infants, and Children (WIC), 397

Xanthomas, 313

Zinc, 26
    infant formulas, 241
    infant intakes of, 226
    needs during pregnancy, 61
Zygote, 49